Amazon
4/14
$30

The Johns Hopkins
Guide to Diabetes

A Johns Hopkins Press Health Book

Christopher D. Saudek, M.D., was Professor of Medicine at the Johns Hopkins University School of Medicine and Director of the Johns Hopkins Diabetes Center.

Richard R. Rubin, Ph.D., CDE, was Professor of Medicine and Pediatrics at the Johns Hopkins University School of Medicine and a staff member at the Johns Hopkins Diabetes Center and the Johns Hopkins Pediatric Diabetes Clinic. He also had a private practice specializing in counseling people with diabetes.

Thomas W. Donner, M.D., is Associate Professor of Medicine at the Johns Hopkins University School of Medicine and Director of the Johns Hopkins Diabetes Center.

The Johns Hopkins Guide to Diabetes

For Patients and Families

Second Edition

Christopher D. Saudek, M.D.
Richard R. Rubin, Ph.D., CDE
Thomas W. Donner, M.D.

JOHNS HOPKINS UNIVERSITY PRESS   BALTIMORE

Note to the reader: This book is not meant to substitute for medical care of people with diabetes, and treatment should not be based solely on its contents. Instead, treatment must be developed in a dialogue between the individual and his or her physician. Our book has been written to help with that dialogue.

© 1997, 2014 Johns Hopkins University Press
All rights reserved. Published 2014
Printed in the United States of America on acid-free paper
9 8 7 6 5 4 3 2 1

First edition published as *The Johns Hopkins Guide to Diabetes: For Today and Tomorrow*, by Christopher D. Saudek, M.D., Richard R. Rubin, Ph.D., CDE, and Cynthia S. Shump, R.N., CDE

Johns Hopkins University Press
2715 North Charles Street
Baltimore, Maryland 21218-4363
www.press.jhu.edu

Library of Congress Cataloging-in-Publication Data
Saudek, Christopher D.
  The Johns Hopkins guide to diabetes : for patients and families /
Christopher D. Saudek, M.D., Richard R. Rubin, Ph.D., CDE, Thomas W.
Donner, M.D. — Second edition.
     pages cm — (A Johns Hopkins Press health book)
  Includes index.
  ISBN-13: 978-1-4214-1179-8 (hardcover : alk. paper)
  ISBN-10: 1-4214-1179-2 (hardcover : alk. paper)
  ISBN-13: 978-1-4214-1180-4 (pbk. : alk. paper)
  ISBN-10: 1-4214-1180-6 (pbk. : alk. paper)
  ISBN-13: 978-1-4214-1181-1 (electronic)
  ISBN-10: 1-4214-1181-4 (electronic)
  1. Diabetes—Treatment—Handbooks, manuals, etc. I. Rubin, Richard R.
II. Donner, Thomas W. III. Title.
  RC660.J536 2014
  616.4'62—dc23   2013015256

A catalog record for this book is available from the British Library.

Figures 13, 14, and 26–33 are by Jacqueline Schaffer.

Special discounts are available for bulk purchases of this book. For more information, please contact Special Sales at 410-516-6936 or specialsales@press.jhu.edu.

Johns Hopkins University Press uses environmentally friendly book materials, including recycled text paper that is composed of at least 30 percent post-consumer waste, whenever possible.

We dedicate this book to the memory of Christopher Saudek, brilliant scientist, caring clinician, and beloved friend.

We also dedicate this book to people with diabetes. They fight the daily battles great and small. Their courage and perseverance inspire us and teach not just about diabetes but about the human spirit.

Contents

Preface ix

Acknowledgments xiii

The first edition of this book was published in 1997. Much has changed in the years since then, including diabetes care. Three years ago Christopher Saudek and Richard Rubin began working on a new edition reflecting the many advances in diabetes treatment since we wrote the first edition of *The Johns Hopkins Guide to Diabetes*. Tragically, that effort was interrupted by Chris Saudek's untimely death in October 2010. Last year Richard Rubin, with the encouragement of Chris Saudek's wonderful wife, Susan, decided to try again to bring to print the vision that he and Chris had shared. Richard asked Chris's successor as head of the Johns Hopkins Diabetes Center, Dr. Tom Donner, to join him.

The words you read in this edition of *The Johns Hopkins Guide to Diabetes* are those of Chris, Richard, and Tom, supplemented by the following faculty members and fellows at Johns Hopkins: Dr. Nestoras Mathioudakis, Assistant Professor of Endocrinology; Dr. Sharon Solomon, Associate Professor of Ophthalmology; Emily Loghmani, RD, CDE, nutritionist at the Diabetes Center; Drs. Shabina Ahmed, Ilias Spanakis, Reshmi Srinath, and Laila Tabatabai, all clinical fellows in endocrinology; and Dr. Kristin Arcara, clinical fellow in pediatric endocrinology. Others who contributed to the book are Shereen Arent, J.D., Executive Vice President, Government Affairs and Advocacy, American Diabetes Association, and Katie Hathaway, J.D., Managing Director, Legal Advocacy, American Diabetes Association.

This book retains the wisdom, humor, and eloquence that Chris Saudek brought to all his endeavors. We miss him and we are honored to offer you an opportunity to benefit from his gifts.

As we wrote the first edition of *The Johns Hopkins Guide to Diabetes: For Today and Tomorrow*, we included stories we had heard from our patients and other people. These vignettes gradually became a central element of the book, and it dawned on us that, like many teachers, we learn far more from our students than we teach them. This edition includes even more of these personal stories. We have also added "take home messages" to the end of each chapter.

We are sharing what we have learned, and we hope that it's helpful. We know, however, that your "truth" will come from many sources, not only this book. You may jump into the primary literature, reading original research articles. You will almost certainly talk with people, too: family members, people with diabetes, and your health care professionals. We hope you read the diabetes magazines and keep your eyes open for information from many directions, including reliable resources on the Internet. You will need to sort through all these sources of information and figure out what works for you.

You know your own self best. You know how you feel, what you eat, how much you exercise, and how your blood glucose responds. No one else knows you in as much detail as you know yourself. But we provide another perspective, the perspective of professionals who have had lots of experience with diabetes. Actually, we provide three perspectives.

• • •

Chris Saudek was a clinically oriented academic physician. In addition to caring for people with diabetes on a daily basis, he was in charge of teaching medical students at Johns Hopkins about diabetes, contributed to various treatment advances, and held positions in professional diabetes organizations, including a year as president of the American Diabetes Association. It was his business to stay in touch with the literature. He tried to be sure that the information provided here was factually correct and that current research findings were accurately integrated into the text. Mainly, with some 25 years invested in clinical care, he cared for and about people with diabetes.

When Chris died, diabetes lost a hero. "We have lost one of our giants," said Dr. Edward D. Miller, dean of the faculty of the Johns Hopkins University School of Medicine. "He always tried to make things better for patients. His compassion and understanding of the human condition was unsurpassed." Ronald J. Daniels, president of Johns Hopkins University, who was also a patient of Dr. Saudek's, added that "Chris was the best Hopkins had to offer. His death is a huge loss to Hopkins and to medicine in the U.S. and beyond. He was a gentle and caring soul and an absolutely gorgeous human being."

Richard Rubin's professional life was also devoted to diabetes. Like Chris, he served as president of the American Diabetes Association. His sister Mary Sue has had Type 1 diabetes for 54 years, and his son Stefan has had Type 1 diabetes for 34 years. Richard devoted his career over the past 30 years to diabetes research and clinical care.

Richard was involved in several long-term studies of psychosocial and lifestyle issues in the management of diabetes, including the NIH-funded Diabetes Prevention Program (DPP) and Look AHEAD trials. He published many papers on treatment adherence, psychological problems associated with diabetes, and techniques for counseling people with diabetes. He also coauthored several books for people with diabetes and their families. With a handful of others around the country, Richard began teaching what should have been obvious all along: that psychological factors play a definitive role in the success of any treatment.

Finally, Tom Donner, before coming to Johns Hopkins, was director of the Joslin Diabetes Center affiliate at the University of Maryland. His clinical and research interests include prevention of diabetes complications and ways to safely control high glucose levels in all patients with diabetes. Tom worked with Chris Saudek on a multicenter clinical trial using implantable insulin pumps in humans. He was also a co-investigator on the NIH-funded DCCT/EDIC trial, which looked at the long-term effects of intensive diabetes control in patients with Type 1 diabetes, and the NIH-funded BARI 2D trial, which investigated ways to reduce heart attacks and prevent death in patients who have Type 2 diabetes and underlying heart disease. Tom's more recent research work is focusing on ways to prevent the immune destruction of insulin-producing beta cells of the pancreas in persons with Type 1 diabetes.

The Johns Hopkins Guide to Diabetes provides not one but two perspectives, each essential: that of the physician and that of the mental health researcher and counselor. The different views are woven into the whole fabric of the book. The only perspective we have highlighted for special attention, though, is yours. The stories you tell and the concerns, frustrations, and triumphs that are repeated over and over again from day to day, person to person—these are the basis of all our understanding and all our teaching.

Acknowledgments

The authors are indebted to countless people who have taught us and encouraged us over the years. Foremost are our families. We are always grateful for their love and support as we have taken yet more time away to pursue the writing of this book.

We want specifically to acknowledge the help of the following colleagues: G. William Benedict, Charlene E. Freeman, Sherman M. Holvey, Robert H. Knopp, Maria Lim, Lynn D. Mahbubani, Simeon Margolis, David Marrero, Nancy Neville, Margaret O'Neil, Leslie Plotnick, Robert E. Ratner, Gayle E. Reiber, Catherine S. Sackett, Paul J. Scheel Jr., Kristi Silver, and Judith Wylie-Rosett. These experts reviewed portions of the manuscript.

Gloria Elfert not only contributed significantly to the dietary portions of the text but also has been the model teacher of nutrition to generations of participants in the Johns Hopkins Diabetes Center. Likewise, the center's programs, including much of what appears in this book, could not have been accomplished without the central contributions of Joseph Napora, Mark Peyrot, Samuel Zaccari, and the physician-educators from the Johns Hopkins faculty, Division of Endocrinology and Metabolism.

Finally, we especially want to thank our editor, Jacqueline Wehmueller, for having originated the project and for guiding us through it with patience, good counsel, and unwavering support.

Understanding Diabetes

There are enough uncertainties in life without wondering whether you have diabetes. And if you do, you won't want to spend time worrying about what kind of diabetes. Nevertheless, a great many people are confused on these very basic issues. Part I will clear up the confusion. We will consistently reject such phrases as "a touch of sugar," "just in my blood, not in my urine," and "the sugar's just a little high," making it clear that either you have diabetes or you don't. And we will point out the misfortunes that can result from denial.

This is not because we are unsympathetic or like to beat people over the head with the fact that they have diabetes. Quite the opposite. We feel nothing but compassion for and solidarity with our patients, friends, and relatives with diabetes. It's perfectly clear why they would like to deny the disease, wish it away, wake up one morning without it. But we also see every day the effects of living in long-term denial. We see people who for one reason or another didn't come to grips with their diabetes, didn't hear the diagnosis, and paid dearly.

So in Part I we lay out the fundamentals of making the diagnosis. We describe the types of diabetes and set a foundation for understanding what blood glucose measurement is all about. It would be terrific if we could also set out certainties, provide unambiguous criteria, and give definitions that will never change. Unfortunately, this isn't possible. The criteria, definitions, and even names do change from time to time, as scientific evidence evolves. But the basic facts remain: it is crucial to know when you have diabetes, to hear the diagnosis, and to pay attention to it.

1

The Diagnosis of Diabetes

Making It and Hearing It

with Ilias Spanakis, M.D.

- "It hit me like a ton of bricks. How could this be possible? I didn't know a thing about diabetes. Why me? It was never in my family."
- "I'm a doctor, so you would think I'd recognize the symptoms. But when my son started drinking all the time and losing weight, I thought it was just because of summer; and when he urinated it was just all the Cokes he was drinking. It didn't cross my mind that he had diabetes until he was really quite sick. Then it hit me."
- "I had a suspicion, since there is so much diabetes in my family. To tell the truth, I pretty much knew I had it, and told the doctor so."
- "It's strange, but when the doctor told me I had diabetes, I was actually relieved, because I was convinced I had cancer. I'd been losing weight for so long, feeling worse and worse. To my way of thinking, diabetes was a whole lot better than cancer."
- "Looking back, I'll bet I've had diabetes a long time. Sometimes when I'd go to the doctor, he would say something like, 'Your sugar's a little high' or 'You may have a touch of diabetes in your blood test.' But he never made much of it, and I felt pretty good, so I just forgot about it."

As these statements illustrate, when a person first hears the diagnosis of diabetes, he or she may be devastated—or take it in stride. Some people ignore it altogether. For some people, however, the symptoms are impossible to ignore, which brings them to medical attention quickly. In other people the symptoms are mild or nonexistent, and these people may go years without even knowing they have the disease. In fact, about one-third of all the people with diabetes in the United States don't know that they have it.

Doctors may unintentionally encourage a person to deny the diabetes by using convenient phrases that minimize the problems—phrases like "a touch of sugar." We wish everyone would ask the doctor specifically, "Do you mean I have diabetes?" But, as is only natural, people usually don't want to hear the answer. Denial is a potent defense mechanism, and we've seen people deny their diabetes almost to the point of death.

A central theme of this book is that you can live a long and healthy life with diabetes, but it is a dangerous disease to ignore. The first step is to know whether you have diabetes, so that, if you do, you can begin taking care of it. In this chapter we emphasize that the diagnosis of diabetes can and should be clearly made: *either you have it or you don't.* Long before most diabetes is diagnosed, the blood glucose level often runs mildly high, but not to the diabetes range. *This is "prediabetes" and is also important to recognize*, because people who have prediabetes are predisposed to develop diabetes in the future.

We've helped thousands of people come to grips with the diagnosis of diabetes, and we have seen the shock that may go along with learning that diagnosis. So in this chapter we also consider how people cope when their diabetes is first discovered. Then we start the process of understanding what blood glucose values really mean and how they fluctuate in diabetes. Glucose is the form of sugar that is found in blood. In this book we will use the word *glucose* rather than the word *sugar* when we are talking about this form of sugar. Other sugars, including sucrose (table sugar) and fructose (a sugar in honey and fruits), appear in very small amounts or not at all in blood.

Diagnosing Diabetes

The name *diabetes mellitus* is a good description: the word *diabetes* comes from the Greek for "siphon." We recently saw a man who described such bad thirst and frequent urination that he would literally drink water while he urinated—as though he were, in fact, a siphon, the water just flowing in and flowing out. *Mellitus* is from the Latin for "sweet," referring to the glucose in the urine. (*Diabetes insipidus* is another disease altogether, characterized by excess urination but unrelated to blood glucose. It has nothing to do with diabetes mellitus, which is the subject of this book.)

Diabetes has many different causes and involves many different systems and organs in the body. But it is defined very specifically, and that definition depends on only one thing: high blood glucose.

The *blood glucose*, also called *plasma glucose*, refers to the amount, or concentration, of glucose in the blood. The units used in measuring the amount are milligrams per deciliter, or mg/dl; in most countries other than the United States, the units millimoles per liter, or mM, are used instead of mg/dl. (To convert mM to mg/dl, multiply the mM value by 18; to convert from mg/dl to mM, divide by 18. For example, 180 mg/dl equals 10 mM.)

Everyone has some glucose in the blood, usually, in persons who do not have diabetes, about 60–99 mg/dl when fasting and 80–139 mg/dl after meals. The brain needs glucose to function normally; this is why, when the glucose level in the blood drops too low (*hypoglycemia*), a person's ability to reason is impaired and coma may even result. When the blood glucose is found to be too high (*hyperglycemia*), the diagnosis of diabetes is made.

The diagnostic criteria for diabetes are listed in Table 1. Often, the diagnosis is obvious to doctors because the symptoms are so characteristic. The most common symptoms include excessive thirst, frequent urination, blurred vision, weight loss, persistent vaginal infections in women, and general fatigue. In the presence of these symptoms, the diagnosis of diabetes can be confirmed by a "random" test of blood glucose, meaning that the blood is drawn at any time during the day, rather than specifically before you eat breakfast. If the person is thirsty and urinating large amounts, the blood glucose is usually well over 200 mg/dl, sometimes up in the 300s, 400s, or even higher.

Sometimes a person has few or even no symptoms, and a high blood glucose is found on a blood test during a routine physical examination. In this case, the diagnosis is less clear, and it is in this situation that people may not be told specifically that they have diabetes. So let's look more closely at the criteria for diagnosing diabetes when the classic symptoms aren't present and the random blood glucose isn't over 200 mg/dl.

First, a *fasting* blood glucose may be elevated. This means the blood glucose is drawn at least eight hours after a meal, when it is usually at its lowest point in the day. In 1979, when an expert committee agreed upon the criteria for diagnosing diabetes, a fasting glucose (technically, plasma glucose measured twice) of 140 mg/dl or more made the diagnosis of diabetes. In 1997, this level was lowered to the new criterion of 126 mg/dl.

In 2009 an International Expert Committee from the American Diabetes Association, the International Diabetes Federation, and the European Association for the Study of Diabetes concluded that hemoglobin A1c can also be used as a blood test to diagnose diabetes when the level is 6.5% or higher. Measurement of the A1c is an easily performed blood test that accurately shows what the average blood glucose of an individual has been for the pre-

Table 1 Blood Glucose Criteria for Diagnosing Diabetes Mellitus and Impaired Glucose Tolerance in Nonpregnant and Pregnant Adults

---

Diabetes mellitus in nonpregnant adults is defined as:

a random plasma glucose greater than or equal to 200 mg/dl with symptoms of hyperglycemia (thirst, excessive urination, weight loss)

or

a fasting plasma glucose greater than or equal to 126 mg/dl*

or

during a 75-gram oral glucose tolerance test, a 2-hour plasma glucose greater than or equal to 200 mg/dl*

or

a hemoglobin A1c of 6.5% or higher*

Gestational diabetes mellitus is defined as:

a fasting glucose at any time during pregnancy that is greater than or equal to 92 mg/dl and less than 126 mg/dl—a fasting glucose over 126 mg/dl is frank diabetes

or

during a 75-gram oral glucose tolerance test at 24–28 weeks pregnancy, any glucose values greater than or equal to the following:

Fasting	92 mg/dl
1 hour	180 mg/dl
2 hours	153 mg/dl

Impaired glucose tolerance in nonpregnant adults is defined as:

fasting plasma glucose less than 126 mg/dl but greater than 99 mg/dl

or

in a 75-gram oral glucose tolerance test, a 2-hour plasma glucose between 140 and 199 mg/dl

---

*For someone without typical symptoms of hyperglycemia, these test results should be confirmed by repeat testing.

vious two to three months. This is used not only as a screening test for the diagnosis of diabetes mellitus but also for monitoring and assessing diabetes control (see Chapter 4).

If the random blood glucose isn't over 200 mg/dl, the A1c is not 6.5% or higher, *and* the fasting glucose isn't over 125 mg/dl, then one of these findings on its own does not confirm a diagnosis of diabetes. If there is a strong suspicion that you have diabetes or there is an important reason to screen for it (such as pregnancy), an *oral glucose tolerance test*, or OGTT, can be done. In the nonpregnant person, the OGTT consists of taking a blood sample for a fasting blood glucose level, having the person drink a measured amount of glucose (75 grams) as a very sweet drink, and testing blood glucose again at least 120 minutes later, sometimes with in-between samples also drawn. (The OGTT is done slightly differently in pregnancy.) According to World Health Organization criteria, diabetes is diagnosed if the blood glucose value two hours after the oral glucose is 200 mg/dl or higher.

During pregnancy, diabetes is diagnosed by slightly different criteria (see Table 1 and Chapter 29), but it is especially important to know whether you do or do not have diabetes during pregnancy.

Often, there is confusion over whether *urine* testing can be used to diagnose diabetes, without testing the blood. While high blood glucose levels (over about 180 mg/dl) do ordinarily cause glucose to "spill over" into the urine, the presence of glucose in the urine is *not* by itself sufficient to diagnose diabetes. A blood glucose level must be obtained.

Using the specific blood glucose criteria, then, it is possible to say definitely whether you do or do not have diabetes. There are some levels of blood glucose, though, that are not quite high enough to be called diabetes, but nor are they entirely normal. These levels fall into a "prediabetes" range. *Prediabetes* is a condition associated with a high risk of developing diabetes in the future, diabetes being diagnosed at a rate of about 5% per year, if nothing is done to help prevent diabetes from developing. Prediabetes is diagnosed when a fasting glucose value is between 100 and 125 mg/dl, when an A1c level is between 5.7% and 6.4 %, or when the blood glucose level at two hours during an oral glucose tolerance test is between 140 and 199 mg/dl.

We avoid using such terms as *borderline diabetes, a touch of diabetes,* or *chemical diabetes.* If a person actually does have diabetes, these terms tend to minimize it, suggesting that it really isn't very important. And if the person does *not* have diabetes—for instance, if the right diagnosis is really prediabetes—then he or she should not be saddled with the label *diabetes,* since it may have a negative effect on health or life insurance availability, employment, and so on. Again, it's important to get the straight answer: do you or do you not have diabetes?

Another common question is whether a person who has diabetes at one time will *always* have diabetes. It's not so easy to answer this question. If normal blood glucose levels have resulted from an ongoing treatment such as diet or pills, the person still has diabetes, very well controlled by treatment. But in some people, weight loss alone will effectively "cure" the diabetes, at least for the time being. In others, completion of a pregnancy will "cure" it. But anyone who has a previous history of diabetes, even if they don't have it currently, is definitely at greater-than-normal risk of developing diabetes in the future.

Hearing the Diagnosis of Diabetes

The whole range of emotions may pour out when someone hears for the first time that he or she has diabetes. Fear, anger, and feelings of impotence or being out of control are common responses. Some people cry, and others feel the emotional impact hours or even days later. Others minimize the seriousness of the disease and how it will affect their lives. Some people, though, seem almost unnaturally matter-of-fact, accepting the changes they will have to make without apparent concern. Emotional swings occur, even from hour to hour. What causes this spectrum of responses, and is there a "normal" or "abnormal" response?

We don't think that there is any one normal response. An emotional outburst is certainly common, as is an overwhelming concern about how this new diagnosis will affect life and life expectancy. People do better if they feel support and sympathy, both from their health care professionals and from their families. Reassurance is definitely helpful: there *are* effective treatments, you *can* control this very well, and in all likelihood you *will* lead a long and healthy life. There is no need to learn everything about diabetes or self-care in the first few days, although people often want to make a frantic run to the library, the bookstore, or the Internet to learn all there is to know about diabetes immediately. There is time. Self-care can be learned gradually.

How you respond depends, first, on your own personality. If you are an unusually calm, easygoing person with lots of confidence in yourself, you are more likely to accept diabetes in a matter-of-fact way. People who are naturally nervous, or "hyper," will probably have to cope with a series of diabetes-related anxieties. If you tend to be depressed, this news may make things worse.

Some people feel so overwhelmed by the diagnosis of diabetes that they do become clinically depressed. It's important to recognize when a response goes beyond the bounds of normal, tipping over into frank depression. We talk about how to detect and deal with psychological problems in Chapter 16.

The state of your life generally is another strong influence on your emotional response to the diagnosis. If you have a steady job that you like, one that earns you a reasonable income, it obviously helps. If you are otherwise healthy, with no other serious medical conditions and few family problems, you will undoubtedly find that things go easier, since you'll have time to learn about your diabetes, and you'll have the support of family and friends.

We find that the most intensely negative emotional responses to the diagnosis usually pass within a few months, as people move through the period of crisis and adjust to daily life with diabetes, learning that they can, in fact, cope with it. But if you feel that you are suffering too much during this early adjustment period, get professional help. Not only will it make you feel better, but it may start you on the road to better self-care.

Denying the diagnosis altogether is at least as worrisome to us as a highly emotional response. It's one thing to be stoic and another to pretend you don't have diabetes. We feel such sadness when we see people who have willfully ignored the diagnosis until they develop significant long-term complications.

Diabetes is an important illness that will affect your life. If not well cared for, it could shorten your life. There is no use denying these realities or denying the diagnosis. But diabetes is also a disease that can be very well managed, and people often live their full life expectancy with diabetes. It is something you can live with, something you can control

As a start, you should begin to learn what blood glucose values really mean.

Blood Glucose Variations in Diabetes

Andy, who was diagnosed with diabetes not long ago, came to see us because he was worried by the fact that his blood glucose readings were never the same, even when he tested at the same time of day. "One morning it's 80 and the next it's 95," he explained. "One evening after supper it's 110 and another it's 135. What am I doing wrong?"

Sonia, who had had diabetes for more than 15 years, was also worried about blood glucose variations. "I've been taking insulin for an awfully long time," she told us, "but my blood sugars still don't always make sense. Okay, when I eat too much, it goes high. But some days, it can be 300, and then I take some extra insulin, and in almost no time at all it's 30. What's going on?"

Seeing your blood glucose levels bounce up and down in unpredictable patterns can be one of the most frustrating things about having diabetes, especially when you are testing regularly and trying to do your best with your diet and exercise patterns. It is one of the strains we put on ourselves by regular blood glucose testing, wanting to see how the glucose is doing. But if you check your glucose regularly, you *will* see it bounce. The first thing to understand is that no one's blood glucose is constant. The human body isn't made that way. And if the blood glucose readings are within normal limits—as is true for Andy—then there's absolutely no need for anxiety.

What is a normal blood glucose concentration? This is a deceptively simple question, especially since many laboratory result sheets print out the "normal values" for fasting blood glucose, usually about 60-99 mg/dl. Actually, the "normal" value is something like the "normal" speed of a car: it may be 55 miles per hour on a freeway but 10 miles per hour in rush hour traffic. Likewise, the blood glucose level varies depending on the exact situation.

When you haven't eaten for some time, say 8-12 hours, the normal (without diabetes) "fasting" blood glucose is what the lab printout says: about 60-99 mg/dl. (The low side of this range is variable, and what's acceptable here depends on the individual's situation: if the person is taking insulin, a fasting blood glucose in the 60-70 mg/dl range may be too close to hypoglycemia; if the person is not taking insulin and is not bothered by symptoms of low blood glucose, a fasting blood glucose in the 60s may be perfectly acceptable.)

After eating any meal that contains carbohydrate or protein, blood glucose normally rises, often to about 120-130 mg/dl but generally not to more than 140 mg/dl in the person without diabetes. Over two to four hours, the blood glucose returns to baseline. Day in and day out, from hour to hour, the normal blood glucose levels vary (see Figure 1). If you chart blood glucose levels in a person without diabetes, you won't get a flat line but rather a series of hills and valleys. And these are the variations that occur *without* diabetes; the swings are always much wider with diabetes.

To understand *how* and *why* blood glucose varies so much even in a person without diabetes, you have to understand something about insulin. Insulin is the remarkable hormone that comes out of the beta cells of the pancreas. Its purpose is to help the cells of the body *burn glucose* for energy. As the blood glucose rises after a meal, from the carbohydrate being absorbed, this triggers a release of insulin from the pancreatic beta cells. The insulin then opens the doors of the body's cells to glucose, allowing the glucose to

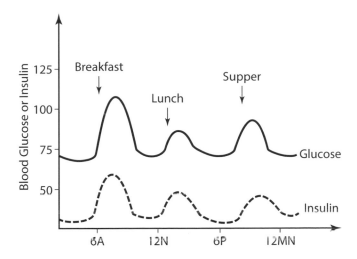

Figure 1. The normal relationship between glucose and insulin levels in the blood-stream. Without diabetes, the pancreas functions like a thermostat for the blood glucose. There are minor variations in level, but overall, blood glucose is kept within a tight range. When the blood glucose starts to go up with ingestion of a meal, the beta cells of the pancreas put out insulin, bringing down the level of glucose in the bloodstream. When the meal is complete, the beta cells put out just a little insulin to take care of the glucose that is made and released by the liver. Thus the blood glucose is kept in the normal range of 70–99 mg/dl before meals and less than 140 mg/dl after a meal.

leave the bloodstream and enter the cells, where it is used as fuel. (Figure 2 diagrams this process.) As glucose enters the cells, the blood glucose level returns to normal. Glucose is fuel for all cellular functions.

When the blood glucose level is relatively low, as happens before a meal, the beta cells are at rest and almost no insulin is secreted. The cells of the body turn to other sources of fuel they have kept in reserve, such as stored fat or carbohydrate.

In the person without diabetes, this is a finely tuned system. Blood glucose is relatively low and beta cells are at rest overnight and before a meal, with body cells burning alternative fuels. As soon as the person eats, blood glucose levels rise, the beta cells wake up and make insulin, this insulin circulates and opens up the cells to glucose, and the cells use the available glucose as fuel, bringing the blood glucose level back to baseline.

The basic problem in diabetes is that not enough insulin is made by the pancreas. Sometimes the beta cells don't make any insulin at all, and the

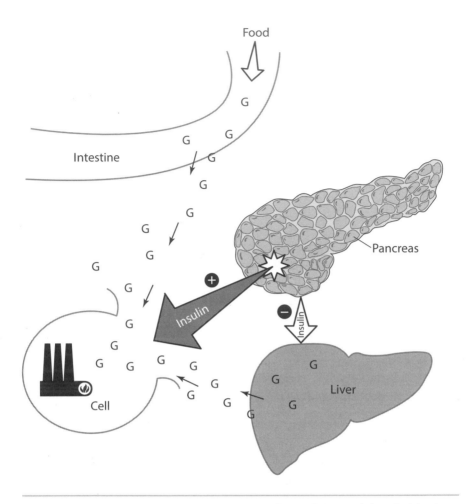

Figure 2. The role of insulin. Insulin reduces the level of glucose (G) in the bloodstream by allowing glucose to enter cells to serve as fuel for the various cellular activities. Insulin binds to a spot on the cell surface called a *receptor*. When this happens, glucose is able to pass through the cell membrane into the cell, where it is used for energy. Some people liken this to a lock and key. Insulin is the key that opens the lock (receptor) so that glucose can pass through the door into the cell. Using this analogy, in Type 1 diabetes, someone stole the keys (no insulin is made by the pancreas); in Type 2, the door won't open fully even with the right key (insulin resistance). At the same time that insulin promotes the uptake of glucose by cells, it inhibits the release of glucose by the liver.

person has to take injections of insulin; sometimes the body is resistant to the insulin that is made, and the pancreas, try as it might, can't put out enough insulin. In either case, if not enough insulin is made, the blood glucose has a strong tendency to rise, since it is not leaving the bloodstream to enter the cells as fuel.

How much, and how quickly, do blood glucose levels rise and fall in a person with diabetes? This is an unanswerable question. There is just too much variability from person to person, from day to day. But let's discuss some generalizations, which are diagrammed in Figure 3. To begin with (Figure 3a), if you don't have diabetes, the blood glucose level starts the day below 100 mg/dl and will not rise above about 140 mg/dl. How high the level goes after each meal, and how soon it returns to baseline, depends largely on what the meal contains.

Figure 3b shows the pattern that might be seen in someone with "stable," well-controlled diabetes, or in a person with diabetes that is mild (the person makes almost but not quite enough insulin). You can see that the blood glucose tends to start higher than normal and rises somewhat higher after meals, returning to normal more slowly. It is less finely tuned than normal, and on average it is higher.

When you look at the pattern in "unstable" diabetes (see Figure 3c), you see the kind of fluctuations that made Sonia throw up her hands in despair. Even though, on average, the blood glucose is well controlled, there are times in the day when it is actually over 300. Sonia also feels the effects of a definite low just before supper. This is frustrating, to say the least. And the

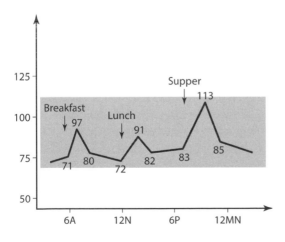

Figure 3a. No diabetes. The blood glucose level fluctuates—rising somewhat after meals—but stays in the normal range, 70–140 mg/dl, throughout the day. The average blood glucose in this case is 86 mg/dl.

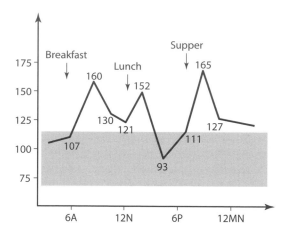

Figure 3b. Stable, well-controlled diabetes is characterized by mild variations in blood glucose levels, which remain in the normal range most of the time. The average blood glucose in this case is 129 mg/dl.

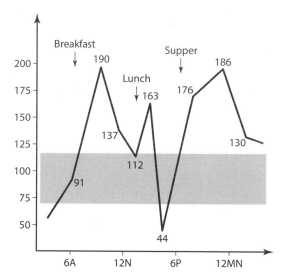

Figure 3c. Unstable, well-controlled diabetes is characterized by more abrupt changes in the blood glucose level throughout the day. At one minute it may be in the 200s and within the hour it may drop to 60. But the average is good in this case, at 136 mg/dl.

pattern she has today may not be much like the pattern she had yesterday or will have tomorrow. But there are reasons for the rises and falls, and if these reasons are understood, the peaks and valleys may be smoothed out. Much of this book is devoted to helping people smooth out their blood glucose control. On a positive note, although Sonia's blood glucose was bouncing from low to high and back again, the average throughout the 24-hour period was actually not bad at all. She has good average blood glucose levels, though her levels are unstable as they vary from hour to hour. She may have difficulty dealing with the highs and lows, but she is doing a good job of reducing her risk of long-term complications.

Finally, Figures 3d and 3e illustrate "uncontrolled" diabetes. In uncontrolled diabetes, the blood glucose level starts high, goes higher, and stays high. The average for this person is 365 mg/dl. She is undoubtedly feeling the symptoms of uncontrolled diabetes: she is thirsty, urinates frequently, has blurred vision, and is generally without energy. What's more, if these levels continue year in and year out, she is very likely to develop serious complications from diabetes. The difference between Figures 3d and 3e is that in Figure 3d the blood glucose is high but stable, not varying much,

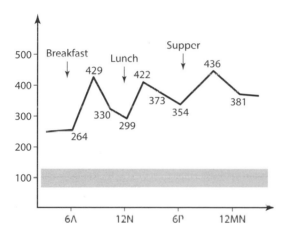

Figure 3d. Stable, uncontrolled diabetes is characterized by persistently high blood glucose. The levels don't fluctuate much but just stay high—in this case, an average of 365 mg/dl.

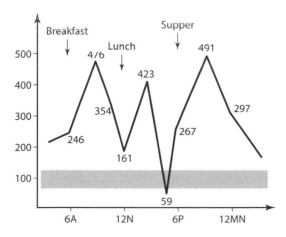

Figure 3e. Unstable, uncontrolled diabetes is characterized by blood glucose levels that fluctuate wildly and are, on average, high. In this case the average blood glucose is 275 mg/dl.

while in Figure 3e it is high and unstable, crashing up and down. This degree of uncontrolled diabetes is not rare; in fact, many people used to live for decades with average blood glucose levels over 200–300 mg/dl. On the whole, these are the people who suffered the worst complications of diabetes.

Few tools were available in the old days to help people control their blood glucose. Fortunately, it doesn't have to be that way any longer. Diabetes is definitely controllable. In this book we'll help you learn how to do it and give you lots of good reasons for following our—and your own doctor's—advice.

Take Home Messages

- Diabetes can be diagnosed on the basis of a random blood glucose test if the value is 200 mg/dl or higher, a fasting blood glucose test if the value is 126 mg/dl or higher, or a hemoglobin A1c test if the value is 6.5% or higher.
- Prediabetes is a condition in which blood glucose levels are higher than normal but not high enough to warrant a diagnosis of diabetes. People with prediabetes have an increased risk of going on to develop diabetes.
- You may feel scared, angry, or overwhelmed when you first learn you have diabetes. For most people these feelings become less intense within a few months.
- It is important to try to keep your blood glucose levels as close to normal as possible, but when you have diabetes, perfect control is *impossible*. Keeping track of your levels and consulting with your diabetes health care team can help you maintain good glucose control.

2

Types of Diabetes

with Ilias Spanakis, M.D.

- "I used to be controlled with diet, and then pills. But now I take insulin, because my sugar went way up. Why do they still say I have non-insulin-dependent diabetes when I definitely need insulin?"
- "People talk about types of diabetes. I'm not sure what type I am. When I talk to doctors, I don't get a straight answer, and I don't see why it matters, anyway."

It is usually easy to diagnose diabetes, but deciding what *type* of diabetes you have can sometimes be far from straightforward for doctors and patients alike. The newer names for diabetes are less confusing than the older ones. Some people just don't fit neatly into the diagnostic "boxes."

In this chapter we look at the different kinds of diabetes. We discuss the rationale behind the formal names and the practical implications of the different types. At the Johns Hopkins Medical School, we show second-year medical students a simple diagram that includes some very complicated theories and debates about diabetes (see Figure 4). The diagram considers diabetes as one disease, defined by high blood glucose (hyperglycemia), with many different primary causes, all leading to an inadequate amount of insulin secreted from the pancreas. The hyperglycemia causes acute (immediate) complications and also long-term complications (which are the subject of Part IV).

Figure 4 is an oversimplification, though, because in reality there are different types of diabetes, and they behave differently in important ways. But diabetes of any type, whatever the cause, may produce any and all of the symptoms or complications. Thirst, fatigue, weight loss, and frequent urination, for example, occur whenever the blood glucose is elevated above about 180 mg/dl, regardless of what kind of diabetes the person has. Long-

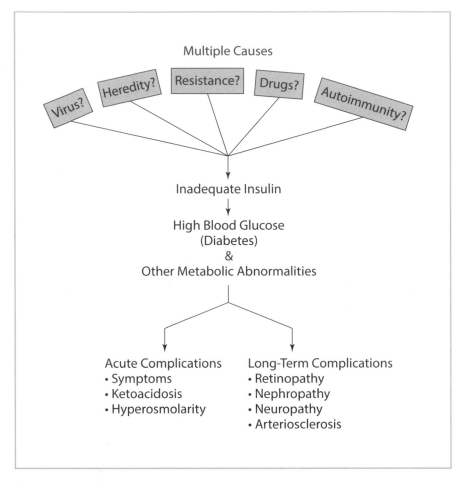

Figure 4. Overall scheme of diabetes.

term complications involving the eyes, kidneys, and nerves have also been found in all kinds of diabetes.

As you will see, the basic distinction made between Type 1 and Type 2 diabetes is that people with Type 1 diabetes get ketoacidosis and those with Type 2 don't. But even this does not always hold. Many people with Type 1 diabetes, adequately treated, have never had ketoacidosis, and some people with Type 2 diabetes do develop ketoacidosis, especially if they are under severe stress.

The Classification System

In thinking about the various kinds of diabetes, you should distinguish four general types:

— *Type 1 diabetes* is due to the complete or almost complete destruction of the pancreatic beta cells (the cells that make insulin) by immune mechanisms.

— *Type 2 diabetes* is due to the body not making enough insulin and also not responding so well to any insulin that is made by the pancreas.

— *Gestational diabetes mellitus* is the type of diabetes that first appears in pregnancy.

— *Other types of diabetes* include those kinds with relatively well-known causes, including cystic fibrosis, medications such as steroids and HIV medications, chronic pancreatitis, surgical removal of the pancreas, some hormone excess disorders, and some genetic syndromes leading to abnormal insulin production or insulin action.

We should emphasize that such diagnoses as prediabetes, borderline results, or a previous history of diabetes mellitus due to illness or medication do not mean that the person has diabetes. As mentioned in Chapter 1, these terms refer to conditions that put a person at *increased risk* of developing diabetes, but that person does not yet have diabetes.

According to the National Diabetes Fact Sheet from 2011, 8.3% of the population in the United States—25.8 million children and adults—have diabetes. Of these, 18.8 million are already diagnosed. But it is worrisome that an estimated 7 million people are currently undiagnosed. Also, 79 million people are considered to have prediabetes. Type 2 diabetes accounts for 90% of all diabetes cases, while Type 1 accounts for 5%–10%. The remaining cases are considered "other types of diabetes."

What difference does it make what kind of diabetes you have? A major difference is how each kind of diabetes is treated:

— *Type 1 diabetes* will need insulin treatment right away.

— *Type 2 diabetes* may not need insulin or pills until weight control through diet and exercise has been given a good try.

— *Gestational diabetes* must be treated aggressively with diet, exercise, and then insulin in order to give the developing fetus every chance to develop normally.

—*Other types of diabetes* may be helped by treating their underlying cause.

An accurate diagnosis does matter. There are differences in the approach to treatment, which we'll discuss in more detail later. First, let's look more closely at the different types of diabetes.

Type 1 Diabetes

- "We were flabbergasted! There was no diabetes on either side of his family, he was a perfectly healthy kid, when all of a sudden he began to lose weight, was thirsty all the time, and spent half the night urinating. Once he started to take insulin, though, he felt much better, settled right down, and it has been very easy to keep his blood glucoses normal for three months now."

Type 1 diabetes was previously called insulin-dependent or juvenile onset diabetes. It is the kind of diabetes that more often comes on in people's early years, usually in childhood, but extending up to about 30 years old and, less commonly, at even older ages. Type 1 diabetes usually occurs in people who are of normal weight or are thin and losing weight, and everyone with this type of diabetes must be treated with insulin, usually right after they are diagnosed. If you have diabetes and you fit these characteristics, the chances are that you have Type 1 diabetes. Most people can determine for themselves whether they have Type 1 diabetes by looking at the typical features of Type 1 listed in Table 2.

The beta cells in the pancreas are the only cells of the body that produce insulin, and in Type 1 diabetes they are destroyed. The beta cells are located in the islets of Langerhans, first discovered in 1869 by Paul Langerhans. Cells in the islets of Langerhans make several other hormones as well, and the islets are located among the acinar cells of the pancreas, which make digestive enzymes.

In 1901, a Johns Hopkins pathologist, Eugene Opie, was the first to discover the key point that beta cells produce an internal secretion needed to avoid diabetes. He noted that if the pancreatic beta cells were absent, the person had diabetes. Twenty years after that, Drs. Banting, Macleod, Best, and Collip, working in Toronto, successfully isolated the substance that those beta cells contain—insulin—and gave it to people with Type 1 diabetes. A marvelous account of this epic discovery, summarized in Chapter 11, can be found in the book *The Discovery of Insulin* by Michael Bliss (Univer-

Table 2   Typical Features of Type 1 Diabetes

Feature	Typical Finding	Comments
Age of onset	Under 40 years old; most common in childhood	Can develop at any age; older people often develop Type 1 more slowly
Body weight	Thin to normal weight	Can be overweight
Presentation	Relatively quick onset, with symptoms developing and worsening over weeks to months	Thirst, frequent urination, and weight loss; may progress to ketoacidosis
Family history	Usually no known history of Type 1 diabetes in the family	Unusually, Type 1 diabetes may be in the family
Risk factors	No major risk factors for Type 1 diabetes; some protective factors such as African American race/ethnicity	Risk increased if strong family history of Type 1 diabetes and mildly increased with a single family member having Type 1 diabetes; eating sugar not a cause of Type 1 diabetes
Insulin treatment	Always needed to control the diabetes and prevent ketoacidosis	Responds to pills for no more than a year or so; in children, insulin usually needed immediately
Blood glucose control	Up and down, harder to keep in the ideal range than in Type 2 diabetes	Blood glucose very sensitive to small changes in diet, exercise, and insulin dose; more frustrating than in Type 2 diabetes!
"Honeymoon period"	Usually starting within a few months of onset, a time when the diabetes is more stable and easier to control	Lower insulin requirements; usually lasts 3–12 months
Laboratory tests	Blood glucose high, usually over 200 mg/dl if thirsty; hemoglobin A1c usually high; islet cell antibodies and/or GAD (glutamic acid decarboxylase) antibodies and/or insulin autoantibodies in about 90%–95% of people at the time of diagnosis	Antibody tests may be done at the onset of diabetes if doubt as to whether Type 1 or Type 2; positive result confirms Type 1
Cause	A combination of heredity and exposure to some factor during life that triggers autoimmune destruction of the insulin-producing beta cells in the pancreas	Details of both the hereditary and the environmental factors not well understood

sity of Chicago Press, 1982). The book was dramatized on television by the Public Broadcasting System in 1993.

In a person with Type 1 diabetes, the beta cells of the pancreas are destroyed by autoimmune processes, so virtually no insulin is produced. (The autoimmune process is discussed more fully later in this chapter.) When no insulin is produced in the pancreas, a person must be given insulin by injection. This is why Type 1 diabetes has been called "insulin dependent": there is an absolute requirement for, or dependence on, insulin treatment. In the absence of insulin treatment or when far too little insulin is given, the result is diabetic ketoacidosis (Chapter 21).

By formal definition, then, Type 1 diabetes is the form of diabetes that, when fully developed, in the absence of insulin treatment, causes ketoacidosis and ultimately death. Today, Type 1 diabetes is entirely treatable, and ketoacidosis is preventable by taking the right amount of insulin.

Since there is no insulin coming from the pancreas, a person with Type 1 diabetes has *labile* blood glucose levels, meaning that the blood glucose tends to shoot up and drop down more easily if insulin, food, and exercise aren't carefully matched. (See Figures 3c and 3e.) *Brittle diabetes* is another term used to describe the same thing—blood glucose bouncing up and down. Sometimes people are diagnosed as having brittle diabetes, as though it were a specific, different kind of diabetes. We think, rather, that lability, or "brittleness," is a spectrum. Even for people on the far end of this spectrum, with very unstable blood glucose levels, glucose can be reasonably well controlled by careful attention to the details of self-management. So we prefer not to consider brittle diabetes as a different form of diabetes.

To understand what causes lability, consider the following metaphor. A thermostat turns the furnace on or off depending on what the room's temperature is, whether too cold or too warm. But if you're using a woodstove to heat the room, you don't have the benefit of a thermostat, and you have to guess how much wood to put in the stove each morning. Unless you guess very well every time, the room may well be too hot or too cold. The healthy pancreas operates under thermostatic control, sensing when the blood glucose goes up and putting out just the right amount of insulin to bring it back to normal. Insulin injections are more like stoking the stove with wood—you have to make your best estimate about how much you will need as the day progresses.

The normally functioning pancreatic beta cell does its job with great precision, secreting just the right amount of insulin to keep the blood glucose in its normal range, no matter the diet, the exercise, or the stress level. Insulin by injection rarely achieves this precision, even with the best intentions. (Insulin pumps, discussed later in the book, also lack the feedback control of a normal pancreas, because current "glucose sensors" are not able to tell a pump how much insulin to give to keep the glucose in normal ranges.) Lacking the natural feedback control of a normal pancreas, the person with Type 1 diabetes is always struggling to estimate how much insulin to take and how much food to eat, and to factor in exercise and stress as well. Treatment is more difficult and imprecise. As the person with Type 1 diabetes knows, the great and wonderful discovery of insulin was not, in fact, a cure for diabetes.

What Causes Type 1 Diabetes?

This common question is very hard to answer. We do know certain things:

—Type 1 diabetes occurs in people with a genetic susceptibility, even when (as is usually the case) there is no known family history of Type 1 diabetes.
—It requires exposure to something in the "environment," so it is not entirely hereditary.
—Most important, it is an autoimmune disease.

Each of these facts requires further discussion, and each can be hard to comprehend fully, mainly because a lot more research is necessary before we really understand the causes of Type 1 diabetes.

Consider, first, the hereditary factor. The best way to find out if heredity is involved in a disease is to see whether the disease tends to run in families. The final proof is to see the disease occurring more often in both identical twins than in both non-identical twins. If the condition were 100% genetic, then if one identical twin had Type 1 diabetes, the other, having exactly the same genes, would have it too. Studies show that, indeed, the "concordance rate" in identical twins is high: in 50% of identical twin pairs, if one twin has diabetes, the other twin does too. But it is not 100%, so Type 1 diabetes is not entirely genetic. If a mother has Type 1 diabetes, there is about a 2%–4% chance of one of her children developing the disease. For a father, the risk in his children is about 5%–8%. If one child has diabetes, there is about a 5% chance that a brother or sister will develop Type 1 diabetes.

It is unusual for several people in the same family to have Type 1 diabetes, but most people who have a child with Type 1 diabetes want to know what the chance is that another child will get it. Table 3 provides the best available figures. Blood tests for autoimmunity, including islet cell antibodies (see below), can be run on first-degree relatives of people with Type 1 diabetes to see whether they show a risk of damage to their islet cells and therefore are likely to develop Type 1 diabetes.

Several studies have attempted but failed to prevent progressive damage of the islet cells once it has started, using insulin by injection, by mouth, or in the nose, or using drugs that block the immune system from attacking the beta cells (Chapter 31). People wanting to have the islet cell antibody test done (for instance, in brothers and sisters of a child with diabetes) must understand that, as yet, there is no known way to prevent the development of Type 1 diabetes if the test results are positive. TrialNet is a multinational group of diabetes centers that are screening family members of patients with Type 1 diabetes for the antibodies that appear before the blood glucose becomes elevated. Those who test positive for the antibodies are monitored closely for signs that they are going to develop diabetes, and they may be able to enter studies using new drugs or other techniques aimed at prevent-

Table 3　Risk of Developing Type 1 Diabetes if a Relative Has Type 1 Diabetes

Population Group	Risk*	Comments
Entire U.S. population	Less than 0.2%	Lower in African Americans, higher in Scandinavians
Type 1 diabetes in second- or third-degree relative	Less than 1%	Grandparent, cousin
Type 1 diabetes in mother	2%–4%	Higher risk if mother developed diabetes before age 11
Type 1 diabetes in father	5%–8%	Higher risk if father developed diabetes before age 11
Type 1 diabetes in one sibling	3%–15%	Most studies find 3%–10%
Type 1 diabetes in identical twin	35%–50%	Risk for non-identical twin equals that of having one non-twin sibling with Type 1 diabetes

*Percentages represent a range of figures drawn from various studies, with factors such as age and racial/ethnic heritage factored out. The exact numbers vary from study to study.

ing Type 1 diabetes or preserving remaining islet cells to allow them to continue secreting insulin. If you are a family member of someone with Type 1 diabetes and are interested in screening for the Type 1 diabetes antibodies, visit the TrialNet website at www.diabetestrialnet.org to locate the nearest TrialNet research center.

Another way of looking at the identical twin data—a perspective that concentrates on the good news—is that even with exactly the same genes, only half of the unaffected twins ever get Type 1 diabetes. This suggests that something in the environment plays a role. It isn't all in the genes. Precious little is known about just what this factor is, what a susceptible person is exposed to that sets off the reaction that damages beta cells and eventually causes diabetes. It may be a virus, although exposure to any particular virus has not been regularly found in people with Type 1 diabetes. It could be a toxin of some sort in the diet or in the air. There is no evidence that emotion or stress causes Type 1 diabetes or that it is caused by excess sugar intake. The fact is, we still don't know what triggers Type 1 diabetes in the susceptible person.

Somewhat more is known about what happens once the genetic predisposition and the environmental factor are established. The path to Type 1 diabetes is an *autoimmune* destruction of the pancreatic beta cells. This means that the body's immune system, which is responsible for recognizing and destroying outside invaders such as viruses or bacteria, begins to think that its own pancreatic beta cells are "foreign" and sets off a response that ends up destroying them. This destructive process is detected by laboratory tests using what are known as islet cell autoantibodies. Several antibodies are known to be associated with Type 1 diabetes, including antibodies to insulin, glutamic acid decarboxylase (GAD), insulinoma associated autoantibody (IA-2), and ZnT8 (zinc transporter). These antibodies may be either the cause or the result of the autoimmune process going on in the pancreas—we don't know which. But either way, a positive test result is evidence of the autoimmune process and the potential to develop Type 1 diabetes.

A positive Type 1 antibody test, which is evidence that beta cells are being destroyed, shows up several years before Type 1 diabetes does. This means that the problem develops for quite some time, not just over the first few weeks the person has symptoms of diabetes. While the stress of a recent cold or other virus may bring out Type 1 diabetes for the first time, it is not the *cause* of Type 1 diabetes. If the person had been tested before the cold or other virus, the test result would have been positive for islet cell antibodies.

Another typical feature of Type 1 diabetes is the "honeymoon period." Just after a person comes down with Type 1 diabetes, and after insulin is given to quickly lower glucose levels, the pancreas seems to recoup, and the person may be very stable or even not require insulin at all for a period of a few months to a year. It's been shown that 20%–30% of a person's beta cells are still functioning shortly after their Type 1 diabetes diagnosis. Both the early phase of Type 1 diabetes, when the antibody tests are positive but diabetes has not actually developed, and the honeymoon period provide "windows of opportunity" in which, if we could safely interrupt the autoimmune process, we might save enough beta cells for the pancreas to deliver adequate amounts of insulin. In other words, if the process that is destroying beta cells could be headed off, we might prevent the appearance of Type 1 diabetes altogether. Research is focusing on these time frames when Type 1 diabetes is destroying beta cells.

Type 2 Diabetes

- "My feet were becoming more and more numb, and I was having real problems performing sexually. I attributed it to aging, but then my doctor told me, 'It's your diabetes.' Well, to be perfectly honest, I didn't even know I had diabetes. He may have said something about a little sugar, but it had never sunk in. This was the first time I really heard that I had diabetes."

Type 2 diabetes, or non-insulin-dependent diabetes—previously called adult onset or maturity onset diabetes—is very different from Type 1 diabetes, even though it is capable of causing all the symptoms and all the complications found in any other form of diabetes. The typical features are listed in Table 4.

Type 2 diabetes is much more common than Type 1: 90% of diabetes is Type 2, while less than 10% is Type 1. Type 2 diabetes is more common with increasing age. In the United States in 2010, about 11% of adults aged 20 or older had diabetes. This increases to about 27% of adults aged 65 or older. Type 2 diabetes is much more common in overweight people and is influenced more by heredity than is Type 1. Certain groups, including African Americans, Hispanics/Latinos from Mexico or Puerto Rico, Asians and Asian Americans, and, particularly, Native Americans, have especially high rates of Type 2 diabetes. The best predictor of the frequency of Type 2 in a given population, however, is obesity.

Table 4 Typical Features of Type 2 Diabetes

Feature	Typical Finding	Comments
Age of onset	Over 40 years old; most common in older adults	Not always over 40; can occur in younger people and even children, particularly those with a strong family history who become overweight and are inactive
Body weight	Overweight	Occasionally occurs in normal-weight people
Presentation	Usually slow onset, with symptoms developing over months to many years	Thirst, frequent urination, and weight loss may not be noticed; can be a "silent disease"
Family history	Usually Type 2 diabetes in the family	The more family members who have diabetes, the greater the risk
Risk factors	Clear, well defined risk factors that put people at increased risk of Type 2 diabetes	Risk increased for those who have a history of diabetes during pregnancy, are overweight, have a strong family history of Type 2 diabetes, or are of Native American, African American, Hispanic/Latino, or Japanese American descent
Insulin treatment	Often needed to control the blood glucose	Treatment usually starts with diet and exercise, then progressing, if needed, to pills and later to insulin
Blood glucose control	Usually easier to control, without the ups and downs found in Type 1 diabetes	Blood glucose may get very high, and lows also seen, but fewer peaks and valleys than in Type 1 diabetes
"Honeymoon period"	Not seen in Type 2 diabetes	
Laboratory tests	Blood glucose may be very high, but typically only mildly to moderately elevated; hemoglobin A1c mildly or moderately elevated; negative for islet cell antibodies, GAD (glutamic acid decarboxylase) antibodies, and insulin autoantibodies	Antibody tests may be done at the onset of diabetes if doubt as to whether Type 1 or Type 2; a positive result confirms Type 1
Cause	A poorly understood combination of heredity, insulin resistance, and deficiency of the insulin-producing beta cells of the pancreas	Not due to autoimmunity

Type 2 diabetes was once thought to be extremely rare in children and adolescents. However, as obesity rates and physical inactivity are increasing globally, the rates of Type 2 diabetes in children and adolescents are also increasing. This is especially true in children who have one or both parents with Type 2 diabetes.

The typical person with Type 2 diabetes, then, is older, is overweight, and has a strong family history of diabetes. Unlike Type 1 diabetes, which usually shows up abruptly (even though, as discussed above, it has been developing for several years), the high blood glucose in Type 2 diabetes may develop very slowly, over many years. It is usually virtually impossible to discover exactly when the diabetes began. This is why we stressed in Chapter 1 that exact criteria do exist to determine whether or not a person has Type 2 diabetes. We believe that a person should not be monitored for years with a vague diagnosis—a "touch of glucose" or "just a little diabetes." With its gradual onset, Type 2 diabetes can easily be ignored or minimized. But to do so is dangerous, since serious long-term complications can occur before people are even aware that they have diabetes.

For many, many years the name *non-insulin-dependent diabetes* has been synonymous with Type 2 diabetes, but it is a confusing name for the simple reason that about 25% of people with Type 2, "non-insulin-dependent," diabetes actually *do* take insulin. Does taking insulin transform the person who previously had Type 2 diabetes into a person with Type 1 diabetes? Absolutely not. We have already mentioned some features that make Type 2 diabetes a fundamentally different disease from Type 1 diabetes, and we will mention more below. Just remember that many people with Type 2 diabetes do, in fact, take insulin.

By formal definition, Type 2 diabetes is the form of diabetes that does not require insulin treatment to avoid ketoacidosis. Except under unusual stress, the person with Type 2 diabetes should not get ketoacidosis even when a needed insulin treatment is withdrawn. The reason for this is really quite simple and basic to Type 2 diabetes: the pancreas of the person with Type 2 diabetes does make some insulin, just not enough. With even a small amount of insulin, the uncontrolled breakdown of fat that causes ketoacidosis (Chapter 21) is prevented. And, most important, the edge is taken off the rises and falls in blood glucose. The longer someone has Type 2 diabetes, however, the less insulin the pancreatic beta cells produce. Therefore, it's common for someone with Type 2 diabetes of longer duration to require insulin injections.

Relative stability, then, is a feature of Type 2 diabetes. Whatever amount of insulin is secreted by the pancreas, it is released at just the right time, when the blood glucose rises, and stops at the right time, when the blood glucose falls. This normal pancreatic insulin secretion is a big advantage, providing some underlying stability to blood glucose levels, even if they are persistently too high (as in Figure 3d).

Finally, although any of the long-term complications can occur in Type 2 diabetes, the frequency of specific complications is quite different from that in Type 1 (these complications are discussed in more detail in Part IV). Such complications as circulatory problems, stroke, heart attacks, and hypertension are more common in Type 2 diabetes than in Type 1. Part of the reason for this is simply the age factor: people in their 60s, 70s, and 80s are much more prone to hardening of the arteries than people in their teens, 20s, and 30s. (As noted earlier, Type 2 diabetes usually begins in people older than 40.) Insulin resistance, a feature of Type 2 diabetes, also leads to changes in cholesterol and in clotting factors in the blood that cause blood vessel disease. The importance of this is that special attention has to be paid to preventing hardening of the arteries in people with Type 2 diabetes. Physicians therefore aggressively treat high blood pressure and high cholesterol in these patients with medications, in addition to treating their high blood glucose levels. Treatment of hypertension and high cholesterol levels has been shown to prevent heart attacks and strokes in people with Type 2 diabetes.

What Causes Type 2 Diabetes?

As with Type 1 diabetes, our understanding of what causes Type 2 diabetes is far from complete. We know certain facts, some already mentioned:

—Type 2 diabetes runs in families and in certain racial/ethnic groups.
— It occurs far more often in people who are overweight.
—The pancreas does make some insulin in Type 2 diabetes, but not enough.
—The cells of the body are resistant (respond less well) to insulin.

A discussion of these basic facts about Type 2 diabetes provides some insight.

The genetic influence in Type 2 diabetes is much stronger than in Type 1 diabetes. Returning to the identical twin model used above, we find that at least 90% of identical twins will both have Type 2 diabetes if one twin has it. The family history of people with Type 2 diabetes is routinely positive for Type 2 diabetes. Table 5 gives some numbers indicating the risk of other family members developing Type 2 diabetes when one person already has it. This strongly hereditary nature of Type 2 diabetes is partly but not wholly explained by inheritance of obesity. It is best illustrated in the greatly increased risk in specific racial/ethnic groups, regardless of body weight.

The importance of obesity as a cause of Type 2 diabetes cannot be overemphasized. Although we don't know precisely why, it is clear that in obese people, the muscle cells—where most of the glucose breakdown occurs (muscle takes up more glucose than any other tissue in the body)—are far less responsive to insulin than are the muscle cells of thinner people. This condition, called *insulin resistance*, means that a unit of insulin has less effect in lowering blood glucose. The liver is also resistant to insulin in persons with Type 2 diabetes. The signal for the liver not to make glucose becomes weaker, and the liver often dumps up to twice as much glucose into the blood as in persons without diabetes. This is why people with Type 2 diabetes may wake up with a higher blood glucose than when they went to bed, even though they've had nothing to eat. Consider the case of Anne.

Table 5 Risk of Developing Type 2 Diabetes if a Relative Has Type 2 Diabetes

Population Group	Risk*	Comments
Entire U.S. population	8%	5% diagnosed, 3% undiagnosed; higher in Native Americans, African Americans, Hispanics/ Latinos
Type 2 diabetes in father *or* mother	20%–40%	Higher risk if mother has diabetes than if father has diabetes
Type 2 diabetes in father *and* mother	40%–60%	
Type 2 diabetes in one sibling	20%	
Type 2 diabetes in identical twin	Up to 90%	Risk in non-identical twin equals that of having one non-twin sibling with Type 2 diabetes

*Percentages represent a range of figures drawn from various studies, with factors such as age, body weight, gender, and racial/ethnic heritage factored out. The exact numbers vary from study to study.

When Anne was 35, she was of normal weight, nondiabetic, and her pancreas could put out 30 units of insulin a day, enough to do the job. With her last pregnancy, she had gestational diabetes that could be treated with dietary changes and exercise, but the diabetes went away entirely after the delivery. At 50, though, she became overweight and resistant to her own insulin. Now the same 30 units of insulin that her pancreas could put out was not enough. To overcome her own resistance to insulin, she would have to make closer to 50 units of insulin; her pancreas was not able to do so, and Anne developed diabetes. The obesity had caused insulin resistance and had increased the demands on the pancreas, asking it to produce more insulin than it could.

Put yet another way, if a person is obese, his or her pancreas has to put out much greater amounts of insulin to keep blood glucoses normal. (The obese person who does not have diabetes has a pancreas with a great deal of extra capacity to produce insulin.) So, if the pancreas is in any way limited, if it is not able to make this large amount of insulin, diabetes occurs when the person becomes obese. The good news is that if some of that weight is lost, the insulin output of the pancreas may very well be sufficient, and the person may no longer have diabetes.

There are many other causes of insulin resistance, some mentioned above in the discussion of other types of diabetes. Perhaps the most common (other than obesity) is pregnancy. The insulin resistance caused by placental hormones gives rise to gestational diabetes when the woman's pancreas is unable to produce enough insulin to overcome this resistance.

In addition to insulin resistance at the cellular level, some limitation of insulin secretion also occurs in Type 2 diabetes. The debate continues as to which comes first, the pancreatic problem or the resistance problem.

When People Don't Fit Neatly into Type 1 or Type 2

- "I'm 35 years old and recently got diabetes. I am mildly overweight and am responding so far to diet and exercise, although my blood glucose is beginning to creep up. I have one grandparent who may have had diabetes. Do I have Type 2 diabetes or Type 1 diabetes, and how do you know?"

It would be nice if every person with diabetes was easily and obviously classifiable, but this is not the case. Some people, such as the person quoted above, seem to be in between. We cannot, of course, just stop treatment to see whether the person develops diabetic ketoacidosis in order to make the "gold standard" diagnosis (ketoacidosis = Type 1 diabetes; no ketoacidosis = Type 2 diabetes). But considering the case of this person can be valuable in sorting out the most important distinctions between Type 1 diabetes and Type 2 diabetes.

It is clear, for instance, that the age criterion is not very reliable. There are some definite exceptions to the general rule that diabetes occurring in the young is Type 1 and diabetes occurring in older people is Type 2. There is a form of diabetes called maturity onset diabetes of the young (MODY), for example, that comes on during the teenage years but is not Type 1 diabetes. MODY is seen more often in African Americans and is now known to be due to specific genetic defects, unrelated to Type 1 diabetes, that cause the pancreas to secrete insulin only when the glucose is considerably higher than normal.

Likewise, we are increasingly aware that when older people get diabetes, it is not always Type 2. Even in the elderly, Type 1 diabetes, with autoimmune destruction of the pancreas, can occur. When much older individuals develop Type 1 diabetes, the destruction of their insulin-producing cells proceeds much more slowly, so they may initially respond to pills used to treat Type 2 diabetes. Eventually, though, as more insulin-producing cells are lost, insulin is required. This condition has also been named latent autoimmune diabetes in adults, or LADA. Scandinavian studies have shown that as many as 7.5%–10% of patients with diabetes in Scandinavia have LADA. This rate is believed to be much lower in the United States. So age alone is not a reliable way to distinguish Type 1 from Type 2 diabetes, and the older terms "juvenile onset" and "adult onset" are better left in the archives.

We have emphasized that taking insulin does not mean you have Type 1 diabetes. Even obesity, so characteristic of Type 2 diabetes, is not a sure diagnostic sign of Type 2. There is nothing to suggest that a person with Type 1 diabetes can't become overweight or that some people with Type 2 diabetes can't have normal body weight.

One of the most reliable indicators of Type 2 diabetes, as we have pointed out, is relatively stable blood glucose levels. This gets at the fundamental difference between Type 2 and Type 1 diabetes, which is at the level of the pancreas: people with Type 1 diabetes are not making any insulin, while those with Type 2 diabetes are. The pancreatic insulin, secreted at just the right time, produces more stability in blood glucose levels in people with

Type 2 diabetes. Only when a person with Type 2 diabetes has had the disease for a long time and the pancreas has lost its ability to make much insulin do blood glucose levels vary more.

If it is necessary to determine whether someone is making insulin, pancreatic insulin can be measured in the blood directly, either by testing the insulin level if the person is not taking insulin by injection or by testing a substance called C-peptide in the blood if the person is taking insulin. The level of insulin or C-peptide will help show how much insulin the pancreas is making. This may help determine whether non-insulin treatments for diabetes are likely to work.

Early in the course of diabetes, the best way to distinguish Type 1 from Type 2 is probably to look for autoantibodies in the blood as the indication of Type 1 diabetes. About 5% of people with Type 1 diabetes do not have a positive autoantibody test at the time of diagnosis, however, so a negative test result is not as helpful as a positive result in making this distinction.

So there are some people for whom, at the start, we can't make a definite diagnosis of Type 1 or Type 2 diabetes. But if we wait several years, beyond any "honeymoon period," it usually becomes much clearer: the blood glucose is either quite stable (Type 2 diabetes) or quite labile (Type 1 diabetes), and the person either responds well to diet and pills (Type 2 diabetes) or, within a year or so, clearly needs insulin (Type 1 diabetes).

Gestational Diabetes Mellitus

- "Diabetes came on toward the end of my pregnancy. The doctors seemed very concerned, but after I delivered a healthy little girl, it just went away altogether."

Diabetes during pregnancy is so important that it is discussed in a chapter of its own (Chapter 29). Here we will just say that gestational diabetes mellitus (GDM) refers to new diabetes that is first discovered during pregnancy (as opposed to established diabetes in a woman who then becomes pregnant). The reason it is so important to diagnose and treat GDM properly is that, if the disease is left untreated, the pregnancy is at greatly increased risk of ending unsuccessfully.

Gestational diabetes signals that the pancreas can't make enough insulin and that the woman has a high chance of developing permanent diabetes later (about 50% of these women do so). The woman with a perfectly normal pancreas overcomes the stress of pregnancy and does not develop diabetes. The woman with a borderline pancreas, however, develops diabetes during pregnancy.

Other Types of Diabetes

- "I had diabetes in my family but never had it myself until I started using prednisone for my asthma. Is there any relationship?"

The answer is yes. Prednisone and other glucocorticoids are a classic cause of increased blood glucose, and prednisone-induced diabetes is a classic form of "other type" of diabetes with a known cause. In fact, all the "other types" of diabetes are those for which the cause is known. If the entire pancreas is surgically removed because of a serious abdominal injury or tumor, that person will have diabetes, since there is no other organ that can make insulin. Severe chronic pancreatitis (in which the pancreas is persistently inflamed, causing chronic pain), cystic fibrosis, or hemochromatosis (a disease of overabsorption of iron) can also damage the pancreas to the point that it cannot make insulin.

More examples of other types of diabetes are diabetes brought on by drugs such as protease inhibitors for HIV disease, cyclosporine, or steroids such as prednisone, as mentioned above. In these cases it is more a question of the drug bringing out diabetes, since the person probably would not have developed diabetes from taking these drugs if he or she did not have an underlying predisposition to diabetes.

There are some very uncommon diseases, such as Cushing's syndrome and acromegaly, in which high steroid or growth hormone levels cause diabetes by counteracting insulin's effect. Finally, there are also some very rare hereditary conditions in which all the cells of the body lack receptors for insulin. This is like having the door key (insulin) but not having the lock (the receptor).

Take Home Messages

- Diabetes of any type produces the same symptoms—especially high blood glucose levels—and may produce the same complications.
- Most people with diabetes (about 90%) have Type 2 diabetes. Their

bodies don't make enough insulin and are resistant to the insulin they do make. Type 2 diabetes is more common in people over the age of 35–40, those who are overweight, and those who are African American, Hispanic/Latino, Asian or Asian American, or Native American.

- About 5%–10% of people with diabetes have Type 1 diabetes. Most people who develop Type 1 diabetes develop it before the age of 30 and need to take insulin right away.
- Gestational diabetes mellitus (GDM) first appears during pregnancy. About 50% of women who develop GDM eventually develop Type 2 diabetes.
- Prediabetes is a condition in which blood glucose levels are higher than normal but not high enough to warrant a diagnosis of Type 2 diabetes. About half of people with prediabetes will eventually develop Type 2 diabetes.

PART II

Controlling Diabetes

It's all a balancing act. You don't want the blood glucose to go too high and you can't let it get too low. You don't want to eat too much or too little. Every medication you take must be in the right dose, not underdosed or overdosed.

To be successful in this balancing act requires a pretty good understanding of what you're doing. We'd be the first to agree that knowledge isn't everything, but you wouldn't get behind the wheel of a car without knowing the brake from the accelerator. Likewise, you can't take good care of your diabetes if you don't have a clue how you feel when your blood glucose is high or low, if you don't know what the pills or insulin you are taking do, or if you wouldn't know a carbohydrate if it jumped off the plate at you.

In fact, there are some fine points to managing your diabetes, things you may not have thought much about. Part II goes through all the important information you might need so you can take care of your diabetes. Some of it may be too basic for you, some may not be relevant to you. But the information is there, simply stated. If you pick up only a few pointers that make a difference for you, then it's all worthwhile. So, use what you can, and come back for more later.

Being successful in the balancing act of self care, in the long run, allows you to live a full and healthy life with diabetes. It does not mean perfection, especially if that perfection comes at the cost of being obsessed with your diabetes. Remember that you control your diabetes, it does not control you.

3

Goals of Treatment and How to Reach Them

with Nestoras Mathioudakis, M.D.

- "I want to enjoy my life."
- "I just want to be healthy so I can see my grandchildren grow up."
- "Low blood sugars scare me, so I let myself run a little high."
- "I'm going to jog 50 minutes, seven mornings a week. I swear I am!"

A goal is where you would like to be—a destination, an objective. Reaching the goal implies planning and action: you have to set the goal, and then you have to act to get there. Three things can prevent you from reaching your diabetes treatment goals. You might set unrealistic goals (like the person who swears he'll jog for 50 minutes every day). You might be trying to reach a goal set not by you but by someone else, perhaps your doctor. Or you might not even know how to set a goal.

We talk a lot about goals in our diabetes management program at Johns Hopkins, from the most general, like having the best possible quality of life, to the most specific, like avoiding potato chips or giving up smoking.

We find it helpful to think of four broad categories of goals:

—Quality-of-life goals: how you feel about your life
—Health goals: how healthy you are and what you can do
—Blood glucose goals
—Self-care behavior goals

Quality-of-Life Goals

Having a good quality of life is about as general a goal as you can imagine, but it is also the worthiest goal of all. Each of us defines a good quality of life differently. For some it means spending lots of time with family or engaged in favorite activities. For others it means having a satisfying job. For still others it means having plenty of money, a nice home, and things we enjoy.

In many ways, your quality of life can be just as good with diabetes as it would be without it. But there is one big possible exception. If, for you, good quality of life means relaxing in front of the television, drinking beer and eating fast food, or doing as little exercise as you can get away with, your definition of good quality of life might need adjusting.

We are not here to tell you that this adjustment is easy. We don't downplay the pleasures of fast food and relaxation. And only you can define your own quality of life, so only you can choose your quality-of-life goals. Still, most people tell us that when they think about it, they recognize that the truly meaningful things in life, the things that really define a good quality of life, have little to do with eating anything they want or avoiding exercise. Some people come to see healthy eating and regular activity as part of a quality life. And even those who find these healthy activities a challenge do them anyway, in order to reach the health goals we discuss below. They eat well and stay active so they can stay as healthy as possible and are able to do the things they want and need to do for as long as possible.

Health Goals

Health goals are about how you feel physically and the things you are physically able to do. Here are some examples of health goals: "I want my energy back. I don't want to be tired and running to the bathroom all the time." "I want to be healthy as I get older, able to climb the stairs, able to play with the grandchildren."

Everyone wants to feel well, and everyone wants to be physically able to do the things they want and need to do for as long as possible.

Feeling well when you have diabetes means avoiding the immediate symptoms of high or low blood glucose and avoiding long-term complications or keeping them from progressing. We believe that avoiding the acute symptoms of diabetes is achievable for virtually everyone. Freedom from high blood glucose symptoms like thirst, frequent urination, and vaginal infections and freedom from low blood glucose reactions is the minimum health goal you should set. If you suffer from these symptoms of high or low blood glucose, reevaluate your treatment. For a first health goal, tell yourself, "I want to be free of the symptoms of diabetes. On a day-to-day basis, I want to feel well."

Another health goal we are sure you share is avoiding the long-term complications of diabetes: kidney disease, visual impairment, nerve damage, blood vessel disease, and so on (described in Part IV). This is a more complicated goal, requiring better blood glucose control than just enough to avoid symptoms. Keeping blood glucose always between 150 and 200 mg/dl, for instance, will keep you free of symptoms but may not be good enough to avoid long-term complications. Along with blood glucose control, healthy habits such as not smoking, exercising regularly, and controlling blood pressure and cholesterol levels are important in controlling long-term complications.

If you already have some long-term complications from diabetes, the health goal should be to keep them from progressing and becoming disabling. Specific ways to manage complications are described later in this book; the good news is that most long-term complications can be effectively treated.

Some of your health goals are not specific to diabetes. You might want to feel well enough to enjoy your favorite activities, like playing with the grandchildren, gardening, dancing, or bowling. Reaching these goals clearly depends on taking the best possible care of your diabetes and protecting your health today and in the years to come. Keeping in mind the rewards of good health can help you stick with the hard work of effective diabetes self-care.

Blood Glucose Goals

One of the most common questions we are asked is, "What should my blood glucose be?" This is certainly a fair question, but there is no single right answer. To determine the right answer for you, raise the question with your own health care professional. Here we talk about factors that affect what that right answer could be.

A person who does not have diabetes has blood glucose levels of about 70–100 mg/dl before eating and up to about 140 mg/dl after eating. These are what we call "normal" levels. In general, the goal for someone with diabetes is to be as close to these normal levels as possible. But that's an ambitious goal, one that's very difficult to reach for almost anyone who has diabetes. This is because when you have diabetes, balancing all the factors that influence blood glucose levels, day in and day out, is a monumental challenge.

This balancing act is especially challenging if you have Type 1 diabetes.

Even with the most intensive treatment and the best of self-care, the blood glucose levels of a person with Type 1 diabetes will vary more than those of most people with Type 2 diabetes, with more highs and more lows. That's a fact of life. Fortunately, as far as we know, it is the blood glucose *average* that mostly determines the risk of long-term complications, not whether you have periods of highs and lows. The hemoglobin A1c (glycated, or glycosylated, hemoglobin) test, which we describe in Chapter 4, provides an estimate of your average blood glucose level over two to three months. This is the test that you and your diabetes health care provider can use to tell whether you are reaching your long-term blood glucose goals and whether your treatment plan needs adjustment. The American Diabetes Association (ADA) recommends that people with diabetes keep their A1c levels at 7% or lower. Checking the average on your blood glucose monitor can also provide valuable information.

Your blood glucose goals may vary from time to time. Glucose targets can change from time to time for the same person. Let's look at some examples.

> *Sam is 38 and has had Type 1 diabetes since he was 12. He works hard to keep his glucose levels as close to normal as possible and is quite successful: he rarely goes above 200 mg/dl and quite often is less than 100. He prizes his tight control, but lately he has had a series of severe lows. His wife and children are alarmed, and so are his coworkers. Sam's doctor suggests that he "back off" a bit, trying to keep his levels always above 100, even if he is over 200 some of the time. He reminds Sam that for at least a few days after a severe low, another severe low is much more likely, because a severe low makes it harder to tell that another low is coming on. So for the moment, the lows are more of a threat than running a bit high. It's hard for Sam to give up his efforts to keep his levels as close to normal as possible, but right now it's the right thing to do.*

Circumstances change, and what was good for Sam earlier now has to be modified, at least for a while. Most likely, he will regain his hypoglycemia awareness and be able to go back to even tighter control. But for now, loosening up is necessary.

Sometimes individual circumstances dictate trying for tighter control, not for looser control as in Sam's case.

> *Stephanie also has Type 1 diabetes. She is taking two injections a day and doing okay. Her last A1c was 7.6%, higher than the ADA's recommended level,*

but not by much. She has some highs and lows, and her levels before dinner are variable. She would like to become pregnant. What do we think?

Stephanie should definitely consider a regimen that will get her blood glucose levels closer to normal. Her goal should be an A1c level below 6.0%. That will almost certainly involve more frequent insulin injections, frequent blood glucose monitoring, and hard work on other aspects of her diabetes care plan. Fortunately, planning a pregnancy is a time when most women with diabetes are motivated to work the hardest. If Stephanie is one of those women, she will be doing everything she can to ensure she has a healthy baby.

Glucose levels are generally easier to control when you have Type 2 diabetes. As we've mentioned, balancing all the factors that influence blood glucose levels is more challenging for people who have Type 1 diabetes. It's easier for most people who have Type 2 diabetes because they are generally still producing some of their own insulin. This means their bodies are still doing some of the work of blood glucose control that people with Type 1 diabetes have to do completely with insulin injections. People with Type 2 diabetes rarely have low blood glucose, unless they are taking insulin or a class of diabetes drugs called sulfonylureas. And because they generally still have some insulin "buffer," their glucose is less likely to go really high.

So, this makes blood glucose control somewhat easier for people with Type 2 diabetes, especially in their early years with the disease, but blood glucose control is just as important for them as it is for people who have Type 1 diabetes. Keeping levels as close to normal as possible has the same benefits regardless of the type of diabetes you have: immediate benefits such as having more energy when your levels are not too high and avoiding the problems associated with lows, and long-term benefits such as living a life free of diabetes complications.

Reasons to think about trying for tighter control. Tighter control may be needed if you:

—Have symptoms of high blood glucose (feeling tired all the time, frequent urination, blurred vision)
—Have noticed your A1c level or average glucose level creeping up
—Are thinking about pregnancy
—Are more "into" actively managing your diabetes, for whatever reason

—Don't mind the glucose monitoring or injections as much as you used to and are ready to step up to another level of control

Reasons to think about trying for looser control. On the other hand, less-tight blood glucose targets may be needed if you:

—Have lost your awareness of hypoglycemia and are increasingly prone to severe blood glucose lows

—Have other serious medical problems, such as coronary heart disease, a psychiatric disorder, or substance abuse, that increase the risks of hypoglycemia

—Are elderly, with relatively recent-onset diabetes, and not so concerned about long-term complications that may occur 20 years down the road

—Have something coming up, such as an important meeting, exam, presentation, or long drive, when the most important thing is not to let your blood glucose go too low

—Are recovering from surgery and not eating much, so it's more important not to have your glucose go too low

. . .

We have talked about some things to consider when setting your own blood glucose goals. Be sure to talk with your diabetes health care provider to decide what the right goals are for you, now and in the future.

Self-Care Goals

Behavior is where the rubber meets the road. To reach your other goals—your quality-of-life, health, and blood glucose goals—you have to set diabetes self-care goals. For example, if you want to be able to do the things you love to do and need to do for as long as possible and to stay as healthy as possible today and in the years to come, you have to set self-care goals that increase your chances of reaching these quality-of-life and health goals. And, thinking very specifically, if you want to keep your blood glucose levels between 100 and 150 mg/dl before bed, you have to check your levels before you go to sleep.

Setting self-care goals requires thought, motivation, and commitment. Other people, including your doctor, can help you set these goals, but if anyone else sets them for you, it isn't likely to work. That's because self-care goals are personal. You and you alone know what your goals are for your quality of life, your health, and your blood glucose, so you and you alone must decide what you can commit to and sustain when it comes to diabetes self-care.

The goals most likely to help you succeed are what we call SMART goals. These goals are:

—*Specific.* You have to be clear exactly what you are going to do. For example, exercising more is not specific, but walking more is. Checking your glucose levels more often is also a specific goal. So is switching from whole-fat dairy products to low-fat ones.

—*Measurable.* If your goal is to walk more, you have to be clear how much you plan to walk. So a measurable goal would be to walk for 30 minutes five days a week. Other measurable goals would be to check your glucose levels before each meal and before bed or to switch from whole-fat milk to 1% milk.

—*Ambitious.* Your goal should usually be to do more than you are doing now. If you are already walking for 30 minutes five days a week, your goal should be to increase that.

—*Realistic.* While your goals should be ambitious, you don't want to make them too lofty, especially at first. If you haven't gotten off the couch in years, walking for 30 minutes five days a week is a great long-term goal. But you are more likely to eventually reach that goal if you set some more realistic short-term goals, like walking for 15 minutes twice a week the first week, then adding 15 minutes and one day a week until you reach your long-term goal.

—*Timely.* Set time frames for your goals. Even ambitious goals can be boosted once you are able to achieve them for a while. For example, after three months of success with your goal of walking for 30 minutes five times a week, consider adding a few minutes to each walk or adding another aerobic activity you enjoy. Or after several months of checking your glucose levels before each meal, consider checking occasionally after a meal. This could give you valuable information about your control, help you adjust your treatment regimen, and improve your health.

The most effective self-care goals are not only SMART, they are inspiring. We have found that people are much more successful at sticking with the hard work of diabetes self-care when they keep in mind what inspires them to do that hard work. In fact, you might say that being inspired is the key to successful diabetes self-management. So before you set self-care goals, think of your personal reasons for committing to the challenging work involved in reaching those goals. The best reasons are personal (they are your reasons, not the ones your doctor or your spouse might have for you). The best reasons are also proximal (that means they are things you can experience day to day). Avoiding long-term complications can motivate your self-care efforts, but you are likely to draw more motivation from the immediate benefits of active self-care (and consequent better blood glucose control), like having more energy and being able to sleep through the night because you don't have to get up so often to urinate. The best reasons to set SMART self-care goals are also positive, reasons like feeling well enough to play with the grandchildren, work in the garden, or go dancing with your partner.

Here are a couple of stories of people with various goal-setting issues.

Seymour's doctor told him his A1c level had gone up quite a bit, and she told him it was time to switch from his diabetes pills to insulin. She showed him how to give himself shots. She also told him he should start checking his glucose after every meal, not just once a day as he had been doing, and should start walking for 45 minutes most days of the week. These were big changes for Seymour, and he felt overwhelmed. He started taking insulin, and it was easier than he had imagined. He also began checking his glucose levels more often, but not as frequently as his doctor had recommended. And he started walking, but he fell far short of the goal his doctor had set for him. He sat nervously in the waiting room before his next appointment, expecting a lecture from his physician about his self-care failures. Her response was very different. She congratulated him on his improved A1c, his success taking insulin, and the steps he had taken toward reaching his other self-care goals. Then she helped him set a more realistic step-by-step plan to reach those goals.

It's almost impossible to make lots of big changes all at once. Seymour was fortunate to have a physician who realized she had asked too much of him at first and who was able to recognize what he had accomplished and help him take further steps toward his goals.

Laura's husband was a charter member of the "diabetes police." He was always after her to eat more carefully and to exercise more. He did it out of love, but it made Laura feel guilty and angry. Besides that, it interfered with their relationship, and it didn't seem to do much for Laura's self-care efforts. One evening when they were out to dinner with friends, Laura ordered dessert, and her husband gave her the evil eye. She didn't say anything then, but when they got home she let him have it. He apologized but added that he was worried about losing her and didn't know what else to do. Laura said, "I have to have my own reasons for doing the right thing; your pushing doesn't help." As soon as she said those words, she realized how true both statements were. Her husband's pushing didn't help, and she did have to have her own reasons for taking better care of herself. They talked, and she saw that she did want to take better care of herself and that, if she did, she would be able to enjoy many things that she currently didn't have the energy to do, like take long walks when she and her husband went on vacation and get down on the floor and play with her nephew.

Stress and Diabetes

Stress can undermine your efforts to keep your blood glucose levels as close to normal as possible, no matter how effective your self-care regimen. Physical stress, such as surgery, illness (a cold or the flu), or, for women, the normal hormonal variations of the menstrual cycle, can send glucose levels out of control. Fortunately, these physical stresses tend to pass, so their effect on blood glucose control is temporary. But emotional stress also can destabilize blood glucose levels.

Mike uses an insulin pump. He was having problems with glucose control and was often under tremendous stress at work. His supervisor, he said, was "the boss from hell," a screamer, not just insensitive but positively boorish, a bully, inconsistent, and stupid as well. The only good news was that the boss was on the road about half the time, so people in the office could get things done. It finally dawned on Mike that when the boss was in the office, his glucose levels shot up. He had to double the amount of insulin his pump delivered. When the boss was out of town, down the levels would come, stabilizing on less insulin every time.

Emotional stress can hit in two ways: by pushing blood glucose up, through stimulation by adrenaline (the "fight or flight" hormone), and by keeping you from practicing effective self-care. Mike is a classic example of the former. An example of the latter is the person who feels a need to eat every time there is any stress. One thing you can do is identify the source of stress that is affecting your glucose control. Then do what you can to avoid the stress or, when you can't avoid it, adjust for the effects of stress on your glucose levels.

How to Tell Whether Your Treatment Is Working

Once you have set goals for yourself, the question becomes how to know when your treatment is working and when it is not. This isn't as easy as it might seem at first glance, but here are some guidelines. First, are your "numbers" in a good range? Second, do you feel well day to day and are you helping yourself avoid or manage complications? And third, do you have the sense that diabetes is not running your life?

Since there are no absolute standards for good blood glucose control, and since no one with diabetes can achieve perfectly normal levels, we recommend individual targets, such as, "I want to be in this range a certain percentage of the time." For example, you may decide that your target is having 50% of your readings under 140 mg/dl and 90% under 200 mg/dl.

Next, your treatment is working if you are feeling well day to day, enjoying the benefits of blood glucose levels that are rarely too high or too low, and doing your best to avoid disabling complications or to manage any complications you may already have: taking good care of your feet, having an annual eye examination, and so on (see Chapters 23 and 26).

Finally, if the treatment plan is working, you will feel that your diabetes is kept in perspective, at least most of the time. You will generally feel that diabetes is in its place in your life and that your life has a place for diabetes, and much more.

If your treatment plan is not working in any of these ways, check out the suggestions in this chapter again. They may be helpful. And be sure to discuss any concerns with your diabetes health care providers.

Take Home Messages

- Treatment goals include goals related to quality of life, health, blood glucose control, and self-care behaviors.
- All treatment goals are personal; you and you alone must choose your goals, though others can help you do this.
- Self-care goals are the key to achieving other diabetes treatment goals.

- The best self-care goals are smart: specific, measurable, ambitious, realistic, and timely. They are also inspiring.
- Physical and emotional stress can make reaching your goals more difficult, so you must identify sources of stress and deal with them or adjust for them.
- Your treatment plan is working if you are reaching your quality-of-life, health, and blood glucose goals.

4

Blood Glucose Monitoring

- "I think I can tell when I am high or low. Do I really have to check?"
- "I have Type 2 diabetes. Does it matter if I monitor my blood glucose?"
- "What's the best blood glucose monitor for me?"
- "I want to know my blood glucose levels throughout the day, but I don't want to have to stick my finger all the time. Are there tools that could help?"
- "What's the A1c test my doctor does?"
- "I check my blood glucose every morning. How can those numbers be fine and my A1c level be high?"

When you have diabetes, especially if you have Type 1 diabetes, your blood glucose varies from hour to hour, sometimes almost from minute to minute. It might be 90 mg/dl before dinner and 240 mg/dl a couple of hours later, or 200 mg/dl after breakfast and 70 mg/dl before lunch. To find out what's happening with your blood glucose—whether it's high, low, or just right—you need to know about monitoring.

The symptoms of very high blood glucose and very low blood glucose are usually obvious, though not everyone has the same symptoms. When your level is very high, you might feel thirsty, dry, and tired; when it is very low, you might feel shaky or sweaty or have other telling symptoms. Unfortunately, the symptoms don't come on until your glucose is very high (over 200–250 mg/dl) or very low (under about 60 mg/dl). If people experienced symptoms earlier, they would be able to take corrective action before the blood glucose went very high or very low. As it is, symptoms appear only when blood glucose is at the extremes.

There is a wide range—too wide a range—of blood glucose levels that don't produce any symptoms at all. On the high side, you may "get used to" blood glucose levels in the 200s or even 300s. You can feel okay. But you are probably experiencing some of the immediate consequences of high blood glucose, especially less energy, and these levels dramatically increase your risk of diabetes complications. On the low side, the problem is that if your glucose is regularly near-low at a particular time of day, then every now and then, maybe one day in ten, it will go very low at that time. Three serious insulin reactions a month is way too many. So don't count on your symptoms to tell you when you're out of control. Poor control can be a "silent disease." Check your blood glucose.

Monitoring provides accurate, dependable answers to two questions: "What is my blood glucose right now?" and "How am I doing, on average, over time?" There are several different tests for monitoring blood glucose. We discuss them in this chapter, beginning with self-monitoring, which provides much more reliable and useful information than simply watching symptoms.

Self-Monitoring of Blood Glucose

Mary, 45 years old, came into the office with a medical mystery. She monitors her blood glucose three times a day, and everything seems fine. Her usual evening routine consists of exercising on a stationary bike, eating a small snack and taking her bedtime insulin, and then going to bed. Lately, however, she has been having nightmares, and she sleeps restlessly, with drenching sweats. She doesn't understand these nightmares. Naturally, she wonders about menopause. Mary asked us, "Are the nightmares related to my blood glucose and, if so, am I high or low?" Together, we decided that Mary should find out. She sets her alarm for 2:00 a.m. three nights in a row and finds that her glucose readings at that time are 65, 53, and 60 mg/dl. So there's the answer: she's low! No amount of estrogen replacement therapy or air conditioning is going to help that. Mary reduces her evening insulin dose and does fine.

Mary's case is a simple example but a telling one. With blood glucose monitoring, you can find out if your glucose is high or low, you can find out what makes it go high or low, and you can find out how you're doing, day in and day out. It's hard to overestimate the importance of this tool.

Most experts believe that anyone with diabetes can benefit from checking their blood glucose, and this is the recommendation of the American Diabetes Association (ADA). There has been some debate about whether this applies to people with Type 2 diabetes who don't take insulin, but recent research makes clear that they also benefit. This research reinforces a very important point that applies to anyone who is monitoring blood glucose: it's not the monitoring itself that helps, it's what you do with the monitoring information. You could monitor 10 times a day and it would do you no good unless you changed something—your medication, activity level, or eating—when your blood glucose levels were too high or too low.

The study involved people with Type 2 diabetes who were not taking insulin. Half the people in the study were assigned to a structured testing group (STG), and STG participants were taught to use a system that helped them record their blood glucose levels seven times a day (before and after breakfast, lunch, and dinner and before bed) for the three days before their regular diabetes appointments. STG participants were also taught how to modify their eating and activity level based on their glucose levels. Control group participants continued with their regular monitoring approach.

Physicians caring for the STG participants received training in interpreting their patients' monitoring results. These physicians received a practical manual describing various changes in medication and lifestyle they could use with STG patients whose glucose levels needed correcting.

The results of this study are impressive. Hemoglobin A1c levels among STG participants dropped from an average of 8.9% at the beginning of the study to 7.7% 12 months later, a significantly greater improvement than among the control group participants. And STG participants actually used fewer blood glucose monitoring strips during the 12 months of the study than control group participants did. This makes it clear that the key to success for the STG was the quality of monitoring, not the quantity.

The tools that STG participants and physicians used in this study are available at behavioraldiabetes.org/Studies/STeP-Study/html. Take a look at these tools. You can use the patient tool yourself, and you can ask your physician to use the physician tool.

How the Meter Systems Work

All the glucose monitoring systems available today use an enzyme (either glucose oxidase or hexokinase) to react with the glucose in the drop of blood you put on the strip. In most systems, a color develops once the blood is applied to the strip. The more glucose, the darker the color. The colored strip is then measured by the meter, which translates the measurement into a blood glucose reading. Some of the systems have strips that don't develop a color but instead measure the electrical current generated by the enzyme.

Developing this bit of chemistry and making it practical was no small technological feat. By now, many companies are producing dependable systems, so there are some competing products to choose among. More than 75 meters are currently available in the United States. (See Figure 5 for an illustration of a meter.) Each has its own advantages, so when you select a meter, think about the features that matter most to you. These include:

—*Cost.* The retail price of the meter is probably a poor indicator of what using the meter will actually cost. First, your insurance may pay for part or all of the cost, or you may even get a meter free of charge. Second, the major cost of monitoring is the cost of test strips. Meters can be used only with compatible strips, so once you buy a meter you are locked into buying those strips. Before you make a purchase, find out which brands of strips your health plan covers, what the strips cost, and how many strips your insurance will pay for each month.

—*Coding or calibrating.* Some meters require coding or programming of the meter to recognize a particular batch of test strips. Most new "auto-code" or "no-code" meters allow you to start right away, without taking this step.

—*Size and shape.* Most meters fit easily into your hand. A few are larger, and some "micro," "mini," or "compact" meters are quite small. Think about how you will use the meter in deciding what size is right for you.

—*Sample size.* Today's meters generally require much less blood than older meters did. Most require a drop about the size of this "o," and some use a drop that's even smaller.

—*Storing and reviewing data.* Most meters can store over 100 results and can track averages over days and weeks. Many meters also allow you to see how variable your glucose levels are, graph results, and upload data to your computer. As we write this chapter, the FDA (the U.S. Food and Drug Administration) has just given clearance for the first blood glucose monitor that connects directly to an Apple iPhone or iPod Touch. We can expect more such devices for Apple and other operating systems in the near future.

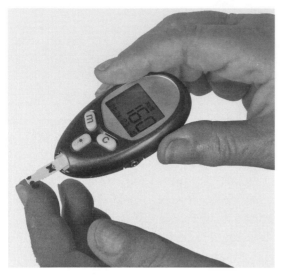

Figure 5. Example of a blood glucose meter.

How to Do Self-Monitoring of Blood Glucose

Here are the ADA's recommendations for checking your blood glucose (some steps are illustrated in Figure 6):

1. Wash your hands, then insert a strip into your meter.
2. Use your lancing device to get a drop of blood from the side of your finger. Lancing the side of your finger hurts less than lancing the pad and protects you from the discomfort of sore fingertips later, when you are typing or doing other work.
3. Gently squeeze or massage your finger until you get a drop of blood as big as your meter requires.
4. Touch and hold the edge of the test strip to the drop of blood and wait for the result.
5. Your blood glucose level will appear on the meter's display.
6. With some meters you can also use your forearm, thigh, or the fleshy part of your hand. Note that even if, with your meter, you are able to use a site other than a fingertip, glucose values from alternative sites are not as accurate as fingertip values when your blood glucose level is rising or falling quickly.
7. Spring-loaded lancing devices make sticking yourself less painful.

Blood glucose results can trigger strong feelings. Near-normal results can make you feel very happy or relieved. High or low results can make you feel confused, frustrated, angry, or discouraged. This is understandable, but it's really important to avoid feeling that your blood glucose values are a reflection on you. That's why we never talk about "good" numbers or "bad" numbers, just high, low, or near-normal ones. Your blood glucose numbers are a way to track your diabetes control and an aid in helping you make ad-

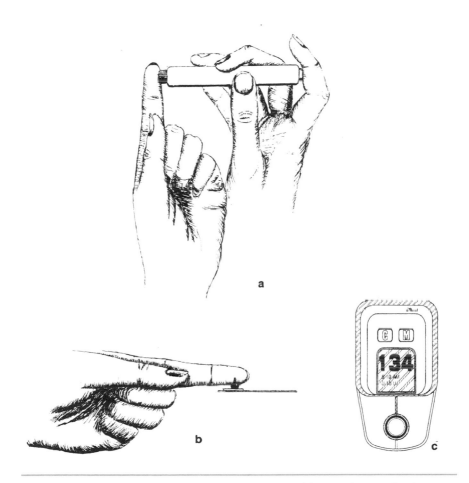

Figure 6. The technique of blood glucose monitoring. (a) Prick the outside of your finger with a lancing device—using the outside of your finger decreases the pain. (b) Milk the finger if necessary to get a large drop of blood to appear on your fingertip. Apply the blood to the glucose reagent strip. (c) The blood glucose reading appears on the meter screen.

justments to reach your diabetes management goals. The numbers are not a judgment of you as a person.

Can You Trust Your Meter Reading?

If the meter is used properly and with reasonable expectations, you can trust the reading. The FDA requires that all meters generate readings that are within ±20% of (that is, within 20% above or below) the actual blood glucose level, but most meters do better—they register ±10% of the actual level. This means that if the most accurate of laboratories found a blood glucose of 100 mg/dl, your meter should read between 90 and 110 mg/dl. At the extremes of glucose—say, over 400 mg/dl or under 50 mg/dl—the meters are less accurate; in those cases the reading will not tell you *exactly* what your number is and can be counted on simply to tell you that you're too high or too low. This should be enough for you to take the appropriate action.

That said, we must admit that several things can go wrong in the technique, so a healthy level of skepticism is needed. Consider Jerry's experience.

Jerry's blood glucose levels were always unstable but in a reasonable range. All of a sudden, he began to get crazy readings. When he was pretty sure he was low, the meter read 180 mg/dl; when he felt definitely high, it read 60 mg/dl. He knew something was wacky. First, Jerry bought new strips. This didn't seem to make any difference. So he got an old meter out of the closet, cleaned it up, and compared the results. The old meter was much closer to what he thought was his reading. He sent the defective meter to the manufacturer through his pharmacy. He never heard what the problem was, but he received a gleaming new meter in the mail shortly after and has not had a problem since.

Jerry knew that it is more common for strips to go bad than for meters to break down, and that's why the first thing he did in troubleshooting was replace the strips. But the main thing Jerry had going for him was that he kept his wits about him: he knew that his readings didn't reflect how he was feeling. Anyone who is self-monitoring needs to be on the watch for odd things like this. After all, if the speedometer in your car suddenly started showing 100 mph when you could see and feel that you were only going about 25 mph, you wouldn't believe the speedometer and slam on the brakes. In the same way, you have to be aware that sometimes the blood glucose monitoring systems break down.

If you are getting results that don't make sense to you, consider the following steps you can take to get things straight:

—Toss damaged or outdated test strips.

—Store strips in their sealed container, away from heat, moisture, and humidity.

—Keep your glucose meter and test strips at room temperature.

—If your meter needs to be coded, be sure the code numbers on your meter and on the strip container match.

—Be sure the test strip is fully inserted into the monitor.

—Apply a big enough blood sample to the test strip. Do not add more blood after the first drop is applied.

- If you're using a site other than your fingertip and you think the reading is wrong, test again using blood from a fingertip. As we've noted, alternative-site values aren't as accurate as fingertip values when your blood glucose level is rising or falling quickly.

What Should I Do with the Blood Glucose Reading?

Meters will automatically store test results for later discussion with your health care professional, or you can keep a written diary of blood glucose (see Figure 7, a and b). It's a good idea to write down the results or print out the results from your meter and look them over for yourself (see Figure 7c). That way you can see the patterns and *adjust your treatment regimen based on the readings you get.*

Did we say adjust your own treatment regimen? We sure did. As you will see in Chapters 11–13, we are strong believers in teaching people how to adjust their self-care, within safe limits, to fit the circumstances. It is especially important to learn to translate blood glucose readings into an action. After all, you're not doing all this finger sticking to make the doctor happy; you're doing it to keep yourself well. So when you find that the reading is especially low or especially high at a particular time of day, *do something about it!* Modify your diet or modify your insulin. If you're not sure what to do, ask your health care professional.

Many research studies have shown that blood glucose testing is most valuable if it leads to rational, thoughtful changes in self-care. Remember the study we talked about earlier in this chapter.

Continuous Glucose Monitoring

In recent years the FDA has approved several types of continuous glucose monitors (CGMs) that can track and record glucose values every few minutes, 24 hours a day, providing hundreds of readings a day. That's clearly a lot more information than even the most devoted person would get with traditional monitoring. CGMs not only provide real-time glucose readings but also display trends, and they sound an alarm when the glucose reaches preset levels for hypoglycemia or hyperglycemia. Many people say the trend graphs on the monitor are especially useful. That makes sense. It's helpful to know your glucose level is 90 mg/dl; it's much more helpful to also know whether an hour or two hours ago it was 70 or 90 or 240 mg/dl. Knowing your glucose level trends helps you make the right decision when it comes to adjusting your regimen (especially food intake and insulin doses). The alarms, of course, can help keep you out of serious trouble.

Clinical trials comparing CGMs with traditional blood glucose self-monitoring have shown that the use of a CGM has an advantage in reducing A1c levels and rates of hypoglycemia in people over the age of 25 and in those who use their CGM consistently. It's not surprising that people who don't use the CGM consistently don't get much benefit, and younger people seem especially likely not to be consistent CGM users.

BLOOD GLUCOSE LOG				
Sunday's Date:				
	Breakfast	Lunch	Supper	Bedtime
Sunday				
Monday				
Tuesday				
Wednesday				
Thursday				
Friday				
Saturday				

Figure 7a (*above*), **b** (*facing page*). Blood glucose logs.

BLOOD GLUCOSE RECORD

DAY	BREAK BG/ MED	MEAL, ACTIVITY, OTHER	LUNCH BG/ MED	MEAL, ACTIVITY, OTHER	DIN BG/ MED	MEAL, ACTIVITY, OTHER	BED BG/ MED	3 A.M. BG/ MED
SUN								
MON								
TUE								
WED								
THUR								
FRI								
SAT								

BLOOD GLUCOSE LOG

Sunday's Date: 2 / 3 / 2013

	Breakfast	Lunch	Supper	Bedtime
Sunday	126 G20 A5	Exer. 52	207 A6	147 G6
Monday	161 G20 A6	102	182 A6	121 G6
Tuesday	107 G20 A5	87 walk	72 A4	133 G6
Wednesday	138 G20 A6	78	140 A5	182 G6
Thursday	209 G20 A7	128	68 A4	100 G6
Friday	111 G20 A5	92	80 A4	158 G6
Saturday	141 G20 A5	70	165 A6	101 G6

Figure 7c. Example of a completed blood glucose log. The record includes blood glucose level, units of aspart (A), and units of glargine (G).

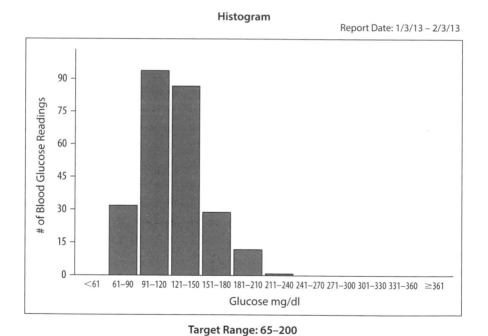

Histogram

Report Date: 1/3/13 – 2/3/13

# of Blood Glucose Readings

Glucose mg/dl

<61 61–90 91–120 121–150 151–180 181–210 211–240 241–270 271–300 301–330 331–360 ≥361

Target Range: 65–200

Figure 7d. Computer-generated printout of blood glucose readings recorded in the monitor memory over a one-month period. The histogram shows the relative number of readings in the specified glucose ranges. This example illustrates excellent blood glucose control.

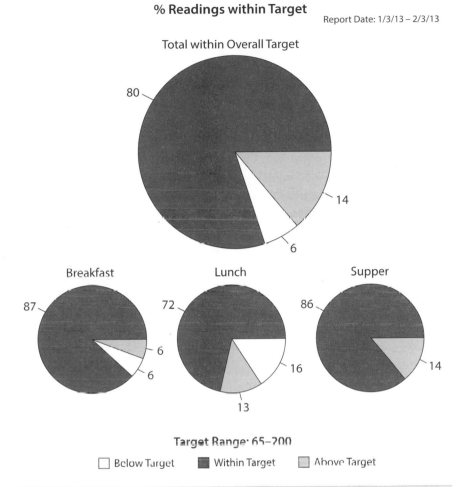

% Readings within Target

Report Date: 1/3/13 – 2/3/13

Total within Overall Target

80

14

6

Breakfast

87

6

6

Lunch

72

16

13

Supper

86

14

Target Range: 65–200

☐ Below Target ■ Within Target ▨ Above Target

Figure 7e. Readings within target: a pie chart illustrating the percentage of readings below target, within target, and above target over a one-month period. This example illustrates very good blood glucose control. Only a small percentage of the readings are above or below the set target.

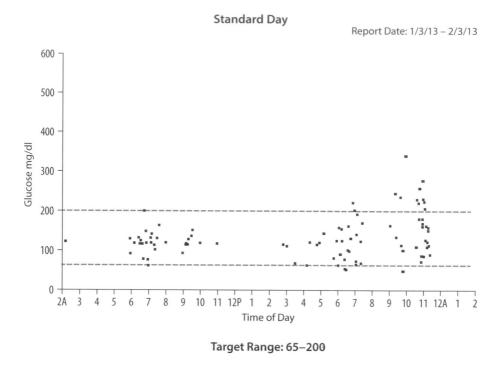

Figure 7f. Standard day. This computer-generated graph plots every reading (the average reading for the month) by value and time of day. It is helpful in spotting trends and visualizing the degree of fluctuation in control. This example illustrates very good blood glucose control with a trend of slightly higher readings in the evening.

CGMs use a tiny sensor inserted under the skin to monitor glucose levels in tissue fluid (called interstitial fluid). These systems don't actually measure blood glucose, but the glucose levels in tissue fluid are very closely related to the levels in blood, with CGM readings lagging about five minutes behind blood glucose values. The sensor stays in place for several days to a week before it needs to be replaced. A transmitter in the sensor sends information on the glucose level to the monitor. Two companies currently sell CGMs in the United States. One company sells a CGM integrated into its insulin pumps. The other monitor is not connected to a pump and fits easily into a pocket. A CGM comes with software that allows the user to download data from the CGM to a computer to track and analyze data in tables and graphs. (See Figure 8 for an illustration of some CGMs.)

If you are interested in a CGM, talk to your diabetes health care provider. While CGMs have many potential advantages, there are some things to keep in mind:

—Glucose monitoring using a CGM can be more expensive than traditional blood glucose monitoring, depending on your insurance coverage. Medicare does not cover CGMs.

—Using a CGM does not mean the end of all traditional blood glucose monitoring. CGMs must be calibrated with traditional blood glucose readings when a new sensor is inserted. Also, all CGM manufacturers recommend that when the CGM shows a high or low reading or one that just doesn't seem right, the reading should be verified with a traditional blood glucose check.

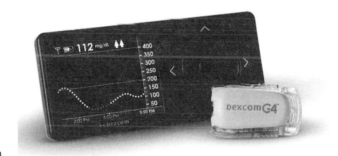

a

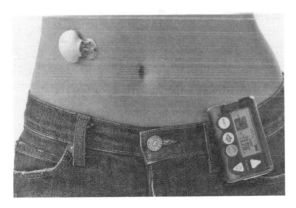

b

Figure 8. Continuous glucose monitoring systems (CGMs). (a) Dexcom G4 Platinum; (b) MiniMed Guardian REAL-Time CGM System. (a) Courtesy of Dexcom, Inc; (b) courtesy of Medtronic Diabetes.

—As we said, the clinical benefits of a CGM are dependent on using it regularly.

CGM technology is developing rapidly. For more information, speak to your health care provider, go to the American Diabetes Association's website (www.diabetes.org) and search for CGMs, or check the FDA website (www.fda.gov/diabetes/glucose.html).

Glycated Hemoglobin and Hemoglobin A1c

Glycated (or glycosylated) hemoglobin and hemoglobin A1c (referred to as HbA1c, or simply A1c) are used to measure the overall control of diabetes in the preceding three months. There are some differences in laboratory technique between the two, but for all intents and purposes they are the same test, and you are most likely to see references to HbA1c or, as we'll use in this book, just A1c.

Here's how A1c monitoring works. The hemoglobin in your red blood cells is what makes them red. Each red cell "lives" for about four months from the time it comes out of the bone marrow, where it is made. During that time, the hemoglobin in the cell becomes more and more *glycated*, meaning that glucose molecules stick to it. The higher the glucose level in the blood over the months, the more glucose is stuck to the hemoglobin and the higher the percentage of glycated hemoglobin. You might think of this process as similar to the sugar that sticks on a glazed donut.

Thus, A1c paints the big picture: it indicates the person's average glucose control over the past few months. As you know well by now, the blood glucose measurement itself gives you information only about blood glucose at that moment, and the reading will be different in a matter of hours. The A1c, in contrast, changes only over a matter of weeks and months.

To understand the meaning of your A1c result, you have to know the "normal value" used by the laboratory doing the test. In many labs, an A1c of 6.5% or higher is used to identify people who probably have diabetes. People with normal blood glucose levels have an A1c of less than 5.7%, and those with blood glucose levels higher than normal but not high enough for a diagnosis of diabetes (what we now call prediabetes) have A1c levels between 5.7% and 6.4%. We now talk about "prediabetes" because about 50% of people with prediabetes will eventually develop Type 2 diabetes unless they do something to reduce their risk. Studies show that losing weight or taking the diabetes medication metformin can reduce diabetes risk for people with prediabetes.

The ADA recommends that most people with diabetes keep their A1c levels below 7% because, as studies show, doing so dramatically reduces the risk of developing long-term diabetes complications. Achieving this goal is very challenging for many people, but the rewards are so great that it's worth striving for. Of course, some people, even some who have had diabetes for a long time, have even lower A1c levels.

Stefan, a 40-year-old man [Richard Rubin's son, and the only person for whom we don't use a pseudonym in our case stories], has had diabetes for 34 years. When he received the results of recent lab tests, his A1c level was 5.7%, with an asterisk next to the result stating, "Your result indicates you may be at risk for developing diabetes." Stefan had to laugh; after 34 years of diabetes, he guessed he was at some kind of risk for developing the disease. Stefan's A1c levels have always been near normal, through a combination of hard work and good fortune.

We should never forget that good fortune, perhaps in the form of good genes, does play a part in blood glucose control and other diabetes outcomes.

Near-normal A1c levels are a good thing, but remember: your A1c level tells you a lot, but it doesn't tell you everything about your glucose control. Your A1c is a measure of your *average* control. For example, if your blood glucose is 140 mg/dl for 24 hours a day in the three months before your A1c is checked, your reading will be about 6.5%. But you would get the same A1c if your level were 240 mg/dl for 12 hours a day and 40 mg/dl for the other 12 hours. Each pattern produces the same excellent A1c, but the patterns are very different when it comes to safety and day-to-day well-being. In the second situation, your glucose is always too high or too low.

Also, research shows that while an A1c of less than 7% is a good target for most people, the target for young children should be higher (less than 8%) because hypoglycemia poses special risks for them. Higher targets probably also make sense for older people, especially if they have only recently been diagnosed with diabetes and so have less risk of developing serious complications. Older people with multiple cardiovascular (heart attack or stroke) risk factors might also consider higher A1c targets. For some people, a target of less than 6.5% might be right as long as reaching that goal doesn't involve significant hypoglycemia or too much treatment burden.

Your glucose variability, which you can check on your meter, can also be important, even if it doesn't go very high or very low. Diabetes experts hotly debate the significance of this variability. Some have found evidence that glucose peaks after meals and fluctuating highs and lows contribute to increased cardiovascular risk. Other researchers report that efforts to show the benefits of controlling these fluctuations have proved fruitless. So the debate continues. But one thing is clear: avoiding really high and really low glucose is a good thing, even if the long-term advantages are not known.

Recently, the ADA established the relationship between A1c levels and average blood glucose levels. It calls this average level "estimated average glucose," or eAG. The ADA did this to assist health care providers and their patients in interpreting A1c values in units similar to those regularly used in self-monitoring. Your health care provider may discuss your A1c level in terms of eAG, and your lab results may do the same. (See Table 6 for a comparison of A1c and eAG values.)

Table 6 Relationship between Hemoglobin A1c and Estimated Average Glucose (eAG)

A1c (%)	eAG (mg/dl)
5	97
5.5	111
6	126
6.5	140
7	154
7.5	169
8	183
8.5	197
9	212
9.5	226
10	240
10.5	255
11	269
11.5	283
12	298

Another type of blood measurement is *fructosamine*, which provides information similar to that obtained by the A1c, except that the "view" provided by fructosamine is shorter—in the range of two weeks instead of several months. This test measures the glucose that is bound to proteins other than hemoglobin, and these other proteins don't have as long a life span as hemoglobin.

Fructosamine assays have not been used very widely, though they can provide useful information, especially if a person's blood glucose control has changed quickly in recent weeks or a short-term average measurement is desirable—for example, during a pregnancy. We usually rely on the A1c instead of fructosamine, but we don't object to having both tests done.

Urine Glucose Testing

The ancient Egyptians, we are told, diagnosed diabetes by putting urine near an anthill. If the ants were attracted, the patient was told that he had diabetes. If that seems a bit crude, it is at least more aesthetically pleasing than the seventeenth-century doctor's approach, which was to taste the urine. Glucose spills into the urine when the blood glucose reaches a certain level, usually about 180 mg/dl, and testing urine for sweetness, as these examples show, is a time-honored procedure.

> Athalia was brought up testing her urine glucose, and naturally she prefers it to measuring blood glucose: there's no finger stick involved. Her diabetes has become more unstable lately, though. She finds, for example, that she feels low before lunch, but when she checks her urine, it is 2+ for sugar. She complains to her doctor that her urine no longer reflects her blood glucose, and she worries that her kidneys are bad.

In fact, Athalia's kidneys are fine, as her doctor points out. What's happening is that her blood glucose is going up after breakfast (spilling glucose into the urine) and then crashing down before lunch (causing her to feel a glucose low). So when she tests her urine before lunch, it is really showing her the after-breakfast rise. Athalia will be much better off when she begins checking with blood glucose monitoring.

For many years, urine testing was the only way to monitor blood glucose. We consider urine glucose testing to be history. It's time to put this time-honored test to rest. As a measure of diabetic control, it has several limitations:

—Since the urine is formed slowly, when you empty your bladder, the urine you are testing was made several hours earlier. As you know, your blood glucose can be very different now than it was then. So the urine reading could be low at the time the blood glucose is going high.

—Urine testing is imprecise. The *renal threshold* (the blood glucose level at which glucose is spilled into the urine) varies markedly from person to person and from time to time.

—You can't tell if your blood glucose is normal, low, or near-low. Testing urine glucose only tells you if it's been high.

—Finally, the concentration of your urine makes all the difference in urine testing: if you drank two glasses of water and diluted your urine, the glucose level in the urine would seem to be lower, when in fact your blood glucose hasn't changed.

Adding up these limitations, we conclude that urine testing can provide only a rough measure of glucose control. There are much better ways of monitoring blood glucose levels.

Testing for Ketones

Ketones can signal danger. They can be a sign that your diabetes may be badly out of control and approaching the medical emergency called *ketoacidosis* (explained more fully in Chapter 21). On the other hand, urine ketones may *not* be an indication of trouble. Ketones reflect fat breakdown for use as fuel. When you haven't eaten any carbohydrate and you don't have much insulin circulating, the body turns to fat as a source of fuel and produces ketones as the fat is broken down. In a normal fast—for instance, when you skip breakfast and haven't eaten in 12–16 hours—some ketones may spill into your urine, but this doesn't mean you are in danger of going into diabetic ketoacidosis.

Testing for ketones, then, is a way to tell how far out of control your diabetes is and whether a true emergency exists. Traditionally, urine ketone testing was the only available approach, but now some companies sell monitors that let you check your blood glucose and blood ketone levels. If there are moderate or large amounts of ketones in your urine (or your blood) *and* your blood glucose is high, you need medical help quickly. Don't be fooled into complacency by blood glucose levels that are only moderately high, since some people develop ketoacidosis with glucose levels only in the 200s.

When should you check for ketones? Though you should always keep up-to-date test strips on hand at home, there is no reason to test for ketones every day; the test will be meaningful only when you are really approaching trouble, and you should know when that is happening: your symptoms or your blood glucose levels will warn you. Test ketones if you're sick or if you think your diabetes is way out of control. If you test positive for ketones, be sure to take at least your usual amount of insulin and *seek help.*

Take Home Messages

- You should definitely know the symptoms of highs and lows in your blood glucose. But knowing the symptoms is not a substitute for actual blood glucose monitoring.
- Regular monitoring provides accurate, dependable information about where your blood glucose is right now; this helps you make immediate adjustments in your treatment plan.
- Continuous glucose monitoring can also tell you about glucose trends and can warn you when your levels are high or low.
- A1c readings, done two to four times a year, can tell you what your average glucose levels have been over the previous three months; this helps you make long-term adjustments in your treatment plan.
- Ketone monitoring when your blood glucose levels are high or you are sick can help you avoid serious problems.
- Combining regular blood glucose monitoring and A1c testing with ketone monitoring, as needed, is the best way to stay healthy today and in the future.

5

Hypoglycemia

with Kristin Arcara, M.D.

- "When I go low I don't have any control over anything—what I'm doing or saying or whatever's going on around me."
- "When I think my husband is low, I'll suggest that he test his blood. If he jumps down my throat, I know he's having a reaction."
- "Hypoglycemia used to come on slowly; I'd have lots of warning so I could deal with it. Now I get blindsided: one minute I'm fine and the next I'm completely out of it."

You may know it as an *insulin reaction*, a *hypo*, a *reaction*, a *low blood sugar*, or simply a *low*. By whatever name, hypoglycemia means trouble. It is by far the most common complication of insulin treatment, estimated to occur and cause symptoms an average of once or twice a week in people taking insulin. For many people, unrecognized mild hypoglycemia is even more common. Most hypoglycemia is fairly mild, but it can be serious enough to cause coma or a seizure. It is more common in people with Type 1 diabetes but can also occur in people with Type 2 diabetes who take insulin or pills. Although most of the pills used to treat diabetes do not cause hypoglycemia, some of the oral medications *can* cause hypoglycemia. These include *sulfonylureas*, including chlorpropamide (Diabinese, Insulase), tolbutamide (Orinase), glibenclamide or glyburide (DiaBeta, Glynase, Micronase), glimepiride (Amaryl), glipizide (Glucotrol), gliquidone (Glurenorm), and gliclazide (Glizid, Glyloc, Reclide, Diamicron); and *meglitinides*, including mitiglinide (Glufast), repaglinide (Prandin), and nateglinide (Starlix).

Hypoglycemia is often unpleasant. It can interfere with your thinking, making normal activities—such as driving a car, riding a bicycle, or operating machinery—dangerous or impossible. Fear of hypoglycemia can cause a person to maintain high blood glucose levels all the time, increasing the risk for long-term complications. Finally, hypoglycemia that causes antagonistic behavior or results in a medical emergency is not just a momentary problem. It can affect family relationships, friendships, or even employment.

In this chapter we describe the symptoms of different levels of hypoglycemia, identify its common causes, and discuss more fully the potential consequences of low blood glucose. Then we review the steps for avoiding, recognizing, and treating hypoglycemia, including suggestions for family members and friends who must deal with a loved one's hypoglycemia.

Before going any further, let's define hypoglycemia. Technically, in laboratory reports, hypoglycemia often is defined as a blood glucose level below 60 mg/dl. We resist the notion of defining hypoglycemia solely by a specific blood glucose level, however, because the clinical effects of low blood glucose occur at very different levels from person to person. In fact, rapidly falling blood glucose can cause people to have symptoms of hypoglycemia even though blood glucose may be in the normal range on testing. We define hypoglycemia as a blood glucose low enough to make you *feel* or *act* hypoglycemic.

Symptoms of Hypoglycemia

The common symptoms of hypoglycemia are quite typical, even though each person may have his or her own "personal" symptom. It is very important for everyone at risk of hypoglycemia (generally, everyone taking insulin or some types of pills or injectable medications for diabetes, as listed above) to know the symptoms, what they mean, and what to do about them. Hypoglycemia causes symptoms that come and go rapidly, usually within a matter of several minutes. These symptoms fall into three categories: physical, mental, and emotional.

Physical Symptoms

When your blood glucose goes low, part of your body's response is to release what we call *counterregulatory hormones* such as those involved in the "fight or flight" response, which we will discuss shortly (see Figure 9). Many symptoms of hypoglycemia are caused by these hormones. The most common physical symptoms of hypoglycemia include:

—Trembling (sometimes a visible fine tremor, sometimes described as an "inner trembling")

—Lightheadedness or dizziness

—Sweating

—Becoming pale

—Pounding or rapid heartbeat

—Poor coordination

Less common physical symptoms of hypoglycemia include:

—Visual disturbances

—Sudden hunger

—Sudden, severe fatigue

In addition, there are what we call each individual's "personal symptoms." One person tells us he feels a tingle in his little finger, another describes a feeling of unease, yet another talks about a feeling of being "distant from the world." One man reported that his most reliable sign of hypoglycemia was a sudden twitch in his left eye. He might be the only person who ever had this symptom, but it helped him know when he was hypoglycemic, and that was all that mattered. It is important to recognize that hypoglycemia

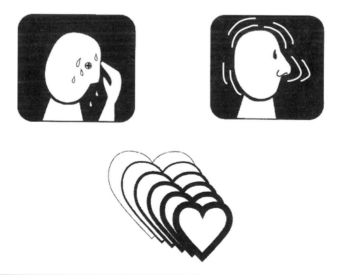

Figure 9. Hypoglycemia: adrenergic signs. For most people, when the blood glucose falls into the low range (hypoglycemia), the body produces adrenaline—the "fight or flight" hormone. This hormone produces characteristic *adrenergic signs*: sweating, shaking and nervousness, and rapid heartbeat. The symptoms are uncomfortable and are a clear sign that something is wrong. Action (eating a sugar) should be taken.

can simply cause someone to "feel different" from how he or she normally feels, and that might be reason enough to suspect and test for hypoglycemia.

Mental Symptoms

If your blood glucose level goes very low, you will develop the mental symptoms of hypoglycemia. These are much more serious than the physical symptoms because, at a minimum, they impair your ability to think clearly, and sometimes they cause a level of confusion that keeps you from recognizing your own hypoglycemia. In the worst case, they cause coma or seizures. They result from your brain not having enough glucose to function at its best (see Figure 10). The mental, or "cerebral," symptoms of hypoglycemia include:

—Difficulty concentrating
—Headache
—Dizziness

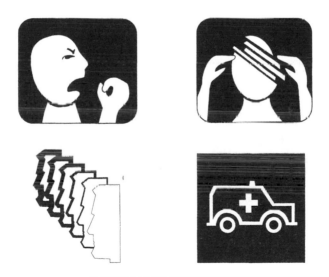

Figure 10. Hypoglycemia: neuroglycopenic signs. Other symptoms of hypoglycemia are caused by the lack of glucose to the brain. When the brain doesn't get enough glucose, the following symptoms may develop: crankiness, confusion, trouble speaking or thinking clearly, and even loss of consciousness. These are called the *neuroglycopenic signs*.

—Confusion
—Slurred or slow speech
—Extreme fatigue
—Lack of coordination
—The feeling of being out of your body

Emotional Symptoms

Some people, and many spouses of people with diabetes, report that low blood glucose affects the mood. It can cause a person to feel irritable or start to "act funny." Family members often tell us that mood changes are the first sign the person is hypoglycemic. Emotional lability (sudden crying, inappropriate giggling, anger, or becoming argumentative) is very commonly associated with hypoglycemia.

The Pitfalls of Using Symptoms as a Guide to Blood Glucose Levels

Unfortunately, counting on symptoms to identify hypoglycemia can be tricky and unreliable at times. First of all, people differ in their symptoms of low blood glucose. Second, many of the symptoms are so nonspecific that they could be caused by any number of other situations besides hypoglycemia.

> Joanna, a 19-year-old college freshman with Type 1 diabetes, was about to go into a big exam at 10 o'clock one morning. She had taken insulin that morning but was so anxious about the test that she couldn't really remember what she had eaten for breakfast. As exam time approached, Joanna's heart felt as though it were beating out of her chest. She had sweaty palms. Almost as a kneejerk reaction, she reached for the glucose tablets in her purse. But then, Joanna thought, "Hey, I'd better just check, to be sure." Two minutes and one finger stick later, she had the answer: her blood glucose was 140 mg/dl—not low, not high, just right. The blood glucose check reassured her that her rapid heartbeat and sweaty palms were probably no more than the nervousness that all her classmates were feeling as they headed into this test. Even more important, it also kept Joanna from taking a lot of sugar to treat a nonexistent hypoglycemic reaction. Her mind relieved, Joanna did well on her exam.

The most serious problem with counting on warning symptoms is that they may not occur until it's too late—until you are too confused to treat yourself. We discuss this situation, called *hypoglycemia unawareness*, in more detail later.

What Causes These Symptoms?

To keep you functioning well, your body has strong defenses against hypoglycemia. As mentioned earlier, when your blood glucose goes too low, your body releases certain hormones, called counterregulatory hormones, that stimulate your liver to make glucose, bringing the blood glucose back to normal. In other words, the counterregulatory hormones bring or hold the blood glucose *up*, acting in opposition to insulin (which, of course, lowers blood glucose).

Glucagon, cortisol, and *growth hormone* are all counterregulatory hormones, released in response to hypoglycemia. Another is *epinephrine,* also called *adrenaline.* Adrenaline, you'll recall, is the same hormone your body releases when you are in any stressful situation ("fight or flight"). This all makes sense when you think about it: if you are about to enter a fight or flee at top speed, you want lots of available fuel (glucose) in the blood, and adrenaline will raise the blood glucose. But it also means that the symptoms of hypoglycemia and the normal "adrenaline rush" in response to stress are identical because they are caused by the same hormone—adrenaline. Joanna's dilemma, described above, was that she *did* have adrenaline pouring out—she just couldn't tell, without checking her glucose, whether the adrenaline rush was due to hypoglycemia or simple stress.

The mental, or cerebral, symptoms of hypoglycemia occur because the brain needs a certain amount of glucose to function normally. When blood glucose falls too far, the incredibly complicated functions we call consciousness begin to break down. It is actually quite remarkable that almost the moment the blood glucose is brought back to normal, the brain recovers (assuming there was no severe, prolonged hypoglycemic coma).

Severity of Hypoglycemia

Insulin reactions vary in severity from a minor nuisance to a major disaster. Many people we know "feel a little low" at some point on most days and simply treat the feeling with a little food. For others, insulin reactions are not a medical danger but can be a significant embarrassment—having to excuse yourself abruptly so you can go get something sugary in the middle of an important meeting, for instance. Then there are the true medical emergencies, when a person is confused, having a seizure, or even in a coma, when someone is dependent on another person for treatment.

We are often asked whether hypoglycemia can be fatal. The answer is yes, but very, very rarely. Usually, the danger is due not to the hypoglycemia itself but to what happens as a result of the hypoglycemia. These dangers include motor vehicle accidents (the number one danger), seizures, and breathing into the lungs any fluid mistakenly given to a comatose or near-comatose person (called *aspiration*).

Because the range of severity of hypoglycemia varies so enormously, it is now broadly classified into three categories:

—*Mild hypoglycemia.* When you are mildly hypoglycemic, the symptoms are mainly physical: sweating, trembling, and so on. You can recognize them. You may notice that you aren't thinking as clearly as you usually do or that you aren't behaving quite normally, though others might not notice these subtle changes. Even mild hypoglycemia can be distressing, but most people don't find these episodes terribly upsetting.

—*Moderate hypoglycemia.* When you are moderately hypoglycemic you may become confused or act inappropriately, but you can still treat the low blood glucose yourself.

—*Severe hypoglycemia.* When you are severely hypoglycemic you are no longer able to self-treat. You are too confused to know what's going on. You may even fall into a coma or suffer a seizure. On very rare occasions, a low blood glucose can be fatal if it stays very low for a prolonged period or if it occurs during an activity in which disordered thinking poses serious dangers.

Common Causes of Hypoglycemia and How to Prevent It

Hypoglycemia is usually caused by one or more factors: too tight diabetes control, too much insulin, too little food, or too much exercise. Other, less common causes include alcohol consumption, use of other medications, changes during the menstrual cycle, or slowed absorption of food from the stomach. A condition known as hypoglycemia unawareness can further complicate blood glucose control.

Tight Blood Glucose Control

There's no doubt about it: intensive regimens designed to keep your blood glucose levels as close to normal as possible do increase your risk of hypoglycemia. That's because there is a much smaller margin of safety if you are aiming for near-normal blood glucose levels than if you are at higher levels. You are driving down a narrow road with plenty of curves. You have to be especially careful. The Diabetes Control and Complications Trial (DCCT) found three times as much hypoglycemia in participants who practiced "intensive" treatment. We should note, however, that newer, rapid-acting and long-acting insulin regimens are associated with a lower risk of hypoglycemia than the older, less flexible regimens used during the DCCT.

This increased risk of hypoglycemia does not in any way mean that you should give up on good blood glucose control. It just means that you should be aware of the risk and should stay alert. Be aware of your near lows. If your blood glucose always tends to run 60–75 mg/dl during the day or at night, once in a while it'll be 50 mg/dl, and you may not have symptoms if you have low blood glucose frequently, as we discuss later. Don't try to cut it too close. If you are noticing patterns of blood glucose levels that are near-low, you should talk to your doctor; this may indicate the need for a decrease or adjustment in your doses of diabetes medications.

There are also times when it makes sense to ease up a little on your blood glucose control. Let the situation guide you. If you have been having lots of lows, talk to your doctor. You may decide together to decrease your insulin doses for a few days. There will also be certain times when a low blood glucose would be so unwelcome that you might choose to run a little high: a key meeting, a long drive, an athletic event, or a camping trip.

We thought it was time for David to go on an "intensive" regimen, by which we meant taking short-acting insulin (NovoLog [aspart], Apidra [glulisine], or Humalog [lispro]) with breakfast, lunch, and dinner and a longer-acting insulin (Lantus [glargine] or Levemir [detemir]) at bedtime. David agreed. For the first month he found himself always on the verge of hypoglycemia at lunchtime—if he didn't eat by noon, he felt low   and again at about 4 o'clock. He checked his glucose for a few days at about 11 a.m. and 4 p.m., on days when he was not actually having symptoms, and found it to be between 60 and 70 mg/dl. David called us, and the morning and lunchtime insulin doses were cut significantly. It was clear that even though the glucose levels he tested were not frankly low, the complete picture—an intensified regimen, quite frequent symptoms late in the morning and in mid-afternoon, and borderline glucose levels at that time—put him at risk of severe hypoglycemia if we did not change things.

Too Much Insulin

In one sense, if you are someone who takes insulin and you become hypoglycemic, then, by definition, you took too much insulin. The fact that you skipped a meal, or exercised more than usual, or did something else that resulted in a low might be the immediate reason why the insulin was too much. But there are certain things you should consider very carefully with regard to your insulin dose and hypoglycemia.

The most common insulin-related cause of daytime hypoglycemia is taking too much fast-acting insulin—for example, Humalog, NovoLog, Apidra, or Regular insulin. Hypoglycemia overnight is usually due to too much pre-supper or bedtime insulin. (These issues are discussed in Chapter 12.) But bear in mind that we don't like to think of an insulin dose as one constant amount, day after day and year after year, especially when the blood glucose control is at all unstable. Frequent hypoglycemia or a pattern of hypoglycemia at one time of day should prompt you to talk with your health care provider about changing your insulin dose, just as you would for frequent hyperglycemia.

Hypoglycemia may also be the result of erratic or altered absorption of insulin. Sometimes you can control this—for example, by picking a nice fleshy spot to inject rather than a hard, tough area of the skin. You should also try to avoid injecting insulin into exactly the same site on your body too frequently, as fatty tissue can accumulate and cause unpredictable insulin absorption when it is injected at that site. You can certainly use the same physical part of your body, such as your abdomen, but it is best to use a different specific spot each time you inject.

Unpredictability of insulin absorption is not entirely controllable, however. If you actively exercise a part of your body where you've just injected certain types of insulin, the more rapid absorption may trigger hypoglycemia. This generally is not true for Lantus or Levemir or the rapid-acting insulins (NovoLog, Humalog, Apidra).

Other medication-related factors that can contribute to hypoglycemia include switching from an old bottle of insulin, which has lost some of its potency, to a new bottle, even though you are taking the same dose. One way to try to keep insulin from losing its potency is to make sure you keep it away from heat—for example, if you are on the beach or at a summer picnic. You may want to keep your insulin in a small cooler if you plan to be out in the heat for any extended time.

If you vary your dose of insulin according to your blood glucose (*sliding scale*), think clearly about the specific times when lows occur. Do low blood glucose levels tend to occur more often after you've had a high level that required a larger dose of insulin to bring your blood glucose down? Or do lows generally occur after blood glucose levels are in your goal range but you've taken insulin to cover a meal? These two scenarios would require different approaches to adjusting your insulin doses. In the first example, when a low occurs after an insulin dose to correct a high blood glucose, maybe the dose of insulin to bring the blood glucose down, or the upper end of the sliding scale, needs to be decreased. In the second case, with low blood glucose levels following normal levels at a meal, the dose of insulin to cover the carbohydrates in the meal, or the lower end of the sliding scale, may need to be decreased. The specific pattern of low blood glucose levels can be very useful in helping you and your doctor decide how to prevent them.

> *George is told to take 6 units of NovoLog before breakfast if his blood glucose is under 100 mg/dl, 9 units if 100–200 mg/dl, and 12 units if over 200 mg/dl. He finds that the 12 units work, bringing him down to a reasonable range by noon, but that if he takes 6 units when he's under 100 mg/dl, he is sure to be symptomatically low by 11 a.m. Solution? Cut down the low end of his scale, so he takes only 4 units if his blood glucose is under 100 mg/dl.*

> *Tammy, when given the same sliding scale for her insulin doses, finds she goes low when she takes 12 units, even if her blood glucose is over 200 mg/dl. Solution? Cut down the upper end of her scale so that she never takes more than 10 units.*

Too Little Food

In the days before the use of the newer insulin preparations (NovoLog, Humalog, Apidra, Lantus, and Levemir), skipping meals, delaying meals, or eating meals with insufficient amounts of carbohydrate would often result in hypoglycemia. The reason was that some of the older formulations of insulin, especially NPH insulin, would reach their peak activity several hours after injection. People with diabetes who took NPH would have to be sure to eat at around the time the NPH was exerting its peak effect, otherwise they would risk having hypoglycemia. Fortunately, many newer insulin formulations do not have this delayed onset of action, so they do not require such strict timing of meals. This is discussed in greater detail in Chapter 12. Lantus and Levemir are long-acting forms of insulin that have almost no peak, and so their effect has little relation to meals and does not require meals to be eaten at particular times. The short-acting insulins (NovoLog, Humalog, Apidra) work very quickly, having an onset within 20 minutes of injection, so they can be taken at mealtimes, whenever those meals occur. Thus, these newer insulin formulations have given people with diabetes much more flexibility with regard to mealtimes and may help to decrease some of the risk of hypoglycemia.

Too Much Activity

Unplanned physical activity and prolonged or high-intensity activity can also make you hypoglycemic. As we discuss more fully in Chapter 9, the hypoglycemic effect of exercise can be immediate or delayed. It may last for as long as 16 hours. So if you are planning to exercise, test your blood first. If there is a reasonable chance your blood glucose will go low during your activity, eat something before you start, or reduce the amount of mealtime insulin by 1–3 units if you plan to exercise shortly after a meal. People with diabetes who use insulin pumps can also temporarily decrease their basal insulin rate during activity. Always have a source of fast-acting carbohydrate available when you exercise, in case you start to become hypoglycemic.

Given the potential for hypoglycemia, it might be tempting to avoid physical activity altogether. Not a good solution! Regular exercise is a very important part of a healthy lifestyle and is especially beneficial for people with diabetes. Learning how your blood glucose reacts to physical activity and trying different strategies to find the best way to manage it will help you safely incorporate this very important aspect of your health into your routine.

Alcohol

One of the less common causes of low blood glucose is drinking alcoholic beverages (even as little as one beer or one glass of wine). Alcohol suppresses glucose release from the liver and in this way increases the risk of hypoglycemia. If you are planning to drink alcohol, be sure you have recently had something to eat. That way you won't be depending on the glucose reserves in your liver to protect you from hypoglycemia. Keep in mind too that drinking enough to impair judgment can make you less conscious of symptoms of hypoglycemia so that you may not be able to recognize and treat it quickly, which can be quite dangerous. As we mentioned earlier in this chapter, prolonged hypoglycemia can, in rare cases, lead to death. So please be careful not to drink to the point that you become less aware of low blood glucose symptoms: it's too much of a risk for a person with diabetes. Remember also that some symptoms of hypoglycemia, such as confusion and slurred speech, can easily be mistaken for drunken behavior. People have ended up in jail for inebriation when, in fact, they were hypoglycemic.

Oral Antihyperglycemic Agents

We have so far talked almost exclusively about hypoglycemia due to insulin. But what if you don't take insulin? What if you take pills for diabetes? Many of the pills and injections used to treat diabetes do not cause hypoglycemia—for example, metformin; thiazolidinediones such as pioglitazone (Actos) and rosiglitazone (Avandia); and alpha-glucosidase inhibitors such as acarbose (Precose), miglitol (Glyset), and voglibose (Voglib). Some types of pills, however, such as sulfonylureas, meglitinides, glucagon-like peptide 1 (GLP-1) agonists, and dipeptidyl peptidase 4 (DPP-4) inhibitors (rarely), can do so. Glyburide is the oral diabetes drug most notorious for causing hypoglycemia. Most often, hypoglycemia may occur when beginning or increasing the dose of one of these drugs, when decreasing the amount of food or, specifically, carbohydrates eaten, or when increasing exercise. Doses of these drugs may need to be decreased or not taken at all on days of significantly increased activity or fasting. They may need to be decreased in the long term if someone makes a more permanent dietary or physical activity change. The fact is, however, that hypoglycemia is much less common with pills than with insulin.

Other Medications

Drugs such as beta-blockers (propranolol, metoprolol, atenolol) may mask some of the counterregulatory warning signs of hypoglycemia. However, as shown by a recent large study, beta-blocker use itself is not associated with severe low blood glucose. We think that beta-blockers can be safely taken by persons with diabetes, should they need them. If you are taking a medication that masks symptoms of hypoglycemia, you may need to test your blood glucose more often or pay closer attention to other signs of hypoglycemia to keep you out of trouble.

Menstrual Cycle

Insulin requirements can fluctuate with the phases of a woman's menstrual cycle. For a few days before a menstrual period begins, insulin needs may increase; they may then drop dramatically when the period starts. These fluctuations seem to be the result of hormonal shifts: just before the menstrual period begins, a woman's body secretes increased amounts of progesterone (another counterregulatory hormone). Once the period begins, progesterone levels go down again.

If you notice that your blood glucose levels tend to fluctuate with the phases of your menstrual cycle, you should keep very close track of the pattern. That way, you can raise your insulin doses at the earliest possible moment and avoid hyperglycemia just before your period, then lower your insulin to prevent hypoglycemia once your period starts.

Gastroparesis

A form of diabetic nerve damage called *gastroparesis* delays the emptying of the stomach contents into the intestines after a meal. If you have this complication, your food will be absorbed more slowly, and any insulin you have injected may get into your system faster than the food. This increases your risk of hypoglycemia.

Gastroparesis is not common, but it can cause havoc with blood glucose control. If you have gastroparesis, try to work out an insulin regimen with your health care professional that takes into account the slower rate at which you absorb your food. You can use slower-acting insulins such as Regular insulin or medications that help the stomach empty.

Hypoglycemia Unawareness

The key to managing your own hypoglycemia without undue problems is to be aware of your symptoms and pay close attention to them. But what if you don't have symptoms any more? What if you are completely unaware that your blood glucose is low until you become confused, disoriented, and unable to care for yourself? This is called *hypoglycemia unawareness*.

Hypoglycemia unawareness usually develops after many years of diabetes. However, it can also occur in the short term, even after only one or two episodes of hypoglycemia. A single low blood glucose in the previous 24 hours has been shown to lessen low blood glucose symptoms should another low occur. In mild forms, people just notice that the insulin reactions "sneak up" on them with less warning than before. There may be recognizable symptoms such as dizziness, lack of coordination, tiredness, visual disturbance, and difficulty concentrating. But if you *start* with confusion, you may not be able to treat your own hypoglycemia. It may progress to the point where there really are no symptoms at all before total confusion sets in.

The condition of hypoglycemia unawareness is thought to result from frequent hypoglycemia that causes the brain to make more glucose transporters. This means the brain can take up more glucose even when the blood glucose is low, allowing it to function more normally at mildly low blood glucose levels. This is dangerous because the usual brain-stimulated release of adrenaline may not occur with mildly low blood glucose levels, and the early warning signs that normally accompany mildly low blood glucose levels may therefore be lost. With defective glucose counterregulation, you may no longer have symptoms of hypoglycemia such as sweatiness, a pounding heart, trembling, and nervousness that are normally triggered by the release of adrenaline. You may have only the mental (cerebral) signs, due to your brain not getting enough glucose when the blood glucose becomes very low.

The treatment for hypoglycemia unawareness involves rigorously avoiding low blood glucose levels for a period of days or weeks. This seems to rejuvenate some of the ability to detect hypoglycemia. If you have hypoglycemia unawareness, be sure to test your blood glucose before performing activities such as driving, during which hypoglycemia can be very dangerous. Frequent, repeated testing during such an activity is a good idea, especially if the activity is going on for a long time.

Blood Glucose Awareness Training

A technique called blood glucose awareness training (BGAT) holds promise for people who are not good at recognizing when their blood glucose is going low. In essence, BGAT teaches people to increase their ability to avoid, detect, and rapidly treat hypoglycemia, using internal and external cues such as the ones discussed above. The internal cues for BGAT include physical symptoms, performance cues, and moods and feelings. The goal of the training is to teach you to identify and react to the first symptom of low blood glucose and to test your blood or simply to treat for hypoglycemia if a glucose meter (glucometer) is not immediately available. Typical of the external cues are the combination of insulin dose, time of day, and last blood glucose reading or the combination of food intake, time of day, exercise, and last blood glucose reading.

The results of BGAT research are impressive. People who completed the training program improved their ability to detect low and high blood glucose levels and had fewer lows, fewer episodes of nighttime hypoglycemia, fewer automobile accidents, fewer traffic violations, and no deterioration in long-term blood glucose control.

Treating Hypoglycemia

If you are taking insulin or even taking hypoglycemic pills, you are at risk for hypoglycemia and should certainly know how to treat it. In theory, treatment is simple: at the earliest sign, you should quickly take in some food—specifically, quickly absorbed carbohydrates or *simple sugars*. In reality, many people get themselves in trouble by either undertreating or overtreating.

All too often, people ignore the early warning signs of hypoglycemia or tell themselves they can hold out another 10 minutes (or 30 or 60 minutes). This mistake can lead to a severe reaction or, at least, a more severe reaction. The answer, of course, is to *treat early symptoms immediately*. Don't be caught anywhere without fast access to quickly absorbed carbohydrate. Always be prepared for hypoglycemia. Have glucose tablets or other sources of sugar in your pocket or purse, in your car, at your office, and by your bed at night.

Overtreating is also a common problem. In the midst of an episode of hypoglycemia, there is an almost irresistible urge to eat everything in sight. The result can easily be to careen from a blood glucose that is too low to one that is too high. You may then take more insulin to bring the glucose back down, and off you go on a roller-coaster ride of too low, too high, too low.

There are a few things you can do to avoid overtreatment of lows. First, remember that it takes a few minutes (often 15-20 minutes) for anything you eat or drink to be absorbed through your stomach and raise your blood glucose level. So eating continuously until the level comes up does not help. You might be able to curb the tendency to overtreat if you prepare a "hypoglycemia first aid package" in advance. Set out exactly the right carbohydrate in the right proportion to treat your hypoglycemia (usually 10–15 grams of carbohydrate; see below). You may use commercially prepared glucose tablets and gels, which are less appetizing than many foods and so you are less likely to overuse them. Or you may pack just enough food to do the job. You might also consider the approach one of our patients uses. As she waits for the food she has eaten to bring her blood glucose back up, she repeats to herself, "You took the right amount. Just wait until it works. You'll feel fine in a few minutes." She tells us that this simple, reassuring message really works to keep her from overtreating.

Specific Suggestions to Treat Hypoglycemia

Mild and even some moderate hypoglycemia can be treated with 10-15 grams of fast-acting carbohydrate. Some examples are:

—2 or 3 glucose tablets (5 grams each)
—⅓-½ of a 30-gram tube of glucose gel
—4-6 ounces of orange juice
—4-6 ounces of regular soda
—¼-⅓ cup of raisins
—5 Lifesavers candies
—4-5 Starburst candies (3 grams each)
—4 sugar packets (3-4 grams each)
—2-2½ packets of Smarties candies (6 grams per packet)

Repeat this treatment after 15-20 minutes if your low hypoglycemic symptoms persist or if your blood glucose level is not above 60 mg/dl. Food that contains fat in addition to sugar is not as good a choice for treating low blood glucose as food containing primarily sugar. Fat slows the absorption of the sugar you need to treat your hypoglycemia. Hence, foods like chocolate or ice cream, with a high fat content, are bad choices for treating hypoglycemia.

Moderate hypoglycemia requires the same treatment as mild hypoglycemia, though it may take more than one treatment and take longer for the person to fully recover.

If you are severely hypoglycemic, by definition you cannot treat yourself. That's why it's essential that your family, friends, and coworkers know what to do. It is always frightening to see someone severely hypoglycemic, especially for people who have not seen it happen before. So even if you are not especially prone to low blood glucose levels, it would be a good idea to rehearse with your family what to do if hypoglycemia should occur. It's like a fire drill: it's better to practice and be prepared, even if the fire never happens.

It is very important that *no one put anything in your mouth unless you are sitting up and able to swallow*. The consequences of trying to pour something sweet into the mouth of a semiconscious person can be tragic. Most people can be coaxed into eating or drinking something sweet, even if they are severely hypoglycemic. If not, *don't force anything into the mouth*. Call 911 or inject glucagon.

Glucagon is to be given only when the hypoglycemic person is unresponsive, so it is always given by another person, someone trained and prepared to do the injection. Be sure glucagon is available and that a family member or roommate knows when and how to give it to you. The injection is not difficult, since it can go into any muscle. Glucagon is not glucose; it is one of the hormones, mentioned earlier, that cause the liver to release glucose into the bloodstream.

Glucagon is safe to use and is available by prescription. When stored in the refrigerator, it is good for several years. Since you probably won't need it very often, be sure to check the expiration date now and then, and periodically review the instructions for administering glucagon with the person or people who might be doing the injection. You should also feel free to review with your physician, nurse, or pharmacist how to give glucagon properly. Here are some guidelines for using glucagon:

—Make sure the person administering the glucagon knows to call for emergency assistance if you don't respond to treatment within 15–20 minutes.
—Your stomach may be upset after you have received glucagon; you may even vomit.
—As soon as you are alert and able to swallow, you should have something light, such as soda or crackers. Eating will restore the glucose supply in your liver.
—As soon as you are able to hold down food, you should eat something more substantial such as a sandwich or some milk.
—If nausea persists, follow your plan for sick days and contact your health care provider.
—Even if you are feeling well after receiving glucagon, always contact your physician; your recent need for glucagon may indicate a need to decrease your insulin or other diabetes medication doses.

Finally, in preparing to manage severe hypoglycemia, make sure everyone in your family, even children as young as 4 years old, knows how to call 911 if you become unconscious or are otherwise unable to care for yourself. We know of cases in which preschoolers have saved their parents from serious hypoglycemic peril by calling for emergency assistance.

When you are away from home, always wear a medical alert identification bracelet or necklace or carry an identification card to inform anyone coming to your aid that you have diabetes and take insulin. Medical alert bracelets now come in all sorts of designs, so you don't necessarily need to wear an old-fashioned one that you may remember your older relatives wearing. Search for different styles and find one that you will feel comfortable wearing every day. It can't help you if you don't wear it!

Nighttime Hypoglycemia

More than half of all episodes of severe hypoglycemia occur during the night. This is the most dangerous time, because you're asleep and not aware that you need to treat the condition immediately. In addition, the insulin requirements of most people are lowest in the middle of the night (often 20%–30% lower than at other times). Finally, if you are on an insulin regimen that includes NPH insulin at dinnertime, its effect generally peaks during this time. To avoid nighttime hypoglycemia, test your blood before you go to bed and perhaps eat a snack if the reading is less than 100–120 mg/dl, especially if you were unusually active during the day. Alternatively, you could check your blood glucose again in an hour or two to be sure it is not falling lower. If you have eaten something and taken short acting insulin close to bedtime, you may want to set an alarm to check your blood glucose two to three hours after the insulin dose. It's also a good idea to check your predawn levels from time to time. If you find that your blood glucose is consistently dropping more than 30 points overnight when you haven't taken short-acting insulin close to bedtime, your long-acting insulin dose may need to be reduced.

Psychological Impact of Hypoglycemia

In addition to the physical, mental, and emotional effects of hypoglycemia in the short term, it can also cause other challenges in diabetes management. Fear or concern about the potential for hypoglycemia can be a significant challenge for people with diabetes and their families. It can lead to anxiety and decreased levels of overall happiness for people with diabetes. It can interfere with optimal treatment and cause people to keep their blood glucose levels higher overall to avoid episodes of hypoglycemia. In some short-term situations, keeping blood levels slightly higher than the target range might be advantageous, as we mentioned earlier (an important meeting, driving, a sporting event), but over the long term—as we know from studies such as the DCCT—the closer to normal the blood glucose levels, the lower the risk of complications from diabetes. Fear of hypoglycemia may make it even more challenging to meet the goal of good glucose control.

You are not alone if you have these feelings and fears. It is important to talk about them with your physician so that you can come up with a strategy that allows you to achieve the best glucose control without causing undue stress and anxiety. Be sure that you understand the effects of each of the medications you are prescribed, especially your diabetes medications, including the timing and duration of medication action. You should be checking your blood glucose levels regularly, recording them, and paying attention to patterns, including the effects of meals, exercise, and alcohol, among other factors. Don't be discouraged by hypoglycemia; be proactive, prepared, and educated to prevent and manage it.

Continuous Glucose Monitors

If you have frequent hypoglycemia or persistent hypoglycemic unawareness, or if you've had severe hypoglycemia requiring assistance, you should discuss with your health care provider whether a continuous glucose monitor (CGM) would be helpful for you. CGMs have a subcutaneous catheter or filament that measures the glucose content in the interstitial fluid, the fluid between cells (see Chapter 4). A new glucose reading appears every 2–5 minutes on a receiver. This glucose measurement lags about 15 minutes behind the actual blood glucose level but is usually pretty close to what the blood glucose level is, unless the blood glucose is changing very rapidly. Depending on the type of sensor used, the receiver needs to be within 5–20 feet or so of the transmitter, which is on the surface of the skin. When you push a button on the receiver, the most recent glucose reading is displayed, the last three hours of readings are shown on a graph, and an arrow indicates whether the level is unchanging or is slowly or rapidly rising or falling. What this device provides, then, is not just the glucose reading but also the direction in which the blood glucose is heading. This allows you to see if it's heading toward a low in the near future and alerts you to eat extra calories to prevent a low glucose before it happens. There are also vibrating and beeping alarms that can be set to alert you to low or soon-to-be-low glucose readings. These devices have helped patients reduce how often their glucose is low and how severely low it goes, and they provide reassurance that a low blood glucose can be better detected.

For Family and Friends

If you have a family member or close friend with diabetes, you are probably already aware that low blood glucose causes changes in behavior. Often, it starts with just a little change in the person's voice or speech pattern or a look in the eye that only you are aware of. The person may become negative, stubborn, irritable, or even verbally or physically abusive. Severe hypoglycemia may make him disoriented, causing him to bump into things, aimlessly pick things up and put them down again, or just sit and stare into space.

When you see this happening, try to keep two things in mind: first, you are probably right that it is hypoglycemia; second, like it or not, you are the person on the spot with a clear head, responsible for doing the right thing. The hypoglycemic person is really out of control.

It is often difficult to convince a person who is mentally confused or emotionally charged to treat her low blood glucose. She may refuse to cooperate or may even fight you, stoutly maintaining that there's no problem, telling you to mind your own business. But you have to trust your own instincts. At the very worst, treating with something sweet won't hurt, so have a plan and the means for treatment.

Dealing with the person whose emotions are spilling out can be especially trying. None of us likes to be called names, be accused of things we didn't do, or have to deal with someone emotionally out of control. The natural tendency is to fight back, to argue, to be defensive. But just keep telling yourself, "He's not himself. This is a person under the influence of hypoglycemia. He doesn't mean it." You must find a way to deal with your own feelings when this responsibility is thrust upon you. Resist the natural temptation to lash out or to walk away. Remember that you are the one with a normally functioning brain, so you need to use it.

Probably most importantly, you need to know how to administer glucagon. It's frightening to think of being responsible for giving your loved one a shot, not knowing if you will succeed in bringing her back to consciousness. But prompt use of glucagon can provide your loved one with the fastest possible treatment and potentially save her life. It can also allow you to avoid the trauma and expense of dealing with emergency medical personnel and hospital staff.

•••

Hypoglycemia is inconvenient at best and frightening or even life-threatening at worst. We hope that what you've learned from this chapter will help you to better avoid low blood glucose levels and to treat them more quickly and effectively when they do occur.

Take Home Messages

- Hypoglycemia is the most common side effect of insulin therapy; it can also occur if you take certain oral diabetes medications.
- When you are hypoglycemic, you may experience physical, emotional, and mental symptoms.
- It is important to recognize symptoms of hypoglycemia while your hypoglycemia is still mild. Checking your blood glucose level is the only way to be certain you are hypoglycemic.
- Mild or moderate hypoglycemia is uncomfortable and sometimes embarrassing; severe hypoglycemia (when you need the help of another person to bring your blood glucose levels back up) can be dangerous, especially if you are driving a car.
- Common causes of hypoglycemia include tight blood glucose control, too much insulin, too little food, and too much activity. Drinking alcoholic beverages may also make hypoglycemia more likely.
- For some people, continuous glucose monitors may reduce the risk of hypoglycemia.
- Family and close friends should be able to recognize the symptoms of hypoglycemia and know what to do if it happens to you.

6

Introduction to Nutrition Therapy
Planning and Understanding the Diet

with Emily Loghmani, RD, CDE

- "None of my favorite foods are on the list of what I should eat. What are they thinking?"
- "I don't understand carbohydrate counting. Just tell me what to eat."
- "Now that I'm eating healthy, I feel so much better."

Eating is a central part of life. It makes us feel comfortable, safe, and warm. No wonder, then, that when your diet becomes medicalized—when what you can eat is dictated by a medical condition—you're likely to put up some resistance. You're not the first person to think, "End my midnight snack and you end life as I've known it!"

We can't deny that to maintain your good health with diabetes, you'll need to make some changes in your way of eating. But these changes don't have to spell the end of the good life—on the contrary. Nutrition therapy means treating disease or illness at least in part through diet. The goals of nutrition therapy these days include planning a diet just for you, one that will keep you healthy *and* have you eating the foods you like, or most of them. Your food preferences, traditions, and preferred seasonings, your ethnicity, and your social patterns of eating—these are factors that a skillful nutritionist will build into your diet plan. If you add your own understanding about foods to the guidance provided by the nutritionist, you can manage your diet and your diabetes and still enjoy your food to the fullest.

The American Diabetes Association's position statement "Nutrition Recommendations and Interventions for Diabetes" of 2008 stated the goals for nutrition therapy as follows:

1. Achieve and maintain
   —blood glucose levels in the normal range or as close to normal as is safely possible

—a lipid and lipoprotein profile that reduces the risk for vascular disease

—blood pressure levels in the normal range or as close to normal as is safely possible

2. To prevent, or at least slow, the rate of development of the chronic complications of diabetes by modifying nutrient intake and lifestyle

3. To address individual nutrition needs, taking into account personal and cultural preferences and willingness to change

4. To maintain the pleasure of eating by only limiting food choices when indicated by scientific evidence.

In this and the following two chapters, we'll explain how the food you eat and the times when you eat it can help you feel better and achieve good blood glucose control. We start here with background information, by looking at food categories: carbohydrate, fat, protein, and the "micronutrients" such as vitamins and minerals. Then we'll talk about how to put this information together into a good, healthy diet.

What Do You Eat, and What Do You Need?

Calories, protein, fiber, chromium, monounsaturated fats, macronutrients, sugar, carbohydrates—there are so many words used to describe food, it's enough to give you indigestion! In truth, though, the terms used to describe what's in food aren't that hard to understand. A calorie, for example, is the energy value of food—how much energy you get when you "burn" that amount of food. The problem is that you don't always burn the calories right away, and if you consume more than you burn, the excess is stored in your body as fat. That's why calories count: too many calories and you gain weight, too few calories and you lose weight. Calories are generally found in three kinds of food: carbohydrate, fat, and protein.

Carbohydrate

Carbohydrates include such foods as pasta, potatoes, grains and cereals, and the sugar in fruit, candy, milk, and cookies. The building blocks of all carbohydrates are sugar molecules, such as glucose, fructose, and galactose (found in lactose, or milk sugar). *Complex carbohydrates*, on the other hand, are very long, branching chains of sugar molecules. They do not taste sweet, and they have to be digested in the stomach and intestine before being absorbed.

How many calories do carbohydrates have? It depends, of course, on how much carbohydrate you're talking about. But the rule is, 1 gram of carbohydrate (simple or complex) has 4 calories.

Simple sugars. When a sugar consists of one molecule, such as glucose, or of two sugar molecules held together, as in sucrose (table sugar), the result is called a simple sugar, or a *concentrated sweet*. The effect on the blood sugar is simple: you eat the carbohydrate (say, sucrose), and the process of digestion breaks it into single sugar molecules that are absorbed into the bloodstream, causing the blood glucose level to go up.

Given their sweet taste, it is not surprising that simple sugars show up all over—as table sugar and in candy bars, honey, molasses, and hard candy, for example. You also often hear about "hidden sugars," which usually means sugar that has been slipped into something like spaghetti sauce or salad dressing to make it taste better. When simple sugars are in the form of "fruit sugar" (mainly fructose) or sorbitol, they are digested more slowly.

Complex carbohydrates. These are the carbohydrates that are made of very long, branching chains of sugar molecules. They do not taste sweet, and they have to be digested in the stomach and the intestine before they are absorbed. Examples of complex carbohydrates are starches, pasta, cereals, breads, and so on.

Are carbohydrates good or bad? Many people think that carbohydrates are fattening. Even the innocent baked potato has gotten a bad rap! With only 4 calories per gram (compared with 9 calories per gram for fat), carbohydrates are a pretty good deal in the energy equation. It's the fat that's often loaded on top of the carbohydrate (butter and sour cream on the baked potato, cream or meat sauce on the pasta) that can do you in.

Carbohydrates, whether bread, pasta, candy, peas, rice, cereal, milk, apples, or juice, do make the blood glucose rise after a meal, but this is normal, and the right amount of insulin brings it back down. It is just plain wrong to think of carbohydrates as a forbidden food. In fact, the cells of the body, with the help of insulin, use glucose for energy. Current recommendations are for 50%–60% of our dietary calories to be in the form of carbohydrate, although there is controversy about this. Some specialists think there should be less carbohydrate in the diet, in the range of 35%, with more monounsaturated fat. Their logic is that eating less carbohydrate may reduce blood triglyceride levels. At present, however, this is a minority view. We'll go with the 50%–60% carbohydrate diet, unless individual circumstances, such as high triglyceride levels, dictate otherwise.

The important thing to remember is that insulin, either from the pancreas or by injection, is needed for the body to use carbohydrates; people with diabetes often do better when they learn to monitor the amount of their carbohydrate intake precisely. This approach, called carbohydrate counting, is discussed later in the chapter.

What about sugar (I'm talking sweets)? In 1994 the ADA went out on a limb. It issued a report that emphasized all sorts of important and well-proven dietary recommendations, stressing individualization of the diet to the person. But a small comment slipped in, allowing people some concentrated sweets. Predictably, the press picked up this little tidbit, and many people with diabetes were led to believe that after all these years, it was now okay to eat sweets. At the risk of being spoilsports, we beg to differ. Here's the story.

Several careful studies on hospitalized subjects showed that, gram for gram, there isn't much difference between the blood glucose rise from complex carbohydrates and the blood glucose rise from simple sugars. In other words, 20 grams of carbohydrate from pasta might increase the blood glucose about the same amount as 20 grams of table sugar. But (and here's the kicker) people tend not to eat the same number of grams of concentrated sugar as they do of complex carbohydrate. When you get into foods that contain sugar and/or other sweeteners, you usually eat many more grams of carbohydrate than you would if you were eating pasta or potatoes. For example, one small fast-food milkshake and two medium-size baked potatoes each contain about 60 grams of carbohydrate, and one 16-ounce sweetened soda and about two cups of cooked spaghetti with meat sauce each contain about 60 grams of carbohydrate.

Get the picture? You are a lot more likely to order a small shake or a soft drink than two baked potatoes or two cups of spaghetti. And your blood glucose will show the difference in carbohydrate intake, unless you take just the right amount of insulin to cover the larger carbohydrate load. "So," you say, "I'll take the right amount of insulin to cover the sweet." And we say, "Okay, do that—if you can figure it out." If you check your blood glucose and it is in an acceptable range, terrific. But do you know exactly how much sugar is in this candy bar or that one, this piece of pie or that one, this doughnut or that one? Almost certainly not. It isn't easy to tell.

There are other problems with concentrated sweets: they are usually high in calories so will tend to put weight on you; they don't provide any of the important nutrients (that's why they're referred to as "empty calories"); and, of course, they are bad for the teeth. The upshot is that we don't have a problem with your eating an occasional cookie or scoop of ice cream, if it means a lot to you and, if you take insulin, you can make a reasonable adjustment in your insulin dose. Or you could use the sweets as carbohydrates allowed in a meal plan, trading them off for other foods. You could, for instance, have 1/2 cup of sweetened cereal instead of 3/4 cup of unsweetened cereal. But we strongly recommend that you fight off the notion that you have a "sweet tooth" that depends on a constant flow of sugars, because your blood glucose control will suffer. We would much prefer that you learn to love diet drinks, fruits, and other nonsugary foods. It'll pay off in the long run.

Fat

Fat on your waistline, fat in your french fries, fat in your blood: it's hard to find much good to say about fat. Yet fatness is sometimes considered a sign of prosperity; it's by far the most efficient way for the body to store calories and, at least for primitive human beings, it was a lifesaver. In times of plenty, when there is lots to eat and lots of insulin to burn the carbohydrate ingested, the body stores away the extra calories as fat. When the famine comes, insulin levels in the body drop, and all that fat becomes the main energy source.

The natural purpose of fat, then, is to store calories efficiently. But in an overfed society, storing fat is not much of a benefit. In fact, too much body fat carries definite risks, chiefly an increased risk of Type 2 diabetes. Too much fat in the blood, of course, is also a risk for heart disease and hardening of the arteries (arteriosclerosis or atherosclerosis). So we are back where we started: there's not much good to be said for lots of fat.

What is fat? Technically, fat is the class of chemicals that don't mix with water. Dietary fat is found mainly in meats, dairy foods, oils, butter and margarine, fried foods, bacon, nuts, and seeds. There are two important kinds of fat in food, the blood, and body fat: triglyceride and cholesterol. Triglycerides make up the majority of the fat we eat, as well as the fat in our bodies; these are the fats in a steak, in bacon, in oils, and in dairy products. You probably eat between 40 and 100 grams of fat a day. Cholesterol, found especially in egg yolks and organ meats, comes in much smaller amounts; you eat perhaps half a gram of cholesterol a day.

Cholesterol in the blood has a lot to do with hardening of the arteries. But just like sugar (which comes both from the carbohydrates you eat and from the liver), blood cholesterol does not all come from food: the liver also makes cholesterol. To complicate the issue, there's the "good cholesterol" (HDL cholesterol), high blood levels of which *protect against* hardening of the arteries, and there's the "bad cholesterol" (LDL cholesterol), high levels of which *cause* hardening of the arteries.

Triglyceride also comes in various forms, generally called *saturated*, *monounsaturated*, and *polyunsaturated*. You probably already know that saturated fat (found in butter, lard, and fatty meats) is the bad stuff and that unsaturated fat (found in olive oil, margarine, and vegetable oils, for example) is good for you. It has been known since the 1950s that eating a lot of saturated fat increases the blood cholesterol level, while eating unsaturated fat lowers cholesterol, although scientists still don't know why this is so. We *do* know that having a low proportion of saturated fat in your diet will help keep your blood cholesterol low. Trans fat, a type of fat made when vegetable oil is solidified, also may increase cholesterol levels.

Monounsaturated fat does not raise cholesterol levels. Found primarily in olive oil and canola oil, it is a preferred form of fat. Polyunsaturated fat, found in safflower oil and other soft fats and oils, lowers cholesterol but has gone out of favor in recent years because it may lower HDL cholesterol too. Dietary fat guidelines are summarized in Table 7. Remember that there are 9 calories per gram of fat, more than twice as many as in a gram of carbohydrate or protein, whether it is saturated or unsaturated fat.

Does fat affect the blood glucose? The answer is no. Eating a pure fat meal does not increase or decrease blood glucose. But dietary fat has an indirect effect on blood glucose. Because fat takes some time to be digested, it will delay the glucose rise from the carbohydrate components of the meal. This means that if a portion of bread would cause the blood glucose to rise to a peak, say, 45 minutes after eating, the peak would be delayed to about 60 minutes if the bread were eaten with significant amounts of fat. We don't think of this as a very important effect. We think that dietary fat can strongly affect your total calorie intake, your waistline, and your blood cholesterol level; its im-

Table 7   Recommended Intake of Fat

Type of Fat	Recommended Intake
Total fat	Less than 30% of total calories
Polyunsaturated	Up to 10%, preferably 6%–8% of total calories
Saturated	Less than 10% of total calories
Trans fats	Minimal intake
Monounsaturated	10%–15% of total calories
Cholesterol	Less than 300 mg per day

mediate effect on blood glucose is small, but over time it increases weight, insulin resistance, and blood glucose levels.

The preferred oils are canola and olive, because of their high monounsaturated fat content. When selecting margarines, check to see that the first ingredient is liquid canola, corn, safflower, soybean, or sunflower oil and that saturated fat is less than 1–2 grams per tablespoon. Reduced-calorie or "light" salad dressings definitely require close inspection. They differ greatly in caloric value and often have increased amounts of sodium. Sugar, corn syrup, or other forms of sugar or starch may be added. Each product must be individually evaluated.

Protein

The days are long gone when protein was considered a muscle-building, power-giving, pregame performance enhancer. To be sure, some protein in the diet is necessary, and protein deficiency is a serious problem in undernourished people living in developing countries. But, as with fat, in the overfed populations of prosperous nations, there is more than enough protein in the average diet to meet nutritional needs.

Protein contains 4 calories per gram and is a large component of such foods as seafood, chicken, turkey, beef, milk, cheese, pork, egg whites, peanut butter, and legumes. Egg whites, for instance, are almost entirely protein. In contrast, a medium-fatty hamburger may contain about 88 calories as protein but 130 calories as fat.

The human digestive system breaks protein down into its building blocks, called amino acids. These are absorbed, providing nitrogen to the body. The amino acids are also, to some extent, converted to glucose, in a process called gluconeogenesis. (Gluconeogenesis helps keep the blood glucose normal during fasting. Amino acids are released from the muscle protein and converted to glucose.) In general, dietary protein will not significantly affect the blood glucose level unless it is taken in a large quantity (more than 8 ounces). Protein, like fat, does slow the absorption of carbohydrate somewhat.

For adults with diabetes, 10%–20% of the total daily calorie intake should be in the form of protein (roughly 36–90 grams, depending on the number of calories consumed). There is some evidence that excessive protein intake accelerates the progression of kidney disease (nephropathy) in diabetes, so for someone with nephropathy, dietary protein is usually restricted to between 7% and 10% of total calories, or 0.8 gram per kilogram of body weight. Protein requirements are increased during childhood and adolescence, during pregnancy, and in physical conditioning with exercise. Higher protein intake is also recommended whenever tissue breakdown is likely to occur, such as after surgery, in the elderly, and during weight-loss diets.

Micronutrients

These are the things you eat that don't add significant calories but are nevertheless important parts of a normal diet. Examples of micronutrients are vitamins and minerals, including iron, sodium, calcium, chromium, magnesium, and the so-called antioxidants.

Vitamins. Vitamins have been known to be essential parts of the diet at least since the late eighteenth century, when British sailors in the 1770s learned to avoid scurvy by taking a good supply of sauerkraut and, later on, citrus fruit on long voyages as a source of vitamin C. But vitamins are needed in only very small amounts to avoid the specific diseases caused by vitamin deficiency. And these trace amounts of all the vitamins are found in the foods that make up a normal, balanced diet. Believe us, you will not suffer from vitamin deficiency diseases if you eat a normal American diet.

Where, then, did all the vitamin hype come from? In some cases it is just that—hype without scientific evidence. In a few cases, though, there is some evidence that amounts higher than the minimum requirement may be beneficial. For example, vitamin C is a powerful antioxidant, and some studies have suggested that the symptoms of a cold may be reduced by taking extra vitamin C. In pregnancy, with its special nutritional demands, a single daily multivitamin pill is usually recommended.

Do high-dose vitamins (so-called megavitamins) provide any health benefits? Our answer is to be cautiously noncommittal. We just don't know of any good evidence showing that high-dose vitamins do any good, and we do know that very high doses can sometimes do harm. So, provided the high doses are not extreme, we won't discourage people from taking vitamin pills daily, but we can't say that there is much benefit.

Iron. The body needs iron, particularly for the formation of hemoglobin in red blood cells. Through blood loss, some people, especially women with heavy menstrual periods, can easily become iron deficient and anemic. It's relatively simple to determine with laboratory tests whether your iron level is normal, so if any doubt exists, a few tests should tell you if you need iron supplements. Again, in pregnancy, iron pills are essential.

Sodium. Sodium is one of the micronutrients that Americans seem to have no trouble getting enough of—even too much of—in the form of salt. The minimum sodium needed for the body is only 220 mg per day, while the estimated average intake is 3,400 mg per day and the recommendation is that sodium be restricted to 2,300 mg per day. (One teaspoon of salt contains about 2,300 mg of sodium.) The recommendation is made because sodium can cause the body to retain water, and in people who tend to have high blood pressure, it will worsen that tendency.

Many people just urinate out any excess sodium they take in, but it is not unusual for fluid retention or high blood pressure to be worsened by salt intake. So be sure to cut down your salt intake if you have hypertension; otherwise, consider getting in the habit of not ingesting too much salt. In rare cases, for people who have low blood pressure associated with dizziness, they actually need a high sodium intake.

Calcium. Calcium is an essential nutrient and is usually present in adequate amounts in a normal diet. It is found in foods like dairy products and leafy vegetables. A person who is on a "tea and toast" diet may not take in enough calcium, and anyone who is prone to osteoporosis (thinning of the bones) should be sure to get enough calcium. A supplement is a good idea if there's doubt about the adequacy of your intake.

Chromium. Not a week goes by where we don't have at least one question about chromium and glucose control. The question stems from the observation that in animals that were purposely fed diets deficient in chromium, blood glucose control suffered and then improved with replacement of the chromium. However, chromium supplementation in persons with diabetes has not resulted in improved control. This suggests that most people with diabetes do not have a chromium deficiency, and we believe there is no benefit from routinely taking a chromium supplement.

Magnesium. Magnesium deficiency can be part of an unusual but vicious cycle. Poor control of diabetes can lead to magnesium deficiency, and magnesium deficiency can lead to insulin insensitivity. In people with a documented deficiency, magnesium supplements may improve blood glucose control.

Antioxidants. You may have heard that antioxidants are thought to protect against a variety of diseases. For example, the common antioxidant vitamins C, E, and A (beta-carotene) have been thought to protect against heart disease. Should you be taking them as supplements? The short answer is that the jury is still out. Studies on animals show that these antioxidants inhibit the oxidation of LDL cholesterol and can slow the progression of atherosclerotic disease. In humans, this has not been proven. Two large randomized trials recently failed to show any benefit of beta-carotene and even suggested that for smokers, beta-carotene supplementation may be dangerous. Evidence is lacking to recommend antioxidants to everyone. But consider that vitamin E is found in vegetable oils and cereal grains; vitamin C is found in many fresh fruits and vegetables; and beta-carotene is found in carrots, winter squash, broccoli, and many green leafy vegetables. To us, this sounds like another good argument for a healthy, well-balanced diet.

Fiber. Fiber is the indigestible carbohydrate that comes primarily from plant cell walls. There are two kinds of fiber, water-insoluble and water-soluble. Water-insoluble fiber is found in whole wheat products, wheat bran, and fruit and vegetable skins. Its action is in the large bowel, where it draws water into the feces. This type of fiber is helpful for relieving constipation, diverticulosis, and irritable bowel syndrome. It may also prevent colon cancer.

Water-soluble fiber is found in fruits, vegetables, oats, beans, and peas. There is evidence that large amounts of soluble fiber have a beneficial effect on fat levels in the bloodstream.

Sweeteners. The sweeteners, of course, give a good taste to food. But you have to be careful because there are two very different kinds of sweeteners: those that contain calories (nutritive) and those that do not (nonnutritive).

Table sugar, called sucrose (discussed above), is the classic caloric sweetener and, in our opinion, is one to avoid. You may think that if you choose a "more natural" sweetener such as unrefined sugar, honey, fruit juice, or molasses, you're doing yourself a favor. But it doesn't work that way. There is no evidence that these sweeteners offer any advantage over sucrose when it comes to calories and blood glucose control. They are not "freebies." Other sweeteners that are just about the same as table sugar are corn syrup, dextrose, and maltose. See Table 8 for a list of other sweeteners.

Fructose seems to cause less of a rise in blood glucose than sucrose does, but there is some evidence that if taken in large quantities, it may increase LDL cholesterol levels. There is no reason to avoid fruits and vegetables in which fructose occurs naturally.

Consuming the sugars sorbitol, mannitol, and xylitol may result in lower and slower glucose and insulin rises than consuming glucose or sucrose. However, these sugars are high in calories and may cause cramping and diarrhea if taken in large amounts.

In marked contrast to the nutritive, caloric sweeteners, the nonnutritive sweeteners—saccharin, aspartame (NutraSweet), acesulfame K (Sunett), rebaudioside A (various Stevia products), and sucralose (Splenda)—have no calories and no effect on the blood glucose level. They are therefore considered "free": you may eat and drink as much as you want of them (within reason, of course). They are approved by the FDA and are considered safe for use.

Drinking diet drinks with aspartame is no worse than drinking water, if the labels say the drinks have zero calories. So go for it! We would even suggest that you keep trying different brands until you find one you really like.

Summary of Food Components

Nutrition may seem a complicated science, but if you concentrate on it for a while, you very quickly learn to distinguish a carbohydrate from a fat, a nonnutritive sweetener from a sugar, and a micronutrient from a microchip. Still, it really helps to talk to a professional in nutrition, such as a registered dietitian. Your local chapter of the ADA or the American Association of Diabetes Educators may be able to provide some recommendations about a qualified professional in your area, or you can call the American Dietetic Association.

Table 8 Sweeteners

Caloric: Contains Carbohydrates	Noncaloric: Considered Carbohydrate-Free
Carob powder	Acesulfame K
Dextrin	Aspartame
Dulcitol	Cyclamates
Fructose (fruit sugar, levulose)	Rebaudioside A (rebiana)
Glucose (corn sugar, dextrose, grape sugar)	Saccharin
Glucose syrups (corn syrup, corn syrup solids, sorghum syrup, starch syrup, sugar cane syrup)	Sucralose
High-fructose corn syrups	
Honey (comb honey, creamed honey)	
Lactose	
Maltose	
Mannitol	
Maple syrup (maple sugar)	
Milk chocolate (bitter chocolate, bittersweet chocolate)	
Molasses (blackstrap, golden syrup, refiners' syrup, treacle, unsulfured)	
Sorbitol	
Sucrose (beet sugar, brown sugar, cane sugar, confectioner's sugar, invert sugar, powdered sugar, raw sugar, saccharose sugar, sugar, table sugar, turbinado)	
Sweetened condensed whole milk (sweetened condensed skim milk, sweetened condensed whey)	
Xylitol	

Nutrition Recommendations: General Guidelines

In the next two chapters, we discuss recommendations for people with special requirements, but first it's important to tie together the information presented above on the different foodstuffs with basic information about how much of them you should consume and why you should include them in your diet.

How Many Calories Do I Need?

This depends on your height and activity level. A larger person needs more calories to maintain body weight than a smaller person; a person who has a high level of physical activity needs more calories to maintain weight than a less active person of the same size; and a person who is trying to lose weight needs less than a person who is trying to maintain or gain weight. In other words, to maintain body weight unchanged, you need to take in the same number of calories that you expend; to lose weight, you need less intake than expenditure; and to gain weight, you need to take in more calories than you expend.

Here is one method of estimating the calorie requirements for weight maintenance for a nonpregnant, nonlactating adult: 10 calories per pound of body weight, plus 20% for a sedentary lifestyle, or plus 33% for light physical activity, or plus 50% for moderate physical activity, or plus 75% for heavy activity.

This rough guide does not even take into consideration age and gender, so it must be considered only a rough estimate. Nevertheless, it can indicate more or less what your weight-maintenance calorie intake should be. For example, a 120-pound woman who engages in low levels of physical activity would require 10 × 120 = 1,200 calories, plus 33% (1,200 × 0.33 = 400), which equals 1,600 calories per day to maintain body weight. We emphasize that this is an example and a rough estimate. Pound for pound, women require slightly fewer calories than men to maintain body weight. Also, obese people require slightly fewer calories than lean people to maintain their weight.

Once you have an estimate of how many calories you need to consume every day to maintain your weight, you can calculate how many calories to cut back if you want to lose weight: 3,500 calories represent 1 pound of body weight, so if you eat 3,500 calories less than you require—over whatever period of time you're comfortable with and is healthy for you—you will lose

1 pound. For example, if during a one-week period your diet contains 500 fewer calories a day than your requirement, you will lose 1 pound.

Does Water Matter?

Water is necessary for life, and pure water must be one of the "safest" of all substances to ingest. How much do we recommend? You should be drinking enough fluid to keep from feeling thirsty. Most people drink about 2 quarts a day. If you find yourself unusually thirsty, of course, the first thing to consider is that your blood glucose may be high.

Alcohol

Alcohol is a touchy subject, wrapped in mystique, morality, and merriment. Let's deal with the facts, some of which you may find surprising:

—Alcohol is not necessary. People do very well without it.

—In moderation, alcohol is not intrinsically harmful. A large body of scientific evidence indicates that one or two drinks a day may reduce the risk of heart attacks.

—Alcohol acts to *potentiate* insulin. With insulin, alcohol can cause hypoglycemia. We know one very careful person with Type 1 diabetes who two years in a row had his only significant hypoglycemic reaction on New Year's Day, after imbibing the night before. Rather than reducing the insulin dose, we recommend eating something along with a drink of alcohol.

—In excess, alcohol can not only cause severe insulin reactions but also damage the liver, causing cirrhosis. People with any liver disease, therefore, are routinely counseled to avoid alcohol. Excessive alcohol intake is also the major cause of traffic fatalities and family breakdown, and drunkenness can easily be confused, as we noted in Chapter 5, with an insulin reaction.

The calories consumed as alcoholic beverages can add considerably to your total daily calorie intake, leaving aside the peanuts, cheese, or chips that people tend to munch on as they drink. The number of calories in an alcoholic drink depends on the proof of the alcohol. If you are interested in knowing approximately how many calories you are consuming, try this formula:

0.8 × proof of the drink × number of ounces = number of calories

For example, if you drink two 4-ounce glasses of 86 proof bourbon, that's 550 calories (0.8 × 86 × 8 = 550). One 6-ounce glass of 12.5% alcohol wine (equivalent to 25 proof) contains 120 calories (0.8 × 25 × 6 = 120). Finally, one 12-ounce can of 6% alcohol beer (12 proof) contains 115 calories (0.8 × 12 × 12 = 115).

The bottom line? We stop short of recommending alcohol but are supportive if our patients want to incorporate a liquor drink or a beer or a glass of wine into their regular diet. A moderate amount of alcohol is defined as 1.5 ounces of distilled liquor, 4 ounces of wine, or 12 ounces of beer. Much has been said about red wine being higher in sugar than white wine, but we are not impressed with the data and support a glass or so of either red or white. We recommend strongly against excessive drinking, which we define as more than one or two drinks daily. Pregnant women, people with a history of alcohol abuse, and people with conditions such as gastritis or high triglycerides or a history of pancreatitis may also be well advised to avoid alcohol. Talk with your health care provider to see if he or she agrees.

Carbohydrate Counting

Decades ago, exchange lists were devised to help people with diabetes recognize portions of food that are more or less equivalent. There were lists for six food groups: starch/bread, fruit, milk, vegetables, meats, and fats (see Table 9; we now also include a list of plant-based proteins). A dietitian worked out a meal plan that recommended specific amounts of each food group at each meal. Some people found this very helpful, and some found it totally useless or confusing. In the 1980s, nutrition research focused on carbohydrate intake, since it's the carbohydrates in foods that affect blood glucose levels more than the intake of fat and protein. While the exchange lists are still available to use, learning how to count carbohydrates is the recommended approach to help maintain consistency while varying what you eat. For people with Type 1 diabetes, counting carbohydrates is essential for matching the pre-meal insulin to what you eat. Carbohydrate counting measures the amount of total carbohydrate, not the kind, eaten. Using this system, you can vary your foods from day to day provided the total grams of carbohydrate for that meal are counted, so the right amount of pre-meal insulin can be calculated (see Chapter 11). Food groups with carbohydrate are starches (bread, rice, potatoes, pasta, cereal), fruits, milk, or other carbohydrates (like sweets and desserts). One carbohydrate choice or serving is equal to 15 grams of total carbohydrate, no matter which group it

(text continues on page 117)

Table 9 Exchange List

STARCH LIST
One starch choice equals 15 grams of carbohydrate, 0–3 grams of protein, 0–1 gram of fat, and 80 calories.

Bread

Bagel, large (about 4 oz)	¼ (1 oz)
Biscuit, 2½ inches across	1
Bread, reduced-calorie	2 slices (1½ oz)
Bread: white, whole wheat, pumpernickel, rye, unfrosted raisin	1 slice (1 oz)
Chapatti, small, 6 inches across	1
Cornbread, 1¾-inch cube	1 (1½ oz)
English muffin	½
Hot dog bun or hamburger bun	½ (1 oz)
Naan, 8 inches by 2 inches	¼
Pancake, 4 inches across, ¼-inch thick	1
Pita, 6 inches across	½
Roll, plain, small	1 (1 oz)
Stuffing, bread	⅓ cup
Taco shell, 5 inches across	2
Tortilla, corn, 6 inches across	1
Tortilla, flour, 6 inches across	1
Tortilla, flour, 10 inches across	⅓
Waffle, 4-inch square or 4 inches across	1

Cereals and Grains

Barley, cooked	⅓ cup
Bran, dry	
Oat	¼ cup
Wheat	½ cup
Bulgur (cooked)	½ cup
Cereals	
Bran	½ cup
Cooked (oats, oatmeal)	½ cup
Puffed	1½ cups

Shredded wheat, plain	½ cup
Sugar-coated	½ cup
Unsweetened, ready-to-eat	¾ cup
Couscous	⅓ cup
Granola	
Low-fat	¼ cup
Regular	¼ cup
Grits, cooked	½ cup
Kasha	½ cup
Millet, cooked	⅓ cup
Muesli	¼ cup
Pasta, cooked	⅓ cup
Polenta, cooked	⅓ cup
Quinoa, cooked	⅓ cup
Rice, white or brown, cooked	⅓ cup
Tabbouleh (tabouli), prepared	½ cup
Wheat germ, dry	3 Tbsp
Wild rice, cooked	½ cup

Starchy Vegetables

Baked beans	⅓ cup
Cassava	⅓ cup
Corn, on cob, large	½ cup or ½ cob (5 oz)
Hominy, canned	¾ cup
Mixed vegetables with corn, peas, or pasta	1 cup
Parsnips	½ cup
Peas, green	½ cup
Plantain, ripe	⅓ cup
Potato	
Baked with skin	¼ large (3 oz)
Boiled, all kinds	½ cup or ½ medium (3 oz)
Mashed, with milk and fat	½ cup
French fried (oven-baked)	1 cup (2 oz)
Pumpkin, canned, no sugar added	1 cup
Spaghetti/pasta sauce	½ cup
Squash, winter (acorn, butternut)	1 cup
Succotash	½ cup
Yam, sweet potato, plain	½ cup

(continued)

Table 9 (*continued*)

Crackers and Snacks

Animal crackers	8
Crackers	
Round, butter-type	6
Saltine-type	6
Sandwich-style, cheese or peanut butter filling	3
Whole wheat regular	2–5 (¾ oz)
Whole wheat lower fat or crisp breads	2–5 (¾ oz)
Graham crackers, 2½-inch square	3
Matzoh	¾ oz
Melba toast, about 2-inch by 4-inch piece	4 pieces
Oyster crackers	20
Popcorn	
With butter	3 cups
No fat added	3 cups
Lower fat	3 cups
Pretzels	¾ oz
Rice cakes, 4 inches across	2
Snack chips	
Fat-free or baked (tortilla, potato), baked pita chips	15–20 (¾ oz)
Regular (tortilla, potato)	9–13 (¾ oz)

Beans, Peas, and Lentils
(Count as 1 starch + 1 lean meat)

Baked beans	⅓ cup
Beans, cooked (black, garbanzo, kidney, lima, navy, pinto, white)	½ cup
Lentils, cooked (brown, green, yellow)	½ cup
Peas, cooked (black-eyed, split)	½ cup
Refried beans, canned	½ cup

FRUIT LIST

One fruit choice equals 15 grams of carbohydrate and 60 calories.
The weight includes skin, core, seeds, and rind.

Fruit

Apple, unpeeled, small	1 (4 oz)
Applesauce, unsweetened	½ cup
Apples, dried	4 rings
Apricots	
Canned	½ cup
Dried	8 halves
Fresh	4 whole (5½ oz)
Banana, extra small	1 (4 oz)
Blackberries	¾ cup
Blueberries	¾ cup
Cantaloupe, small	⅓ melon (11 oz) or 1 cup cubes
Cherries	
Sweet, canned	½ cup
Sweet, fresh	12 (3 oz)
Dates	3
Dried fruits (blueberries, cherries, cranberries, mixed fruit, raisins)	2 Tbsp
Figs	
Dried	2 Tbsp
Fresh	1½ large or 2 medium (3½ oz)
Fruit cocktail	½ cup
Grapefruit	
Large	½ (11 oz)
Sections, canned	¾ cup
Grapes, small	17 (3 oz)
Honeydew melon	1 slice (10 oz) or 1 cup cubes
Kiwi	1 (3½ oz)
Mandarin oranges, canned	¾ cup
Mango, small	½ fruit (5½ oz) or ½ cup
Nectarine, small	1 (5 oz)
Orange, small	1 (6½ oz)
Papaya	½ fruit (8 oz) or 1 cup cubes
Peach	
Canned	½ cup
Fresh, medium	1 (6 oz)

(continued)

Table 9 (*continued*)

Pear
Canned	½ cup
Fresh, large	½ (4 oz)

Pineapple
Canned	½ cup
Fresh	¾ cup

Plums
Canned	½ cup
Dried (prunes)	3
Small	2 (5 oz)

Raspberries	1 cup
Strawberries	1¼ cup whole berries
Tangerines, small	2 (8 oz)
Watermelon	1 slice (13½ oz) or 1¼ cup cubes

Fruit Juice

Apple juice/cider	½ cup
Fruit juice blends, 100% juice	½ cup
Grape juice	⅓ cup
Grapefruit juice	½ cup
Orange juice	½ cup
Pineapple juice	½ cup
Prune juice	⅓ cup

MILK LIST
One milk choice equals 12 grams of carbohydrate and 8 grams of protein.

Milk and Yogurts

Fat-free (skim) or low-fat (1%)
Milk, buttermilk, acidophilus milk, Lactaid	1 cup
Evaporated milk	½ cup
Yogurt, plain or flavored with artificial sweetener	⅔ cup (6 oz)

Reduced-fat (2%)
Milk, acidophilus milk, kefir, Lactaid	1 cup
Yogurt, plain	⅔ cup (6 oz)

Whole
Milk, buttermilk, goat's milk	1 cup
Evaporated milk	½ cup
Yogurt, plain	1 cup (8 oz)

Dairy-Like Foods

Chocolate milk
Fat-free	1 cup

Whole	1 cup
Eggnog, whole milk	½ cup
Rice drink	
Flavored, low-fat	½ cup
Plain, fat-free	1 cup
Smoothies, flavored, regular	¼ cup (2½ oz)
Soy milk	
Light	1 cup
Regular, plain	1 cup
Yogurt	
And juice blends	½ cup
Low-carbohydrate (less than 6 grams of carbohydrate per serving)	1⅓ cups (12 oz)
With fruit, low fat	⅓ cup

NONSTARCHY VEGETABLE LIST

One vegetable choice (½ cup cooked or 1 cup raw) equals 5 grams of carbohydrate, 2 grams of protein, 0 grams of fat, and 25 calories.

Amaranth or Chinese spinach

Artichoke

Artichoke hearts

Asparagus

Baby corn

Bamboo shoots

Beans (green, wax, Italian)

Bean sprouts

Beets

Borscht

Broccoli

Brussels sprouts

Cabbage (green, bok choy, Chinese)

Carrots

Cauliflower

Celery

Chayote

Cole slaw, packaged, no dressing

Cucumber

Daikon

Eggplant

Gourds (bitter, bottle, luffa, bitter melon)

(continued)

Table 9 (*continued*)

Green onions or scallions

Greens (collard, kale, mustard, turnip)

Hearts of palm

Jicama

Kohlrabi

Leeks

Mixed vegetables (without corn, peas, or pasta)

Mung bean sprouts

Mushrooms, all kinds, fresh

Okra

Onions

Pea pods

Peppers (all varieties)

Radishes

Rutabaga

Sauerkraut

Soybean sprouts

Spinach

Squash (summer, crookneck, zucchini)

Sugar snap peas

Swiss chard

Tomato

Tomatoes, canned

Tomato sauce

Tomato/vegetable juice

Turnips

Water chestnuts

Yard-long beans

LEAN MEAT AND MEAT SUBSTITUTES LIST
One choice equals 0 grams of carbohydrate, 7 grams of protein, 0–3 grams of fat, and 45 calories.

Beef: Select or Choice grades trimmed of fat: ground round, roast (rib, chuck, rump), round, sirloin, steak (flank, T-bone, porterhouse, cube)	1 oz
Beef jerky	½ oz
Cheeses with 3 grams of fat or less per oz	1 oz
Cottage cheese	¼ cup

Egg substitutes, plain	¼ cup
Egg whites	2
Fish, fresh or frozen, plain: catfish, cod, flounder, haddock, halibut, orange roughy, salmon, tilapia, trout, tuna	1 oz
Fish, smoked: herring or salmon (lox)	1 oz
Game: buffalo, ostrich, rabbit, venison	1 oz
Hot dog with 3 grams of fat or less per oz (8 dogs per 14-oz package) (*Note*: May be high in carbohydrates.)	1
Lamb: roast, chop, leg	1 oz
Organ meats: heart, kidney, liver (*Note*: May be high in cholesterol.)	1 oz
Oysters, fresh or frozen	6 medium
Pork	
Lean	1 oz
Canadian bacon	1 oz
Rib or loin chop/roast, ham, tenderloin	1 oz
Poultry, without skin: chicken, Cornish hen, domestic duck or goose (well-drained of fat), turkey	1 oz
Processed sandwich meats with 3 grams of fat or less per oz: chipped beef, deli thin-sliced meats, turkey ham, turkey kielbasa, turkey pastrami	1 oz
Salmon, canned	1 oz
Sardines, canned	1 oz
Sausage with 3 grams of fat or less per oz	1 oz
Shellfish: clams, crab, imitation shellfish, lobster, scallops, shrimp	2 small
Tuna, canned in water or oil, drained	1 oz
Veal: loin chop, roast	1 oz

Medium-Fat Meat and Meat Substitutes List   *One choice equals 0 grams of carbohydrate, 7 grams of protein, 4–7 grams of fat, and 75 calories.*

Beef: corned beef, ground beef, meatloaf, Prime grades trimmed of fat (prime rib), short ribs, tongue	1 oz
Cheeses with 4–7 grams of fat per oz: feta, mozzarella, pasteurized processed cheese spread, reduced-fat, string	1 oz
Egg (*Note*: High in cholesterol, so limit to 3 per week.)	1
Fish, any fried type	1 oz
Lamb: rib roast, ground	1 oz
Pork: cutlet, shoulder roast	1 oz
Poultry: chicken with skin; dove, pheasant, wild duck, or goose; fried chicken; ground turkey	1 oz
Ricotta cheese	2 oz (¼ cup)

(continued)

Table 9 (*continued*)

Sausage with 4–7 grams of fat per oz	1 oz
Veal cutlet (no breading)	1 oz

High-Fat Meat and Meat Substitutes List *One choice equals 0 grams of carbohydrate, 7 grams of protein, 8 or more grams of fat, and 100 calories.*

Bacon	
Pork	2 slices (16 slices per lb or 1 oz each, before cooking)
Turkey	3 slices (½ oz each before cooking)
Cheese, regular: American, bleu, brie, cheddar, hard goat, Monterey jack, queso, and Swiss	1 oz
Hot dog: beef, pork, or combination (10 per 1-lb package)	1
Hot dog: turkey or chicken (10 per 1-lb package)	1
Pork: ground, sausage, spareribs	1 oz
Processed sandwich meats with 8 grams of fat or more per oz: bologna, hard salami, pastrami	1 oz
Sausage with 8 grams of fat or more per oz: bratwurst, chorizo, Italian, knockwurst, Polish, smoked, summer	1 oz

PLANT-BASED PROTEINS LIST
(with meat and carbohydrate equivalents)

"Bacon" strips, soy-based	3 strips (1 medium-fat meat)
Baked beans	⅓ cup (1 carbohydrate + 1 lean meat)
Beans, cooked: black, garbanzo, kidney, lima, navy, pinto, white	½ cup (1 carbohydrate + 1 lean meat)
"Beef" or "sausage" crumbles, soy-based	2 oz (½ carbohydrate + 1 lean meat)
"Chicken" nuggets, soy-based	2 (1½ oz) (½ carbohydrate + 1 medium-fat meat)
Edamame	½ cup (½ carbohydrate + 1 lean meat)
Falafel (spiced chickpea and wheat patties, about 2 inches across)	3 (1 carbohydrate + 1 high-fat meat)
Hot dog, soy-based	1 (1½ oz) (½ carbohydrate + 1 lean meat)
Hummus	⅓ cup (1 carbohydrate + 1 high-fat meat)
Lentils: brown, green, or yellow	½ cup (1 carbohydrate + 1 lean meat)
Meatless burger, soy-based	3 oz (½ carbohydrate + 2 lean meats)
Meatless burger, vegetable and starch-based patties	1 (2½ oz) (1 carbohydrate + 2 lean meats)
Nut spreads: almond butter, cashew butter, peanut butter, soy nut butter	1 Tbsp (1 high-fat meat)
Peas, cooked: black-eyed and split peas	½ cup (1 carbohydrate + 1 lean meat)

Refried beans, canned	½ cup (1 carbohydrate + 1 lean meat)
"Sausage" patties, soy-based	1 (1½ oz) (1 medium-fat meat)
Soy nuts, unsalted	¾ oz (½ carbohydrate + 1 medium-fat meat)
Tempeh	¾ cup (1 medium-fat meat)
Tofu	4 oz (½ cup) (1 medium-fat meat)
Tofu, light	4 oz (½ cup) (1 lean meat)

FAT LIST
One fat choice equals 5 grams of fat and 45 calories.

Unsaturated Fats—Monounsaturated Fats

Avocado, medium	2 Tbsp (1 oz)
Nut butters (trans fat-free): almond butter, cashew butter, peanut butter	1½ tsp
Oil (canola, olive, peanut)	1 tsp
Olives	
Black (ripe)	8 large
Green, stuffed	10 large
Nuts	
Almonds	6 nuts
Brazil	2 nuts
Cashews	6 nuts
Filberts (hazelnuts)	5 nuts
Macadamia	3 nuts
Mixed (50% peanuts)	6 nuts
Peanuts	10 nuts
Pecans	4 halves
Pistachios	16 nuts

Unsaturated Fats—Polyunsaturated Fats

Margarine	
Lower-fat spread (30%–50% vegetable oil, trans fat-free)	1 Tbsp
Stick, tub (trans fat-free), squeeze (trans fat-free)	1 tsp
Mayonnaise	
Reduced-fat	1 Tbsp
Regular	1 tsp
Mayonnaise-style salad dressing	
Reduced-fat	1 Tbsp
Regular	1 tsp
Nuts	
Pignolia (pine nuts)	1 Tbsp
Walnuts, English	4 halves
Oil: corn, cottonseed, flaxseed, grape seed, safflower, soybean, sunflower	1 tsp

(continued)

Table 9 (*continued*)

Oil: made from soybean and canola oil—Enova	1 tsp
Plant stanol esters	
Light	1 Tbsp
Regular	2 tsp
Salad dressing	
Reduced-fat	2 Tbsp
Regular	1 Tbsp
Seeds	
Flaxseed, whole	1 Tbsp
Pumpkin, sunflower	1 Tbsp
Sesame seeds	1 Tbsp
Saturated Fats	
Bacon, cooked, regular or turkey	1 slice
Butter	
Reduced-fat	1 Tbsp
Stick	1 tsp
Whipped	2 tsp
Chitterlings, boiled	2 Tbsp (½ oz)
Coconut, sweetened, shredded	2 Tbsp
Coconut milk	
Light	⅓ cup
Regular	1½ Tbsp
Cream	
Half and half	2 Tbsp
Heavy	1 Tbsp
Light	1½ Tbsp
Whipped	2 Tbsp
Whipped, pressurized	¼ cup
Cream cheese	
Reduced-fat	1½ Tbsp (¾ oz)
Regular	1 Tbsp (½ oz)
Lard	1 tsp
Oil: coconut, palm, palm kernel	1 tsp
Salt pork	¼ oz
Shortening, solid	1 tsp
Sour cream	
Reduced-fat or light	3 Tbsp
Regular	2 Tbsp

is from. For people on set doses of medications for their diabetes, keeping the amount of carbohydrate in meals similar from day to day helps keep blood glucose levels from varying. For example, one day you may decide to have cereal, milk, and a banana for breakfast for a total of 60 grams of carbohydrate, while the next day you might have a piece of coffee cake and juice for the same 60 grams of carbohydrate.

To use this system, you have to learn to recognize what you normally eat and how many grams of carbohydrate each food contains. A dietitian can get you started with food models and a listing of common carbohydrate-containing foods. Practice for a while, just as you would for a piano recital or a spelling test. Pretty soon, you'll be rattling off the carbohydrate content of foods like a pro.

A more detailed level of carbohydrate counting is known as the glycemic index. Under controlled conditions, dietary researchers measured exactly how high a given quantity of each carbohydrate will raise the blood glucose level. The index compares each food with white bread. For example, if 15 grams of a certain carbohydrate raises blood glucose slightly higher than 15 grams of bread, that carbohydrate has a high glycemic index. Other carbohydrates that don't raise the blood glucose as much as white bread have a low glycemic index.

Frankly, we find the glycemic index to be too detailed for practical use, and the ADA states that it may provide only a modest additional benefit over monitoring total carbohydrate alone.

The carbohydrate counting system adds flexibility to food choices for people using external insulin pumps or multiple daily injections of pre-meal insulin. One unit of insulin is equated with a specific number of grams of carbohydrate. As described in Chapters 11 and 13, we might teach a person to use 1.0 unit of fast-acting insulin for every 15 grams of carbohydrate eaten in a meal, plus 1.0 unit for every 50 mg/dl over her blood glucose target. This is determined by your doctor. More insulin may be needed if the person is insulin resistant, or less may be needed if she is particularly sensitive to insulin.

What's the downside of carbohydrate counting? By focusing on the carbohydrate content only, you may forget other aspects of good nutrition. Going overboard with meat portions, for example, won't affect your blood glucose much but could put you over the recommended amounts for protein and fat. And, if you consume excess calories from foods that don't contain carbohydrate, you may soon find yourself with a weight problem.

Monitoring your carbohydrate intake can be complicated at first, but it is a helpful skill to learn for managing your diabetes. Once you get used to it, the system will become part of your life. Think about all the important and trivial things you routinely think about and do in the course of a day—How much travel time do I have to plan to get to work? Do I have enough cash to do my errands? Adding an awareness of how much carbohydrate is in your meal becomes just as much second nature as any other routine calculation you do in your head. And the reward for paying attention to your food intake is immediate and gratifying: you feel better with less worry.

Reading Labels

No discussion of food would be complete without some comments about food labels. The labeling laws that went into effect in the United States in 1994 and are periodically updated make label reading much easier than it used to be. You'll find that if you bypass the colorful trappings boasting "No cholesterol!" or "No added sugar!" and go right to the Nutrition Facts section of the label, you'll learn a lot about the product. We'll take a look at each part of this label (see Figure 11).

Serving size. Start with the serving size: all the other information is applicable only for that amount. The serving size given on the label may be smaller than what you consider to be a serving, so be aware that if you eat an entire package of something that contains four servings, you've just downed *four times* the amounts listed as "per serving."

Calories. Calories are listed only for the serving size specified on the food container, not for an exchange or for other usual serving sizes.

Percent daily value. This part of the label can be misinterpreted because the single item does not represent all the foods eaten for the day. But it can be helpful if you are adding up how much fat, protein, or other nutrients you consume each day and if you eat 2,000 calories per day. Otherwise, this information is not helpful.

Total fat and cholesterol. You need to keep fat consumption within the recommended guidelines. In interpreting the label, it may be helpful to go straight to the saturated fat grams, remembering that 5 grams of fat equals 1 teaspoon of butter, margarine, or oil and that saturated fat is what raises blood cholesterol level. Foods that contain 5 grams of total fat or less are considered lower-fat choices.

Nutrition Facts

Serving Size 7 wafers (29g)
Servings Per Container About 8

Amount Per Serving

Calories 120	Calories from Fat 30

	% Daily Value*
Total Fat 3g	5%
Saturated Fat 0.5g	3%
Polyunsaturated Fat 0g	
Monounsaturated Fat 1 g	
Cholesterol 0g	0%
Sodium 170 mg	7%
Total Carbohydrate 22g	7%
Dietary Fiber 4g	15%
Sugars 0g	
Protein 3g	

Vitamin A 0%-Vitamin C 0%-Calcium 0%

Iron 8%-Phosphorus 10%

* Percent Daily Values are based on a 2,000 calorie diet. Your daily values may
be higher or lower depending on your calorie needs:

	Calories:	2,000	2,500
Total Fat	Less than	65g	80g
Sat Fat	Less than	20g	25g
Cholesterol	Less than	300mg	300mg
Sodium	Less than	2,400mg	2,400mg
Total Carbohydrate		300g	375g
Dietary Fiber		25g	30g

Calories per gram: Fat 9 · Carbohydrate 4 · Protein 4

Figure 11. A nutrition facts label.

Sodium. Sodium is the part of table salt that some people have to cut down on if they have high blood pressure or ankle swelling. The sodium figure includes sodium from salt as well as other sodium-containing foods in the product. Foods that contain 10% or less of the daily value for sodium are considered lower-sodium choices.

Total carbohydrate. Total carbohydrate is the carbohydrate from dietary fiber, sugars, and other (complex) carbohydrates. Examples of sugars are sucrose, fructose, glucose, lactose, corn syrup, and honey. Other carbohydrates are the complex carbohydrates in the product. This amount may not be indicated on the label but can be calculated by subtracting the grams of dietary fiber and grams of sugars from the total carbohydrates.

Protein. This section lists the total grams of protein.

Calories from fat, protein, and carbohydrate. At the bottom of the label are the figures for the number of calories per gram of fat, protein, and carbohydrate. You can use this information to determine how many calories in the product come from each. Just multiply the total fat grams by 9, the total carbohydrate (minus the fiber) by 4, and the protein by 4.

Putting It All Together

Some people are visual learners. Once we see a picture, it all makes sense. For the visually inspired, the U.S. Department of Agriculture (USDA) has put together a sample plate to illustrate the relative proportions of different kinds of foods making up a healthy meal (see Figure 12). It is consistent with recommendations for persons with diabetes. As you can see, the plate shows how the five food groups can be used at mealtime. Fill half your plate with nonstarchy vegetables and fruits, divide the other half of your plate into the protein portion (lean meat, poultry, or fish) and the starch portion, and choose 1% or skim milk to drink.

. . .

We have covered a lot of material in this chapter—facts, figures, and opinions. It will most likely take you a while to even begin to master nutrition. But remember that you're already very familiar with the foods themselves. We're just asking you to think a little more about the foods you eat every

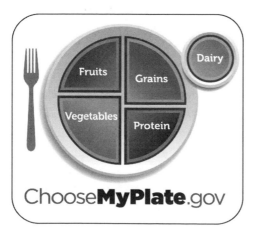

Figure 12. The USDA's recommendations for a healthy meal.

day, to learn what it is you're putting in your mouth. With the help of a good professional nutritionist, you will discover a multitude of healthful foods that taste good too.

Take Home Messages

- Build a healthy plate. Make half your plate fruits and vegetables. Switch to skim or 1% milk. Make at least half your grains whole. Vary your protein food choices.
- Cut back on foods high in solid (saturated) fats, added sugars, and salt. Choose foods and drinks with little or no added sugars. Look out for salt (sodium) in foods you buy—it all adds up.
- Eat the right amount of calories for you. Enjoy your food, but eat less. Cook more often at home, where you are in control of what's in your food. When eating out, choose lower-calorie menu options. Write down what you eat so as to keep track of how much you eat. If you drink alcoholic beverages, do so sensibly—limit to one drink a day for women or two drinks a day for men.

7

Weight Control

Why It Matters and How to Do It

- "Can losing weight reduce my risk of having a heart attack?"
- "I heard losing weight is harder for people with diabetes."
- "I have lost weight lots of times, but I always gain it back."
- "I'm an emotional eater. I eat when I'm bored. I eat when I'm sad. I eat when I'm happy."
- "Are there any diabetes medications that don't make you gain weight?"
- "Do diet pills work?"
- "Can weight loss surgery cure diabetes?"

Americans are getting fatter all the time, and we all hate it. In a recent survey, almost half (46%) of the people who were asked said they would give up a year of life to not be fat. In fact, 15% said they would give up 10 years! That's why we spend $50 billion annually on health club memberships, diet plans, and other programs and potions that promise to peel off unwanted pounds.

Weight Control Is Extra Challenging When You Have Diabetes

Avoiding those unwanted pounds can be especially hard when you have diabetes. For example, lowering your A1c level is a good thing, but when your control improves, your body holds on to more of the calories you consume and fewer calories pass out, unabsorbed, as glucose in your urine. So you may not see the results of your improved control when you step on the scale, unless you compensate by eating less or exercising more.

Other things can also make weight control harder when you have diabetes, like snacking to treat a low blood glucose or to avoid the possibility that it might go low. And some diabetes medications can also contribute to weight gain.

Why Controlling Your Weight Is So Important

There's some bad news but also some good news about being overweight and trying to lose weight when you have diabetes.

Bad news: The fatter you are, on the whole, the *more resistance you have to your own insulin. Insulin resistance* means that a specific amount of insulin doesn't work as well as it should. If you give 1 unit of insulin to a thin person, you might drop his or her blood glucose by 50 mg/dl; give the same 1 unit to an obese person, and the glucose level might drop by only 20 mg/dl. That's resistance to insulin.

You may like to think of insulin resistance with a story.

John's riding a bike. If he's on a nice smooth bike path, the pedaling is easy, no resistance. If he rides off the road onto a beach, though, the wheels sink into sand, and there's lots of resistance. If John is strong, he can push through the sand and keep going. But if he's not so strong, the bike doesn't make it.

What does this have to do with insulin resistance? A slim, physically fit body is like the smooth road, and a little insulin (like a little pedaling) does just fine. Add obesity, and you're in the sand, because obesity causes resistance to the insulin. If you have a strong pancreas that's putting out lots of insulin, it can overcome the resistance. But if your pancreas is weak, it can't make enough insulin, and you have diabetes.

Good news: Losing weight, if you are overweight to begin with, decreases the insulin resistance, like riding out of the sand and back onto the pavement. All of a sudden, your pancreas may be up to the job, and your blood glucose control will probably improve. It might even return to normal.

Bad news: Cardiovascular disease (heart attack and stroke) is the leading cause of death for people who have diabetes. In fact, the risk of heart attack and stroke is two to four times greater in people with diabetes than in the general population. Nearly 75% of people with Type 2 diabetes die from cardiovascular disease.

Good news: If you are overweight, modest weight loss can significantly improve your cardiovascular risk factors, lowering your A1c, blood pressure, and total cholesterol level and increasing your HDL cholesterol (the good cholesterol that cuts your risk of cardiovascular disease). One long-term study found that people who maintained a 5-pound weight loss over 16 years cut their cardiovascular risk factor levels almost in half (48% reduction for men and 40% reduction for women).

Bad news: It turns out that overweight people also suffer more often from sleep apnea. The person who has sleep apnea usually begins to snore heavily soon after falling asleep. After a while the snoring becomes louder, but then he stops breathing altogether (apnea). The apnea is interrupted by a loud snort and gasp, and he starts snoring again. This pattern is repeated frequently throughout the night, leading to a bad night's sleep and feeling tired the next day. Some research suggests that sleep apnea increases the level of proteins called *pro-inflammatory cytokines*; high levels of these protein molecules increase a person's risk for cardiovascular disease.

Good news: Losing weight can reduce your risk for sleep apnea, and reducing your risk for sleep apnea can improve the quality of your sleep and your heart health.

Bad news: Overweight is also a risk factor for urinary incontinence, at least in women. Women entering one study reported an average of 24 episodes of incontinence a week.

Good news: Women in this study who participated in a six-month weight loss intervention lost about 17 pounds, and their average number of incontinence episodes dropped to 13 a week. Not a cure, but a big improvement, suggesting that a decrease in urinary incontinence may be another benefit among the many health improvements associated with weight loss.

People with Type 2 Diabetes *Can* Lose Weight

Look AHEAD (Action for Health in Diabetes) is a 12-year study conducted in 20 medical centers, including our own. The study was designed to find out whether participating in a weight loss intervention protects people with diabetes who are overweight or obese from heart attack and stroke. Remember what we said about the elevated risk for these conditions in people with diabetes.

More than 5,000 people with Type 2 diabetes participated in the Look AHEAD trial. Half of the participants were in an "active lifestyle" group, and the other half were in a "support and education" group, receiving support and education sessions on diabetes. The active lifestyle group received help controlling the number of calories they consumed. They received structured meal plans, and early in the study they also received liquid meal replacements and low-calorie frozen entrees. These participants were also encouraged to be more active, with a goal of 25 minutes of moderately active exercise (such as brisk walking) each day.

The study had to follow participants' progress for a long time because heart attack and stroke (the primary outcomes that were measured in this study) are relatively rare events, even for people with diabetes, so it takes many years to tell for sure if weight loss really helps.

In their first year of Look AHEAD, participants in the active lifestyle group lost an average of almost 20 pounds (8.6% of their average weight when they started the study), much more than the average of less than 2 pounds lost by participants in the support and education group. This is pretty strong evidence that the active lifestyle intervention worked to help people lose weight. And four years after entering the study, lifestyle participants had kept off most of the weight they lost in the first year. On average they weighed about 12 pounds less than they had when they entered the study.

Losing weight was only part of the good news for the active lifestyle participants in Look AHEAD. Their A1c levels dropped from an average of 7.3% at the beginning of the study to 6.6% one year later, while average A1c levels for those in the support and education group barely budged (from 7.3% to 7.2%). And that's not all: blood pressure and cholesterol levels improved much more in the active lifestyle group, and physical fitness—measured by performance on a treadmill test—improved 20% in the active lifestyle group and only about 5% in the other study participants. These advantages for the lifestyle intervention declined somewhat over the next three years, as the average weight increased some, but at the end of four years, improvements in blood glucose, blood pressure, and cholesterol levels were still consistently better in the active lifestyle group.

All these findings were very encouraging. Combined, the results told us that the weight loss intervention dramatically reduced risk factors for heart attack and stroke. But after about 10 years of the study, it was clear that the lifestyle intervention did not reduce the number of heart attacks and strokes in this group compared with the support and education group. We are not sure why this was so. The rate of heart attacks and strokes was low in both treatment groups; perhaps those in the lifestyle group achieved this positive result through weight loss and those in the support and education group achieved this through the additional medication they took to lower blood pressure and cholesterol levels. We'll continue to analyze the Look AHEAD data to better understand our results.

Weight Control: Possible But Not Easy

Look AHEAD tells us that it is possible to lose weight and to keep it off for some years, even if you have diabetes. But as we all know, losing weight is really hard, and keeping it off is often even harder. We've already mentioned some of the reasons this is true when you have diabetes: your body holding onto more of the calories you consume when your glucose control improves, the effects of certain diabetes medications, and the effects of consuming extra calories to prevent or treat blood glucose lows.

Whether or not you have diabetes, consuming fewer calories and burning more calories through exercise will help you lose weight. It can also help you keep it off. But if you lose lots of weight, keeping it off means paying attention to every calorie and exercising at least an hour a day. That's what we've learned through the National Weight Loss Registry, which tracks 10,000 people who have lost at least 30 pounds and kept it off for at least a year. People in the registry weigh themselves every day, they eat the same foods in pretty much the same pattern every day, and they don't "cheat" on weekends or holidays. Registry members are always thinking about their weight.

Even if you are as diligent as the people in the National Weight Loss Registry, we now know that your genes can make it harder to lose weight. It's a fact: when people do lose weight, their bodies fight to gain back some or all of that weight.

Genetics. Obesity tends to run in families, and even the desire to eat higher-calorie foods may run in families as well. People carrying a gene variant known as FTO are more likely to eat high-calorie, high-fat foods, and they have a much higher risk for obesity.

Hormone changes with weight loss. When you lose a lot of weight, your body fights to get you back to your earlier, pre-diet level. For instance, levels of a hormone called *ghrelin*, the so-called hunger hormone, increase. And levels of other hormones decrease, like *peptide YY*, which suppresses hunger, and *leptin*, which suppresses hunger and increases the rate at which your body burns calories. These natural efforts to replace lost weight helped our primeval ancestors, who were often at risk of starving. Today, these hormone changes are a burden, not a benefit.

Scientists estimate that changes in metabolism alone mean that after weight loss, muscles burn 20%–25% fewer calories during exercise.

Changes in how your brain responds to food. A weight loss researcher at Columbia University found that when people lose weight, their brain sends signals that increase their desire for food and reduce restraint for eating that food.

The bottom line. It's not impossible to lose lots of weight and keep it off—those in the National Weight Loss Registry prove that. But it is really, really hard. Food temptations are everywhere, and for most people exercise is not fun. Some genes can make overweight more likely. Add hormone and brain changes that work against your efforts to keep off lost weight, and you have what one scientist called "a perfect storm for weight regain." What helps is to avoid gaining lots of weight in the first place. The hormone and brain changes we mentioned are strongest in people who were very heavy and lost lots of weight. The changes were less dramatic in people who were less heavy and lost less weight. And keep in mind what we said earlier: weight loss of even 5% can lower a person's risk for heart disease and other health problems. Research we are involved in proves this is true.

Losing 5% of your weight (about 10 pounds if you weigh 200 pounds) might not seem like much of an accomplishment, but the health benefits are real. Do yourself a favor: do all you can to gain these benefits.

Weight Control: What Works

Find Your Reason to Lose

One key to success is finding *your* reason for losing weight. We know, there are lots of good reasons to lose weight, and you probably know almost all of them. But none of these good reasons will help you lose weight unless it is *your* reason. People who have found *their* reason say it is like flipping a switch; suddenly eating carefully and staying active are much easier.

Needless to say, most of us have not yet found our reasons for losing weight. We eat too much and we sit too much, and as a result, we often weigh too much. And that extra weight is bad news. There's growing evidence that it hurts us in two ways: it takes years from our lives, and it takes life from our years.

The weight loss masters we have known, patients in our clinical practices and participants in our research studies who have lost weight and kept it off, offer some tips for flipping your weight loss switch and keeping it flipped.

Useful Tips for Losing Weight and Keeping It Off

—*Make it personal.* Jacob said he started losing weight because he wanted to keep up with his grandchildren when they came over to play. Sarah told us her switch flipped with the decision to look her best for her daughter's wedding. Felicia said she had been steadily losing weight since the day she had trouble fitting between desks when she walked down the aisle at the office. Can you think of anything you care enough about to flip your weight loss switch?

—*Accentuate the positive.* As you think about your reason to lose weight, try to focus on positive reasons. We are struck that most of the weight loss masters we know are motivated by the promise of things they want, like feeling better, being able to do more, and feeling in more control of their lives, rather than by things they want to avoid, like diabetes complications. So look for positive reasons to launch your weight loss efforts.

—*Keep track of the benefits.* Staying positive is also crucial once you have started your weight loss program. Keep notes about the good things you see happening as a result of your efforts. Do you have more energy? Are you sleeping better? Do you feel better about yourself? Has anyone complimented you on your appearance? Write down these positive outcomes. Give yourself pats on the back as well. Note the times you go for a walk—even when the weather is bad; note the times you stay at the office and eat the healthy lunch you packed—even when your friends ask you to join them at the local All-U-Can-Eat. Be sure to look at your notes on days when your motivation is low. At those times, seeing what you have accomplished can rekindle your motivation and help you stay on track.

—*Never forget where you were.* Weight loss masters say they never forget what they looked and felt like before they lost weight. Some keep pictures of their heavier selves close at hand and pull them out whenever they are tempted to go back to their old ways. Others say their families help by reminding them how much younger and healthier they look than they used to.

—*Keep in mind that small steps can bring big rewards.* Weight loss masters know the benefits of small steps. Most experts say a healthy rate of weight loss is about 1–2 pounds per week. That's the weight loss goal in two national weight loss studies we're working in.

Avoid Emotional Eating

Few of us eat only when we are hungry. Often we eat to feed feelings, not to fill our stomachs. We eat because we are bored, or stressed, or depressed, or even because we are happy. And the things we are drawn to when we eat emotionally, while undeniably delicious, are rarely healthy choices—the mid-afternoon candy bar at work, or the bowl of ice cream in the evening, for example.

Take this little quiz to see how much of an issue emotional eating is for you.

Emotional Eating Quiz: Do You Feed Feelings?

Eating emotionally means eating when you are not hungry or continuing to eat when you have had enough. How often do you eat emotionally in each of the following situations?

	Never	Sometimes	Often	Always
1. When I'm trying to relax				
2. When I'm sad				
3. When I'm bored				
4. When I'm happy				
5. At home in the evening				
6. At home during the day				
7. At work				
8. In social situations				

The more questions for which you answered "often" or "always," the more you eat emotionally.

Everyone eats emotionally at least occasionally. That's because we all feel stressed, or feel bored, or feel like celebrating from time to time. Eating something tasty when you are feeling any of those things is simply and immediately satisfying. But when you are feeding feelings, the fix is fleeting. Many people say the pleasure is gone almost as soon as the food is. What lingers is guilt and the extra calories you have consumed. Curbing emotional eating, then, can improve your mental and physical health.

Tips for Curbing Emotional Eating

—*Give yourself what you really need.* You can find better ways than eating to relax, to lift your spirits, or to protect yourself from boredom. The first step is to *recognize* when you are eating for one of these reasons and not because you are really hungry. Practice helps you recognize when you are eating emotionally.

When is that most likely to happen to you? Is it mid-afternoons at work when you are feeling bored? Evenings when you are trying to relax? Parties when you want to have a good time? Can you think of anything other than food that might help? Start with anything that has ever worked for you in the past.

—*Experiment.* If you depend on that big blueberry muffin in the afternoon to get you to the end of the work day (and wish you didn't), brainstorm for alternative sources of satisfaction. Could you bring something to work that is just as delicious but healthier, or buy something healthier there? Could you skip food altogether and do something else special during your break, like reading your favorite magazine, calling a friend, or taking a walk? Try every idea that has a chance of succeeding until you find some that work for you. Remember, no plan will *eliminate* emotional eating, but if you experiment you can come up with tricks that will help you curb it, and that's a good thing.

—*Maintain your motivation.* As we said, the goal is *curbing* emotional eating, not eliminating it. We hope some of the tips offered here help you do just that. Keep experimenting until you find a plan that works for you. Keep in mind this story about Thomas Edison: A reporter once asked him why he did not give up after 5,000 experiments had "failed" to produce the first electric light bulb. Edison responded, "I haven't failed once; I'm 5,000 steps closer to the solution." Edison's experiments continued until he reached his goal.

Experimenting will help you reach your goal of less emotional eating, and it probably won't take 5,000 experiments to get there.

Eat Mindfully

Jeff bought his lunch at the office cafeteria every day and quickly gulped it down at his desk while he worked, and every evening he ate dinner in front of the television. If you asked him right after a meal what he had just eaten, he would not have been able to tell you—because his mind was on his work or his favorite television show. Jeff ate mindlessly. And even though he ate a lot, he got almost no pleasure from eating.

Most of us are like Jeff; we don't think about what we are eating, we eat too much, and we eat too fast.

Eating *mindfully* means paying attention to what you are eating and eating more slowly. Eating mindfully can increase your enjoyment of food, protect you from overeating, and help you control your weight, your blood glucose levels, and your risk of diabetes complications. Let's see where you stand when it comes to mindful eating.

Mindful Eating Quiz

1. How often do you eat dinner in front of the television?
   a. All or almost all the time
   b. About half the time
   c. Never or almost never
2. How often do you finish a meal in less than 20 minutes?
   a. All or almost all the time
   b. About half the time
   c. Never or almost never
3. How often do you stop eating as soon as you feel full?
   a. Never or almost never
   b. About half the time
   c. All or almost all the time

If your answer to any of these questions was choice a or choice b, the tips below could help you eat less, enjoy your food more, and live a healthier life.

Tips for Developing Mindful Eating

—*Focus only on food when you eat.* Seventy-five percent of Americans eat dinner in front of the television, and studies show that the more television people watch, the more they weigh. Watching television and mindful eating don't mix. How often have you sat down to watch a favorite show with a bag of chips in hand, determined to "eat just a few," only to find that you emptied the bag without even realizing it? You might not have been aware while you were packing away all those calories, but you packed them away just the same. So it's really important, hard as it might be, to avoid distractions while you are eating. Eat only in the kitchen or dining room, and keep the television off.

—*Eat more slowly and stop when you are no longer hungry.* It takes about 20 minutes for your stomach to tell your brain that you are full. That's why you sometimes end up feeling too full after you eat a meal really fast—you *are* too full. Just like avoiding distractions while you eat, eating more slowly takes practice, but give it a try. Take small bites of food, chew thoroughly, put down your fork, and pause between bites. Very few of us do this naturally, but if you develop the skill—and it is a skill—you will not only eat less, you will also get more enjoyment from what you are eating. You will start to really appreciate the aromas, colors, and textures of your food. Pay attention to your hunger level. When you start to feel full, stop eating. Again, it takes practice to get this right.

—*Shop mindfully.* Mindful eating starts with mindful shopping. Go grocery shopping only when your stomach is full, go with a list, and buy only what is on your list. That way you'll bring home fewer tempting high-fat, high-calorie foods.

—*Put temptations out of sight.* If you do bring home any tempting high-fat, high-calorie foods, put them in hard-to-reach cupboards or in the back of the refrigerator or freezer. Studies show that when these foods are not in plain sight, they are not eaten as often.

—*Keep serving dishes off the table.* This discourages second helpings. Some people take this a step further and put all leftovers in the refrigerator after serving first helpings and before sitting down to eat.

—*Control portions.* Divide big packages of snack foods into smaller, portion-size bags, which helps protect you from eating the whole bag. This is especially important if you can't resist snacking while you watch television.

—*Eat mindfully in restaurants.* This can be a real challenge. Some people say it helps to decide what they are going to order (and what they are not going to order) before they arrive at the restaurant. Others order in stages—this lets them eat only as much as they are hungry for. And a few people we know ask for a "doggy bag" as soon as their main course is served. They pack part of the meal away to take home, which protects them from overeating right then and provides some tasty leftovers for later.

Everyone deserves to really enjoy eating. Eating mindfully can give you more "bang" for your eating "buck"—greater enjoyment with fewer calories. And that's a good thing. In our research studies, participants use suggestions like the ones we have offered here to lose weight, to lower their blood glucose, blood pressure, and cholesterol levels, and to improve their fitness. You can too.

Diabetes Medications That Could Help You Lose Weight

Eating less and exercising more remain the cornerstones of weight control when you have Type 2 diabetes, but a class of diabetes medications introduced a few years ago could help some people.

These drugs are called glucagon-like peptide 1 (GLP-1) agonists. In clinical trials these medications have beneficial effects on blood glucose, blood pressure, and cholesterol levels. In addition, GLP-1 drugs suppress appetite and food intake. In trials lasting at least 20 weeks, people with Type 2 diabetes lost an average of 6.2 pounds. This is not a tremendous amount of weight loss, but we must keep in mind that many other diabetes medications are associated with weight *gain*.

Currently available GLP-1 agonists are exenatide (Byetta and Bydureon) and liraglutide (Victoza). Both are taken by injection, Byetta twice a day, Victoza once a day, and Bydureon once a week.

People who use GLP-1 agonists sometimes experience nausea and occasionally experience vomiting, but these side effects usually pass fairly quickly, and they rarely lead people to stop the medication. If these side effects persist, are very bothersome, or are accompanied by abdominal pain, you should stop taking the medication and contact your physician.

If you think you might benefit from a GLP-1 medication, talk to your diabetes health care provider.

Diet Pills

Everyone is looking for a safe, effective, easy way to control weight. Most people would prefer a pill, assuming it didn't have any serious side effects. In the past, some popular weight loss pills were taken off the market because they turned out to be unsafe. Currently, two pills are available. The first, orlistat (Xenical), works by blocking the absorption of fat in the intestine. It is available over the counter as Alli. In one study, people with Type 2 diabetes who took Xenical for a year lost about 5 pounds more than those who took a placebo pill. The drug seems to have no life-threatening side effects, but it does have some potentially embarrassing ones, including diarrhea, flatulence, and episodes of bowel incontinence. The second diet pill,

Qnexa, was the first new weight loss drug approved in the United States in 13 years. Qnexa is a combination of two existing drugs—the stimulant phentermine, which was part of a previous weight loss drug that was taken off the market when it was found to have serious cardiac side effects, and the epilepsy and migraine drug topiramate, also known by the brand name Topamax. In clinical trials, people using Qnexa lost an average of about 22 pounds (about 10% of body weight) after one year, though some weight was regained in the second year of use. The drug also seemed to have positive effects on blood glucose, blood pressure, and cholesterol levels. But Qnexa also increased heart rate, a danger signal that the drug might increase the risk of heart attack even if it lowers other cardiovascular risk factors. Vivus, the company that developed Qnexa, has agreed to do a large clinical study to see whether the drug causes an increase in heart attacks and strokes. Use of topiramate (one of the drugs in Qnexa) during pregnancy is associated with an increased risk of cleft lips and cleft palates in babies, so women who are pregnant or plan to become pregnant should not take Qnexa.

It's interesting to note that a couple of years ago the FDA rejected Qnexa. The current decision to approve it was based on new evidence about its safety and greater concern about the harm caused by untreated obesity.

Weight Loss Surgery

Weight loss surgery (sometimes called bariatric surgery) for people with Type 2 diabetes is becoming very popular. According to some studies, this type of surgery can actually cure Type 2 diabetes—bringing normal blood glucose levels to many of those who have had the surgery.

Types of weight loss surgery. Almost all weight loss surgery performed in the United States is either *gastric bypass surgery* (typically the Roux-en-Y version of the procedure) or *adjustable gastric banding* (often called lap-banding). (See Figures 13 and 14.)

Bypass surgery does two things. First, it shrinks the size of the stomach to 10% of its original size, limiting the amount of food a person can consume. Second, it changes the path that food takes after leaving the stomach, bypassing part of the small intestine (where most food absorption occurs) and lowering the number of consumed calories that the body absorbs.

In adjustable gastric banding, a fluid-filled band is wrapped around the stomach. Tightening the belt creates a small stomach pouch, which limits the amount of food a person can consume (just as bypass surgery does).

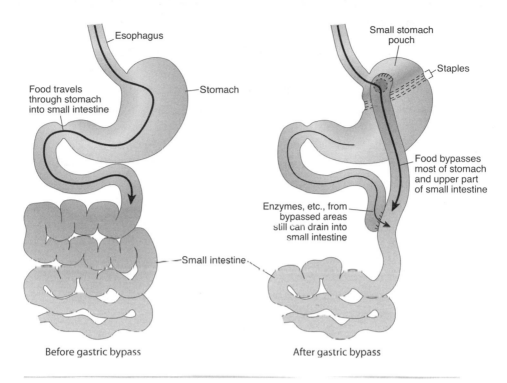

Figure 13. Gastric bypass surgery.

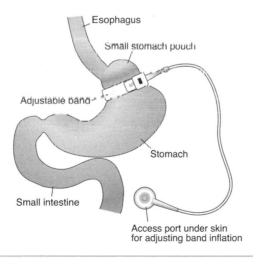

Figure 14. Adjustable gastric banding.

Which type of surgery is more effective and safer? Weight loss is greater and faster with bypass surgery. Studies show that about two years after surgery, the average person undergoing gastric bypass surgery had lost 60% of excess body weight and the average person undergoing lap-band surgery had lost about 40% of excess body weight. So if the person was 60 pounds overweight, she would lose about 35 pounds from bypass surgery or about 25 pounds from lap-band surgery. If she was 100 pounds overweight, the weight loss would be about 60 pounds for gastric bypass and about 40 pounds for lap-banding. Not everyone has this kind of success, partly because some people find ways to defeat the surgeries by continuing to consume lots of calories in liquid form. Liquids pass through their tiny stomachs much more quickly than solid food, so people don't feel full as long.

Complications of the surgery are more common with bypass surgery. People who have had bypass surgery must take vitamins and minerals because the surgery impairs vitamin and mineral absorption. Death from either surgery is rare—about 1 in 200 people.

How weight loss surgery can "cure" Type 2 diabetes, at least for a while. In almost 80% of people treated with weight loss surgery, the surgery leads to normal blood glucose control—to complete resolution of Type 2 diabetes. When you think of the large amount of weight loss that results from these surgeries, this is not surprising—any intervention that produced a 60- to 100-pound weight loss would lead to a resolution of Type 2 diabetes in many people.

What seems more magical is that for many people, diabetes resolves very soon after bypass surgery (but not lap-banding), before substantial weight loss. No one can explain this convincingly, but researchers think changes in hormones associated with bypassing part of the small intestine may be responsible.

Long-term effects of weight loss surgery. Evidence concerning the long-term effects of weight loss surgery is accumulating, but many of the long-term effects of these relatively new surgeries are not yet known. We do already know, as noted above, that gastric bypass surgery leads to vitamin and mineral depletion, so people who have this surgery must take vitamin and mineral supplements for the rest of their lives. Many find life after bariatric surgery less easy than they imagined, with declining psychological benefits after a few years and persistent binge eating and night eating among a substantial proportion of people. Loose skin is another common problem for anyone who loses a very large amount of weight, often leading to expensive cosmetic surgery.

On the other hand, a 2007 article in the *New England Journal of Medicine* reported that obese people who had bypass surgery had 92% fewer diabetes-related deaths than obese people who did not have the surgery. This was not a randomized controlled study, however, so the people who had the bypass surgery might have been different from those who did not have the surgery in ways that could explain part of the advantage for the former group.

Is weight loss surgery right for you? If you are interested in weight loss surgery, talk to your health care provider. The American Diabetes Association recommends considering weight loss surgery if your BMI is 35 or over. For example, a person who is 5' 10" tall and weighs 245 pounds has a BMI of 35. That person weighs about 75 pounds more than someone of "normal" weight, who has a BMI of 24. For an easy-to-use BMI calculator, go to the U.S. government's National Heart, Lung, and Blood Institute website (www.nhlbisupport.com/bmi/bminojs.htm).

Keep in mind that the cost of weight loss surgery is currently $20,000–$25,000 and that many health insurance companies still don't cover these costs.

The bottom line. Weight loss surgery holds great promise for improving health and quality of life for people with diabetes who need to lose a lot of weight. Still, the surgeries are not risk free, and the long-term results are not certain. So you need to think carefully about the place that weight loss surgery might have in your efforts to live a long, healthy life.

Adjusting Your Diabetes Medication When You Lose Weight—However You Lose It

After losing weight, you will probably have less need for insulin and some other diabetes medications—and this is good news. So you will need to make adjustments in your medication regimen to protect yourself from blood glucose levels going too low. Be sure to talk with your health care provider about the best and safest way to make these adjustments.

Take Home Messages

- Most Americans are overweight, and almost one-third are obese.
- Losing weight if you are overweight has many health benefits, including improved blood glucose, blood pressure, and cholesterol control and a healthier heart.
- Weight control can be especially challenging when you have diabetes.
- The Look AHEAD trial proves that people with Type 2 diabetes can lose weight and reduce cardiovascular risk factors.
- When you lose a lot of weight, your body fights to get back some of that lost weight.
- Keys to effective weight control include finding your personal reason for doing it, avoiding emotional eating, and eating mindfully.
- Other tools that can help with weight control include some diabetes medications, diet pills, and weight loss surgery.

8

Special Considerations in Nutrition Therapy

- "First diabetes, then high blood pressure. Now I *know* I won't be able to eat anything."
- "I don't think that dietitian knows what she's talking about. My triglycerides are high, and she told me to cut down on my carbs and increase the monounsaturated fat. That doesn't make any sense. Triglycerides are fat, right?"

No one diet can fit every situation or every person. This is why, in all our discussions of diet, we emphasize individualization. Ethnic and personal preferences are one consideration. Italians don't eat the same foods as people from Ireland; African Americans tend not to eat the way Asian Americans eat. And one member of a couple may love a particular food that his or her spouse just can't abide. But individualization is most important when a person has more than one health problem. This is not uncommon, especially for people with Type 2 diabetes, who very often have high blood pressure or high blood cholesterol.

By discussing nutrition guidelines for special health needs, we are extending the notion that food choices have to be tailored to the individual. If you are healthy except for having diabetes, your diet is constructed in one way; if you have other conditions, they too must be taken into account. An individualized food plan that considers all your health concerns does *not* mean that you "won't be able to eat anything." A skillful dietitian can work all sorts of interesting and good-tasting combinations into almost any dietary restriction. We only ask you to work with the professional, open up your mind and your taste buds, and stick with it.

The specific guidelines we describe here are for people with high blood pressure, kidney disease, high blood fats, and food allergies. (Healthy eating during pregnancy is discussed in Chapter 29.) We know that you may have another problem not covered here; whatever it is, your best bet for getting sound advice on nutrition therapy is to meet with a registered dietitian.

High Blood Pressure

Why do we talk so much about high blood pressure and diabetes? Because any way you look at it, they are closely related. One reason for this is that people with Type 2 diabetes are often overweight and have high blood pressure. Another reason is that if you have diabetes, untreated high blood pressure increases your risk for kidney and eye complications, heart attacks, and strokes. If you have Type 1 or Type 2 diabetes, you should be especially aware of blood pressure control.

There are three nutritional considerations in the treatment of high blood pressure (hypertension): reduce sodium intake, reduce weight, and watch for potassium imbalances in the blood that may result from blood pressure medications.

What, exactly, is sodium? It is a normal part of the blood, where it is found in a concentration very close to that of seawater. Sodium chloride (table salt), which is found in most salty-tasting foods, is the most common source of sodium. There are other salts, to be sure, such as potassium chloride (a "salt substitute"). Because the *chloride* content of sodium chloride is not important to blood pressure, we emphasize the low *sodium* part and allow the use of sodium substitutes such as potassium chloride if advised by your physician.

Why emphasize low sodium intake? Many people with high blood pressure are very sensitive to the salt they take in. Their sodium intake is related to their blood pressure. A high-sodium diet raises their blood pressure; conversely, lowering their sodium intake significantly lowers their blood pressure. The probable reason for this is that when the sodium intake is high, there is a tendency to retain fluid. It may not be enough fluid to show up as ankle swelling, but it is enough to "overfill" the blood vessels and raise the blood pressure—much like putting too much air in a tire.

It is difficult to predict exactly who will be salt-sensitive, so the recommendation for anyone with mild to moderate hypertension is to keep sodium intake below 2,400 mg (2.4 grams) per day. Some people need even more stringent sodium restriction. The 2010 Dietary Guidelines for Americans recommend that African Americans, anyone with high blood pressure, diabetes, or chronic kidney disease, and all adults 51 years or older keep sodium intake to 1,500 mg or less per day.

Making the switch to a low-sodium diet can be hard at first. The sodium content of foods is usually pretty clear from the taste, if not from the label on the package. If you are following a low-sodium diet, you should avoid adding salt to your food from the shaker; you should also stay away from high-salt foods such as most pretzels, potato chips, pizza, pickles, bacon, sausage, soy sauce, and canned foods. You should talk to the dietitian about *your* most common sources of salt and target those for reductions.

Nothing will taste right for a while. But after you get through the first few weeks, believe it or not, you get used to the low-salt diet. You may notice new tastes and natural flavors that you have been drowning with salt (ask a good cook what he or she thinks of the guest who douses the entree in a heavy dose of salt!). After a while, an accidental brush with a high-salt food will actually be unpleasant. Trust us. You're not really physically addicted to salt. The craving will go away.

Losing weight, if you are overweight to begin with, will also help in controlling hypertension. The response of blood pressure to weight loss is variable, but almost everyone benefits to some degree. (See Chapter 7 for nutritional and behavioral interventions for weight loss.) Exercise is especially valuable in both weight loss and control of hypertension.

Blood pressure, like blood glucose, has to be watched regularly. The rare visit to the doctor's office may not be enough. Is there a nurse at your workplace who can check your pressure? A spouse, other family member, or friend? Can you check it at the drug store or supermarket? Or can you learn to do it yourself? When you check your blood pressure, be sure to sit comfortably for a few minutes beforehand, as physical activity and stress can raise the reading, especially the first (systolic) number. If you have been told your blood pressure is high or even "borderline," you should check it regularly.

Quite often, weight loss and reduced dietary sodium will not adequately control hypertension. Medications are often needed. Angiotensin-converting enzyme (ACE) inhibitors are now the favored treatment of hypertension for persons with diabetes (see Chapters 22 and 24). There are several other antihypertensive agents, each with its own efficacy and potential side effects.

Many of the antihypertensive drugs cause changes in blood potassium or sodium content, the "electrolytes" that can easily be measured in a blood sample. So you may want to ask your doctor whether your potassium level should be checked. If it is too high, as can happen with ACE inhibitors or angiotensin receptor blockers (ARBs), you may need to work with your dietitian on controlling high-potassium foods. If it drifts low, as often occurs with the thiazide class of fluid pills, you will need a supplement of dietary potassium, usually in the form of a banana, potato with the skin, orange, or potassium pill. The fact is that these electrolyte imbalances and their dietary implications are hard to predict. You need to know whether you should change your potassium intake, and you should work with a dietitian in designing a plan to accomplish that.

Kidney Disease

Diabetes is one of the most common causes of kidney disease. Blood pressure control can help prevent kidney disease from developing or getting worse. As mentioned above, reducing sodium intake and reducing weight (if you are overweight) are important changes you can make that help control blood pressure. If you do develop early kidney disease, reducing protein in your diet can help slow the rate at which kidney function is lost. If the kidneys are failing, the recommendation is to cut back on protein intake even more. Your dietitian will help you identify exactly where your protein is coming from, but generally you'll want to cut down on red meats, fish, eggs, poultry, nuts, and dairy foods. Certain legumes are especially high in protein, such as green peas and dried beans and peas (kidney beans, black-eyed peas or beans, and so forth).

Failing kidneys also have trouble keeping the sodium, potassium, phosphorus, and magnesium levels in balance, and nutrition therapy may be called upon to help. Your kidneys may not be able to get rid of enough potassium, for example. Meal plans for people with failing kidneys should usually be low in foods that contain potassium.

Another potential issue is your kidneys' inability to get rid of enough phosphorus. High levels of phosphorus cause low levels of calcium, which in turn can cause problems with bone loss and increase the risk of heart disease. In this case, nutrition therapy is aimed at reducing phosphorus-containing foods, initially processed foods and colas, then later certain fruits, vegetables, and dairy products. Individual consultation with a dietitian is essential because you will also want to take in enough calcium, perhaps by including supplements such as calcium carbonate. Controlling dietary phosphorus and calcium definitely requires professional advice.

Does this sound complicated? It is complicated, because you must take into consideration not only the condition of your kidneys but the medications being used to keep your phosphorus and calcium levels in a healthy range. The diet and medication recommendations will be guided by your blood test results. If your kidneys are failing, you have to be sure that your doctor checks your electrolytes, calcium, phosphorus, vitamin D, and parathyroid hormone levels and prescribes a diet that the dietitian can help you implement. Usually, at this stage of progressively failing kidneys, it takes a kidney specialist (nephrologist) to help guide your care.

Dyslipidemia

Several different problems are grouped into the diagnosis of *dyslipidemia*, which means abnormal levels of fat in the blood (discussed more fully in Chapter 22). Hardening of the arteries (arteriosclerosis or atherosclerosis) is the dangerous aspect of dyslipidemia: high fats in the blood increase the chance of accelerated hardening of the arteries, with resulting heart attacks, strokes, or circulatory problems in the legs and feet. All dyslipidemias are not the same, and all dietary modifications should be considered individually. Here, we break the topic down into two basic problems, each with a different meaning for dietary treatment: high cholesterol/high LDL cholesterol and high triglyceride/low HDL cholesterol.

We focus on dietary changes here, but if dietary changes do not normalize your blood level of cholesterol and triglycerides, your doctor will probably recommend medication. Cholesterol-lowering and triglyceride-lowering drugs are now readily available and have relatively few side effects.

High Cholesterol/High LDL Cholesterol

This refers to high total cholesterol and high LDL cholesterol (popularly known as "bad cholesterol," since increased LDL is what increases the risk of arteriosclerosis; see Chapter 22). The total cholesterol can be measured whether or not you are fasting (no food for 12 hours), but it is usually measured when fasting.

When is a blood cholesterol level too high? Guidelines have been established and accepted by various professional associations. These guidelines for people who have diabetes have become strict, since about 70% of Americans with diabetes will die of heart disease or stroke. If people with diabetes were able to lower their blood cholesterol levels, they would live significantly longer, on average. Someone who is at high risk for a heart attack because of other factors such as a family history or heart disease should try to maintain an even lower blood cholesterol than other people. The latest guidelines from the American Diabetes Association recommend an LDL cholesterol level below 100 mg/dl or, in persons with known heart disease, below 70 mg/dl.

If your total cholesterol or LDL cholesterol is high, the first thing to think about is diet. And the first thing to do in changing your diet is to lower your total fat intake, especially saturated fat and trans fats. Remember that saturated fats, in general, are animal fats and dairy fats. The tender steak is tender because it is high in total fat and saturated fats. Hamburger meat, unless specially ground from trimmed meat, is likely to be high in saturated fats.

Read product labels. Other sources high in saturated fats include palm, coconut, and palm kernel oils. In choosing milk, be aware that although low-fat or 2% milk is lower in saturated fat than whole milk, the only really fat-free milk is skim milk.

Monounsaturated fats, mentioned in Chapter 6, are definitely in vogue now. If you can increase their content in your diet, all the better. But not a lot of foods are high in monounsaturated fats. Olive oil, canola oil, some nuts (such as almonds, pecans, pistachios, and cashews), avocados, and olives are all high in monounsaturated fats. None of these are likely to be major ingredients in your diet, however, so increasing the proportion of total calories derived from monounsaturates to 20% or so may be difficult, but worth trying.

What about the polyunsaturated fats that have been so popular for lowering cholesterol? There's no doubt about it: polyunsaturated fats, found in safflower oil and some margarines and fish oils, are effective in lowering total and LDL cholesterol. But they sometimes also lower HDL cholesterol, which is not good. So the polyunsaturated fats are not as highly recommended now as they were in the past. But if your HDL cholesterol is fine, they can still be effective in lowering the LDL cholesterol.

A tricky little subplot has developed of late in the saturated/unsaturated fat story: *partially hydrogenated*, *hydrogenated*, and *trans fats* are all terms used on labels to disguise the fact that these are *saturated fats*. So be on the lookout for these words when you read labels, and definitely choose foods that have zero trans fats. What about dietary cholesterol itself? A lot of foods have a little cholesterol, but just one common food has a lot of cholesterol: egg yolks. In the American diet, the number of eggs you consume, at about 190 mg of cholesterol per egg yolk, will determine your total cholesterol intake. A whole lobster comes close to one egg in cholesterol content, and a crab has about one-third the amount of cholesterol. But, really, how many crabs and lobsters do you eat every day, even if you live in Maryland and vacation in Maine? Moderation is the key! Even 3.5 ounces of cheddar cheese, which has a bad reputation, contains only about one-third the cholesterol of an egg. In the end, the cholesterol content of your diet is likely to come down to how often you eat eggs. So, for the sake of your heart, how about finding a substitute for that daily one or two eggs for breakfast and moving to an egg substitute that uses only egg whites? For home cooking and baking, bananas, tofu, and commercial egg substitutes can be used to replace eggs in recipes.

The National Cholesterol Education Program Step III guidelines define the dietary recommendations for lowering cholesterol: less than 7% of total calories from saturated fat, up to 20% of total calories from monounsaturated fat, up to 10% of calories from polyunsaturated fat, less than 200 mg of cholesterol per day, and 25%–35% of calories from total fat. Other nutrients in food that may help lower total cholesterol and LDL cholesterol are soluble fiber and plant stanols/sterols. Soluble fiber is found in oats, oat bran, dried beans, and many fruits and vegetables. Plant stanols/sterols are found in small amounts in many foods but are now being added to special margarines and some juices.

High Triglyceride/Low HDL Cholesterol

The relationship between high triglyceride levels and low HDL cholesterol is difficult to explain, especially because we have only some hypotheses about why it happens. But as a rule, when your blood triglyceride is high, your HDL cholesterol (the "good cholesterol") is low—and the combination is dangerous. This condition is common in persons with Type 2 diabetes and is due to insulin resistance, meaning that insulin in the body does not work efficiently. It develops most often when people become overweight and are physically inactive. Blood triglyceride levels over 150 mg/dl carry some increased risk of accelerated hardening of the arteries, but the risk is not very high unless it is combined with low HDL cholesterol. Tests for both triglycerides and HDL cholesterol need to be done when fasting, preferably 12 hours after eating.

How do we treat high triglyceride/low HDL cholesterol? The first step is to get your diabetes under control. It is remarkable to see how, when the blood glucose comes down, the triglyceride level also comes down. If the triglyceride level is very high—say, over 500 mg/dl—then you probably have to reduce your fat intake to less than 15% of total calories because severely high triglycerides can cause pancreatitis. Fat intake needs to be less than 25–40 grams daily, and this includes even the healthy fats found in vegetables and nuts. With triglyceride levels that are not so high—say, 150–499 mg/dl—the dietary approach is different. Triglyceride levels may come down with a decrease in calories that promotes weight loss and by cutting back on carbohydrates, especially foods that contain sugar, fruit juices, and high-fructose drinks. Increasing monounsaturated fat to 20% of total calories (a hard thing to do, as noted above), holding saturated and polyunsaturated fat to less than 10% of total calories each, and increasing dietary omega-3 fatty acids may also be beneficial. Since alcohol raises triglyceride levels, men are encouraged to limit alcoholic drinks to no more than two per day, and women to limit drinks to no more than one per day.

Food Allergies

What do food allergies have to do with diabetes? People with diabetes are no more likely to have food allergies than anyone else. But allergies can make following a diet much more difficult, and misconceptions about what constitutes an allergy can further complicate life with diabetes. An allergic reaction to food is a response to food that can start immediately after ingesting the food or some hours later. The allergic response does not occur in the gastrointestinal tract: it is not abdominal upset or pain. It is either a skin response or a whole body response. In mild forms, allergies usually cause some degree of itching, hives, swelling around the eyes, mild wheezing, or a rash. But they can be extremely serious and even fatal if the person has an *anaphylactic reaction*, an allergic reaction so extreme that he or she is in immediate danger of dying if not properly treated.

A food allergy is not just a dislike for a certain food. If you hate lima beans, you have a food aversion, not an allergy. A food allergy, as we've noted, does not mean getting cramps or diarrhea from a food. Even lactose intolerance—a common cause of severe diarrhea and stomach upset after eating milk or other lactose-containing foods—is not an allergy. It is an inability of the intestine to digest lactose, so lactose-containing foods cannot be properly absorbed and used.

If you think you are allergic to a certain food, the best thing to do is not to eat it at home or in a restaurant, at least until you check it out with your doctor. If the signs do point to an allergy, you should avoid the food completely. Sometimes you have to be very careful to determine whether a given dish contains the food you are allergic to. A physician friend of ours knew that he was allergic to shellfish. He did his best to avoid them. But at a restaurant he ordered a fish chowder after being assured that it contained no shellfish, only to find out after he ate it that it had traces of crabmeat. His allergic reaction was so severe that he was in the hospital for three weeks.

Be aware that food allergies do exist. If you have one or more such allergies, be sure your dietitian knows it. Your diet will have to be even more individualized.

Having not just diabetes but diabetes plus [fill in the blank] can be challenging. Special dietary modifications may well be necessary, and if so, you will probably not be able to manage this by yourself. So put the challenge to your treating physician and a professional dietitian. Ask them just what you can eat and how you should structure your food plan. Work with the dietitian to get as many of the foods you like into your diet as is possible, and be willing to try some helpful alternatives.

Changing your diet may mean tossing aside a family tradition of using fatback to season your vegetables; it may mean ending your serious love affair with high-salt, high-carb, high-fat pizza. But you will find that food selections targeted to your health needs as well as your taste buds will keep your system in balance and keep you feeling better and living longer.

Take Home Messages

- Controlling your blood pressure reduces your risk of kidney disease, eye disease, heart attack, and stroke.
- Treatments for high blood pressure include reducing sodium intake, reducing weight, and watching for potassium imbalances that may result from some medications.
- Abnormal levels of fat in the blood (dyslipidemia) increase the risk of heart attacks, strokes, and circulatory problems in the legs and feet.
- You can help control your LDL cholesterol ("bad cholesterol") level by reducing dietary cholesterol, especially egg consumption, and by switching from full-fat to low-fat or no-fat dairy products and monounsaturated and polyunsaturated fats.

9

Exercise and Diabetes

- "I've been a couch potato for 25 years, and now, just because I got diabetes, you tell me I'm supposed to start exercising!"
- "When I first began walking, I couldn't make it to the corner without stopping to catch my breath. Now I walk for 40 minutes, and when I get back I feel better than I did when I left."
- "I never could stick with an exercise program until someone suggested I ride my stationary bike while I watch television. Now I kill two birds with one stone: I stay fit while I keep up with my soap operas."
- "I used to like racquetball as a kid. And you know what? I still do. Picking up the old racquet got me back into exercise."

Exercise has to be a central part of your diabetes treatment plan. Increased activity provides a wide variety of physical, mental, and even social benefits. Exercise is as close to a panacea or "magic pill" as anyone could dream of. In fact, if it were possible to create a medication with the same benefits as exercise, those who owned the patent would be very wealthy. Better mood, more energy, closer to normal blood glucose levels and body weight, and a longer, healthier life—who could ask for anything more?

Still, we're aware that most people don't want to exercise. Our goal is to help you develop an exercise plan you not only can live with but will positively enjoy.

If you follow guidelines specifically tailored to your own condition and your own goals, you can exercise safely regardless of your age or physical condition. In this chapter we take a close look at the benefits of exercise, as well as some cautions, for a person with diabetes. We also help you develop your own exercise plan, help you get started, and discuss rules for safe exercise when you have diabetes. Finally, we offer some suggestions to help you stick with your exercise plan and keep from slipping back into inactivity.

Kinds of Exercise

Let's start by talking about different kinds of exercise, because all exercise is not the same, and different kinds of exercise have different benefits.

First, there's *aerobic exercise*. The goal of aerobic exercise is to get your heart rate up and sustain this for an extended period of time. Aerobic exercise is sometimes called cardiovascular exercise. Typical aerobic exercise activities include:

—Aerobics classes

—Brisk walking

—Jogging

    Swimming

—Bicycling (outdoors or on a stationary bike)

—Dancing

Second, there's *strength (or resistance) training*. The goal of strength training is to improve muscle strength, endurance, and tone. This is a very important goal because we tend to lose muscle mass and strength as we age. Strength training can be done with:

—Weight machines

    Free weights / hand weights

—Resistance tubing / bands

—Calisthenics such as push-ups and abdominal crunches

Third, there's *flexibility training*. The goal of flexibility training is to improve the range of motion around your joints. This is another important goal because, like muscle strength, flexibility tends to decline as we get older. Flexibility can be improved through:

—Aerobics or fitness classes that include stretching

—Yoga or Pilates

—Stretching on your own before and after aerobic exercise or strength training

Benefits of Exercise

All forms of exercise play a major role in keeping you healthy today and in the future. In 2010 the American College of Sports Medicine and the American Diabetes Association published a joint position statement on exercise and Type 2 diabetes (www.guidelines.gov/content.aspx?id=32410). Most of the recommendations in this statement apply to all people with diabetes. One of the authors of this book (Rubin) was a coauthor of the position statement.

For people with diabetes, both aerobic exercise and strength training have immediate positive effects on weight, blood glucose and blood pressure levels, cardiovascular risk factors, bone strength, risk of injury, and quality of life. These activities can also reduce a person's need to take medication to control blood glucose, blood pressure, and cholesterol levels. In the long term, these activities are also associated with longer life. There's evidence that combining aerobic exercises and strength training exercises increases these benefits.

There's less evidence for the benefits of flexibility training for people with diabetes, but that's probably because few researchers have studied flexibility training. It's safe to say that improving your flexibility is a good thing, even in the absence of conclusive evidence. Keep in mind that you should not count the time you spend in flexibility training toward your aerobic activity or strength training goals.

Of course, you have to exercise regularly to get these benefits. The American Diabetes Association recommends that people with diabetes perform at least 150 minutes of moderate-intensity aerobic exercise a week, spread over at least three days of the week with no more than two consecutive days without exercise. The ADA adds that unless your doctor recommends otherwise, people with diabetes should perform resistance training at least twice a week.

Latisha was 47 when she learned she had Type 2 diabetes. When her doctor suggested she start aerobic exercise and strength training to improve her health, she was pretty skeptical. "I haven't done any of that since I graduated from high school," she said. But she decided to give it a try. She started slowly, walking 15 minutes a couple of times a week, and in a few months she was up to 20 minutes four times a week. Good, but not as much as her doctor recommended. At her next appointment the doctor suggested Latisha exercise while

she watched television. That did the trick. Latisha did aerobics three nights
a week while watching her favorite shows, and she did strength training two
other nights using some stretch bands she bought. She was at her exercise goal
and she felt good.

Getting Ready

If you haven't exercised in years or you are considering a dramatic increase
in the amount or intensity of your exercise, talk it over with your health
care provider first. If you take insulin, ask whether you should decrease
your dose on exercise days. If you are older than 50, obese, or have a history
of heart disease, your health care provider may want to check your cardiac
status. Finally, if you have uncontrolled high blood pressure or complications of diabetes, such as severe proliferative retinopathy or neuropathy or
a history of foot ulcers, you should also talk to your health care provider
about the effect of exercise on these conditions. (See the section on exercising safely below.)

If you are reasonably healthy and if you use your head, you needn't be
frightened about starting to exercise. It is safe for almost everyone.

Once you know you can safely exercise, it's important to start slowly and
build up gradually. Experts recommend that you increase your exercise
by no more than 10% a week. That includes the duration and intensity of
aerobic exercise and the amount of weight used in strength training. For
example, if you haven't been physically active in a long time and you get
started by walking 30 minutes three times a week (total of 90 minutes), you
should not increase your total walking time by more than about 8–10 minutes in the second week. If you are a beginning exerciser, you might want to
be more conservative; a 5% increase each week might be best for you.

What activities do you like? Your chance of sticking with activities you enjoy
is good; your chance of sticking with activities you hate is poor. How can
you tell which exercise activities you might enjoy? Maybe you're already
doing something you like but not doing it often enough. Maybe you used to
enjoy a particular activity and you can pick it up again, like the former racquetball player quoted above. Maybe there's an activity you've always wanted to try because it looks like fun, like dancing. Or maybe you want to spend
more time with your best friend. Walking and talking can be a great way to
socialize. Whatever you choose, it should be something you *want* to do.

Do you prefer to exercise by yourself or with other people? Some people like solitude and an opportunity for contemplation or don't want the hassle of always scheduling someone else into their exercise time slot. Some people are embarrassed at the start by how out of shape they are and so avoid exercising with others (this won't last). A work or school schedule could also make exercising alone the best choice. But other people find that company helps them stick to their commitment and makes exercise more fun. Company can also make some outdoor activities safer, such as walking or running. Naturally, the choice of exercising alone or with a partner is not a lifetime decision. You can vary your pattern depending on circumstances and your disposition.

> *Guy could not get himself to exercise. He'd make commitments to himself time after time, but it never worked. Then one day a friend at work told him he had the same problem, and they decided to find a solution together. They had a 45-minute lunch break each day, so they decided to commit 20 minutes of that time to walking together. On days when the weather was good, they walked outside. On other days they walked the halls and added some intensity by taking the steps up and down a few floors. That gave Guy a jumpstart, making it easy for him to fit the rest of his weekly walking time into the weekend.*

Do you like competitive sports? Anything from jogging to swimming can be undertaken in a hotly competitive or totally noncompetitive mode. Which approach do you prefer?

What facilities do you need? If you like the idea of an aerobics class, what's available? What will it cost? If you're planning to swim, where's the pool? If you'd like to ski, how far away are the slopes, and what will you do for exercise when there's no snow? Whatever activity you are considering, you'll need to think through these issues of where, when, how, and how much. There is a very strong relationship between how *convenient* exercise is and how *often* and how *consistently* it's done.

> *Leo found the perfect place to exercise. His local YMCA was close by, the aerobics classes were inexpensive (some were even free), and he enjoyed the people. It was fun to socialize while exercising, especially because he was lonely a lot since his wife died. And exercising with others increased his motivation to stick with his commitment.*

Will you be better off exercising at home, outdoors, or in a specific facility? Some people say they can complete their entire exercise routine at or near home—using an exercise bike, walking, or jogging—in the time it would take them to get to the local health club. If finding time to exercise is a problem for you, this might be the way to go. Other people like the social atmosphere and the wide range of activities and equipment available at an exercise facility. You'll want to think seriously about what's going to work best for you. You may want to pay a visit to a health club, if you think you might enjoy it. Most clubs offer one-time visits or short-term trial memberships free or at very low cost. There is some evidence that people with diabetes who engage in supervised training are more likely than those who exercise on their own to stick with their routine and gain exercise benefits like better glucose control.

How intense an exercise program do you want? The intensity of exercise that is best for you depends on your age, physical conditioning, and motivation. Exercise intensity can be estimated by the pulse rate (which is the same as heart rate) you reach while you are exercising and how long you exercise.

To determine your heart rate while you are exercising, you have two choices: the old-fashioned manual way and the new-fangled way that involves a digital heart rate monitor. To check your heart rate manually, stop several times to check your pulse rate. Use the tips of your index and middle fingers to find your radial artery, on the thumb side of either wrist, just below the base of the thumb. You will feel the pulse when your fingers are in the right place. Hold gently. After locating the radial pulse, begin your count with "zero" on the starting time mark of your watch, then count the pulses for 10 seconds. Multiply the number of pulses by 6 and you will have your heart rate. Check your pulse quickly when you pause your exercise. If you wait too long the pulse rate will not be accurate. Resume exercising immediately after the pulse check so your heart rate does not have time to slow down, out of your training heart rate range.

Digital heart rate monitors have a major advantage—with a quick glance at the watch that's part of the system, you see your heart rate and percentage of target heart rate. You don't have to stop, check your pulse, and calculate. Digital heart monitors consist of the monitor itself, which is strapped to your chest, and a watch that displays the readings. Reliable monitors cost between $30 and $60.

Begin by calculating your maximum heart rate (approximately 220 minus your age). For example, if you're 50 years old, your approximate maximum heart rate is about 220 − 50 = 170 beats per minute. This number is then used in determining a good target zone for your exercise pulse rate.

Arlene's doctor told her to check her pulse rate while exercising to be sure she was in the right zone. The doctor calculated Arlene's maximum heart rate—220 – 60 (Arlene's age) = 160—and suggested she aim for a pulse rate of 100 (about 60% of her maximum rate) while exercising. Arlene went home and practiced getting her pulse rate when she wasn't exercising, to be sure she could do it. After a few tries she found she could. Then she tried while she was walking. Her rate was just a little lower than her target, so she picked up her pace a bit and soon was right where she needed to be.

The ADA recommends that aerobic exercise be at 50%-70% of maximum heart rate. So if your maximum heart rate is 170, your target heart rate should be between 85 and about 120.

If you are looking for higher levels of fitness, your exercise plan needs to be more ambitious, perhaps as high as 80% of your maximum heart rate. At the same time, make sure that it is realistic. Setting your goals too high will almost certainly lead to frustration or injury, and ultimately you probably won't stick with your exercise plan. Start where you are. If you are already fairly active, add a little to your current regimen or make exercise a more regular part of your routine. If you are basically sedentary, start with a modest regimen, maybe walking a few blocks several times a week. See Table 10 for exercise guidelines from the ADA and Table 11 for a list of activities and an account of how much energy you expend when engaging in them.

Getting Started

You're convinced of the benefits of exercise, you have selected an activity you think you will enjoy, and you have encouragement to get started from your health care provider. Now what? Getting started is one of the hardest parts of exercising (sticking with it is another). Most people have lots of excuses (some people call them "reasons") for not exercising regularly. Let's look at some of the most common ones.

I can't find time. We hear this one often, and for good reason. Exercise *does* take time, though probably not as much as you think. As we've mentioned, 30 minutes of moderate-intensity aerobic activity three times a week is a good starting exercise routine from which you can build. Think about how you might fit this into your busy schedule. Here are some tips provided by people with diabetes who have established the exercise habit:

—Schedule your exercise, just as you schedule anything else that really matters to you.

—Think about things you do that you could cut down on or cut out to make time for exercise.

—Plan to exercise when it works best for you. If you are an early bird, try to fit in part or all of your exercise before you start your day's other activities. If you are a night owl, exercise in the evening.

—Take a walk on your lunch break.

Table 10   American Diabetes Association Guidelines for Exercise

General Guidelines

• Use proper footwear and protective equipment.
• Avoid exercise in extreme heat or cold.
• Inspect your feet daily and after exercise.
• Avoid exercising during periods of poor blood glucose control.
• It you have advanced eye disease, balance problems, lightheadedness, or autonomic neuropathy, discuss the safety of exercise with your doctor before starting an exercise program.

Specifically for Those with Type 1 Diabetes

• Exercise is recommended to improve your diabetes control, cardiovascular fitness, and psychological well-being and for social interaction and recreation. Safe participation in all forms of exercise, consistent with your lifestyle, should be the main goal. Participation in competitive sports is possible if you so desire. You need to self-monitor your blood glucose so that necessary adjustments can be made in diet or insulin dosage.

Specifically for Those with Type 2 Diabetes

• Exercise should be part of your diabetes therapy to improve your blood glucose control, reduce your risk of cardiovascular complications, and increase your psychological well-being. An exercise stress test is recommended if you have other risk factors for heart disease and have been inactive. If you take a sulfonylurea type of pill or insulin, you need to self-monitor your blood glucose level before exercising. Your exercise program should include moderate aerobic exercise (50%–70% of maximum heart rate) for 150 minutes per week spread out over at least 3 days. Resistance training (use of light weights, for example) is also recommended at least twice per week.

Source. Copyright 2011 American Diabetes Association. From *American Diabetes Association Complete Guide to Diabetes.* Modified by permission of the American Diabetes Association.

Table 11 Energy Expenditure Associated with Common Exercises

Activity	Calories Burned Each Minute	Calories Burned in an Hour
Light housework; polishing furniture; light hand-washing of dishes, clothes, windows, etc.	2–2½	120–150
Golf, using power cart Level walking at 2 miles per hour	2½–4	150–240
Cleaning windows, mopping floors, or vacuuming Walking at 3 miles per hour Golf, pulling cart Cycling at 6 miles per hour Bowling	4–5	240–300
Scrubbing floors Cycling at 8 miles per hour Walking at 3½ miles per hour Table tennis, badminton, and volleyball Doubles tennis Golf, carrying clubs Many calisthenics and ballet exercises	5–6	300–360
Walking at 4 miles per hour Ice or roller skating Cycling at 10 miles per hour	6–7	360–420
Walking at 5 miles per hour Cycling at 11 miles per hour Water skiing Singles tennis	7–8	420–480
Jogging at 5 miles per hour Cycling at 12 miles per hour Downhill skiing	8–10	480–600
Running at 5½ miles per hour Cycling at 13 miles per hour Squash or handball (practice session)	10–11	600–660
Running at 6 miles or more per hour Competitive handball or squash	11 or more	660 or more

Source. Copyright 2011 American Diabetes Association. From *American Diabetes Association Complete Guide to Diabetes.* Modified by permission of the American Diabetes Association.

—Combine exercise with socializing. Instead of meeting a friend for coffee or lunch, take a walk together.

—Use the stairs. Ten minutes of climbing stairs burns the same number of calories as 10 minutes on a "stair stepper" at the gym.

—Exercise while you are doing things around the house. You can ride a stationary bike, lift weights, use exercise bands, or do other activities while watching your favorite television shows. An added benefit: if you exercise while watching television, you are less likely to snack.

I'm too old and out of shape. Recent studies show that it's never too late to start exercising. Many of the physical consequences of aging are primarily the result of inactivity. Regardless of your age, regular exercise can improve your mobility, strength, and endurance and provide many other health benefits.

We have heard countless stories of people with diabetes who are out of shape, begin to exercise, and go on to reach amazing heights.

Teresa was diagnosed with diabetes at the age of 32. A classic couch potato, she decided to take up running. The first day she couldn't make it to her corner mailbox. But she stuck with it, and within a year she could run a mile without stopping. At this point she really got the running bug and began to train harder and enter local weekend races. Eight years after her diagnosis, just after her fortieth birthday, Teresa completed a 100-mile race!

We aren't advocating this level of exercise, but we do believe that anyone at any age can enjoy the benefits of a healthy, active lifestyle.

Also keep in mind that you don't have to do all your exercise for the day in one session. Researchers found that people who did several short (10 minute) workouts during the day were more successful than people who did the same amount of total daily exercise in a single workout. The short-workout people stuck with their workouts more consistently, exercised more days a week, and lost more weight.

Exercise hurts. If you do it right, exercise shouldn't hurt. Sure, you may get winded and your muscles may stiffen up a bit (when you first get started). Working up a sweat and getting winded are part of exercise. But the expression "no pain, no gain" is just plain wrong—unless, perhaps, your goal is to be a professional athlete. (See below for a discussion of how to keep exercise safe.) Remember, you are trying to develop an exercise program for life. If you are pushing so hard that it hurts, you need to ease up. Rethink your exercise program and consider switching to a less stressful activity, or check with your health care provider.

Exercise is boring. For some people this is a real problem. If you are one, there are several things that might help. First, try to combine exercise with things you like to do, such as walking in a pretty place or watching a good movie on DVD or videotape while you do aerobics. As we said, you might find an exercise partner or take up a competitive sport. We all have days when we just don't feel like exercising. If you have an exercise partner whom you can't let down, you'll be more likely to get out there and exercise even if you don't feel like it.

Another way to avoid boredom is to cross-train, or vary your exercise routine. If walking is your main activity, consider an occasional swim, a bike ride, or an evening of dancing. Cross-training not only cuts boredom, it also gives you a more balanced workout and reduces your risk of overuse injuries.

Benjamin was doing great with his exercise program, walking briskly for 30 minutes five days a week and lifting weights while he watched television twice a week. Then winter came and it was harder to get out five days to walk. He still made it on most days, but some days it was just too cold. His wife suggested he "cross-train" on days when he couldn't walk outside. They downloaded some of their favorite sixties' rock-and-roll hits, rolled up the dining room carpet, and danced until they dropped a couple of nights a week. Good exercise and great fun.

You may also be able to stave off exercise boredom by treating yourself to an exercise-related gift from time to time. If that beautiful sweat jacket would help you stick with your routine, get it.

I just can't maintain my motivation. There are several ways to avoid this pitfall. First, set goals. Those who succeed *plan* for success. Consider writing an exercise contract with yourself. This kind of formal planning may be a big help. Your contract can be a simple one that you draft in a few minutes. It might look something like this:

Exercise Contract

Exercise goal for week of: July 3
Activity: Walking 12 blocks in 30 min. 3 times

Exercise goal for week of: July 10
Activity: Walking 15 blocks in 35 min. 3 times

Exercise goal for week of: July 17
Activity: Walking 15 blocks in 30 min. 4 times

An added benefit of a weekly contract is that it keeps you from getting discouraged by the inevitably slow progress you will make toward your long-term goals. To maximize your motivation, have both short-term and long-term goals.

Notice that the contract states goals in terms of behavior. It's better to set behavioral goals, because behavior is something you can control. In contrast, if you set a goal of, say, losing a pound a week, you might do everything you could to make it happen and still not succeed. Besides, if you meet your exercise (and diet) goals, you will also reach your weight loss goals.

Another way to maximize motivation is to keep in mind why you want to be more physically active. The reason shouldn't be that your doctor or spouse told you that you should—this reason is not likely to keep you on track for the long run. You are most likely to keep on track when you have personal, positive reasons, like being around to see your grandchildren grow up, being able to work in the garden, or being able to do the other things that really matter to you.

Also, keep track of your progress. Pay attention to the personal benefits of being more active, whether it's feeling fitter, feeling better about yourself, sleeping better, or anything else you might notice. Keeping these benefits in mind can help keep your motivation high or rekindle it when it flags.

It also helps to recognize that no one is perfect—not even your most physically fit friend. There will be days, and even weeks, when you don't meet your goals. The key to coping with these rough spots is to see them as lapses or plateaus, not failures. You've simply had a bad day or week (even world-class athletes have slumps). You can put the lapse behind you and get back with the program. If you take the opposite tack and tell yourself you've failed, you create a self-fulfilling prophecy: your motivation evaporates and you continue to slide.

So be good to yourself. Give yourself credit for your hard work and accomplishments. And pay attention to how you feel when you work out regularly. Most people tell us they feel better: stronger, healthier, more energetic, and more confident. Don't lose sight of these benefits, especially if you feel your commitment beginning to flag. That's when you most need to accentuate the positive.

Exercising Safely

We have talked about the importance of not trying to do too much too soon when it comes to exercise. This is not a book on sports medicine, but we can still tell you that pulled muscles and strained ligaments are a definite risk when you take up exercise directly from the couch potato position. So start slowly and work out regularly. If a muscle pull occurs, back off. There are also some cautions about exercise that apply specifically to people with diabetes, which we'll review here.

Exercise and Blood Glucose

Exercise will affect your blood glucose levels; in most but not all cases, it will lower those levels. If you don't take insulin or a class of diabetes drugs called *sulfonylureas*, the risk of your blood glucose going too low as a result of exercise is minimal. If you do take these medications, you may need to adjust the doses. As you become familiar with how exercise affects *your* blood glucose, you'll learn how to reduce your risk of hypoglycemia or hyperglycemia.

As we discussed in Chapter 5, exercise can affect glucose levels for quite a long time—in the range of 6–12 or even 24 hours. When you start to exercise, you may need less insulin or oral antihyperglycemic medication, for example, or you may need more food (see Table 12). Timely self-monitoring of blood glucose is the key to making these adjustments safely and effectively. If you don't check, you'll never know why you feel different.

Especially if you take insulin, you may notice some surprising effects of exercise. For instance, the same amount of insulin may lower your blood glucose more than it used to. This may be especially noticeable the day *after* exercise. Exercise also increases the rate at which insulin is absorbed from your injection site, so your insulin may start to work more quickly than usual. This is particularly true if you injected your insulin in a part of your body that you are exercising vigorously. On the other hand, very strenuous exercise can increase the amount of glucose the liver releases into your bloodstream, so sometimes your blood glucose level actually *increases*, especially right after exercise.

Table 12   Strategies to Avoid Hypoglycemia and Hyperglycemia with Exercise

1. Eat a meal 1–3 hours before exercise.

2. Take supplemental carbohydrate feedings during exercise at least every 30 minutes if exercise is vigorous and of long duration.

3. Increase food intake for up to 24 hours after exercise, depending on intensity and duration of exercise.

4. Take insulin at least 1 hour before exercise. If less than 1 hour before exercise, inject in a non-exercising area.

5. Decrease insulin dose before exercise.

6. Alter daily insulin schedule.

7. Monitor blood glucose before, during, and after exercise.

8. Delay exercise if blood glucose is over 250 mg/dl (over 14 mM) and ketones are present.

9. Learn individual glucose responses to different types of exercise.

Source. Copyright 2009 American Diabetes Association. From *Therapy for Diabetes Mellitus and Related Disorders*, 5th Edition. Reprinted by permission of the American Diabetes Association.

In sum, when you exercise, you have to watch out for both hypoglycemia and hyperglycemia. Try to sort out for yourself what a given type of exercise does to your glucose level. Just be aware that the effect could depend on a combination of exactly how much exercise, how vigorous the exercise, when you took your last insulin shot, and when you last ate. Sorting it all out can be complicated. But you will find patterns, and this will help you make adjustments so that exercising will be safe and you can enjoy all the benefits of an active lifestyle.

Exercise and Long-Term Diabetes Complications

Exercise does not cause long-term complications; on the contrary, there is evidence that it may help prevent them. But several complications, if already at a relatively advanced stage, may be aggravated by exercise. Strength training and vigorous aerobic activity may not be safe if you have serious (proliferative) retinopathy or have had multiple bleeds in your eyes.

Significant peripheral neuropathy (see Chapter 25) increases your risk for soft tissue and joint injuries, since you are less likely to feel the trauma.

You have to be much more careful of footwear. Take measures to avoid blisters or foot trauma, and inspect your feet especially carefully. You may want to choose low-intensity exercise such as walking, using a stationary bike or low-intensity rowing machine, or swimming. Be sure to wear proper shoes and to check your feet daily for blisters or other signs of injury. If you have an open sore, don't do any weight-bearing exercise.

Autonomic neuropathy (see Chapter 25) may reduce your capacity for high-intensity exercise because it can decrease your maximum heart rate and cardiac capacity. In this case, select a lower-intensity exercise.

Exercise training increases physical function and quality of life for people with kidney disease and may even be undertaken during dialysis sessions. Even after kidney or pancreas transplantation, exercise is important. Prednisone, the drug people take to prevent organ rejection, causes weight gain, muscle wasting, and weakness. Aerobic exercise and resistance or strength training are the best ways to fight these side effects of prednisone.

Exercise during Pregnancy

Exercising during your pregnancy helps you stay fit, control your weight gain, increase your strength and stamina, and reduce back pain. Exercise can also help you control your blood glucose levels, which is especially important when you are pregnant. If you already exercise regularly, you can probably continue with your routine as long as you take special precautions. Don't do exercises that involve straining, holding your breath, or making jerky movements or do anything that might increase your core body temperature above 100 degrees (such as exercising in extreme heat or taking saunas or whirlpool baths for longer than 10 minutes).

If you did not exercise regularly before pregnancy, this isn't the time to start a *strenuous* new program. Low-intensity activity, on the other hand, might be a wonderful idea. Check with your health care provider to discuss the best plan for you.

Exercise for Older Adults

Physical abilities inevitably decline with age. Even the serious athlete loses speed and fast reflexes. For recreational athletes or "weekend warriors," much of the decline is a result of simple inactivity. So increased activity in the form of sensible exercise can provide older adults with the same benefits it offers younger people.

Older adults with diabetes should have a pre-exercise physical examination and work out an exercise prescription with their health care provider. Once you begin exercising, you'll need to keep certain precautions in mind. Starting slowly and building up gradually is especially important. Not letting your heart rate rise above about 60%–70% of maximum is also a good idea. You may want to stay away from exercises that require fast movements and quick changes of direction, because coordination and reaction time can slow with age.

There are many aerobic activities to choose from, like walking, water aerobics, swimming, and biking outdoors or using a stationary bike. But don't forget about strength training. Studies show that it is great for older adults. In older men with Type 2 diabetes, progressive strength training improved insulin sensitivity to the same extent as or even more than aerobic exercise. And clinical trials provide strong evidence for the glucose-lowering value of strength training and the additive benefit of combining aerobic and strength training for adults with Type 2 diabetes.

Hannah was 70 years old when she was diagnosed with diabetes. Her doctor told her about the benefits of both aerobic activity and strength training for older adults with diabetes, and Hannah jumped on the advice. She had been an athlete when she was younger and had never completely stopped being active. Getting diabetes just took her motivation to be fit to another level. She joined her local gym (with a senior discount) and was soon enjoying the company, the water aerobics, and the strength training equipment.

You can lift weights, do calisthenics, or use exercise bands at home or at your local Y, health club, community college, or recreation center.

If you have difficulty with balance and standing, chair exercises can help you improve your strength, coordination, and flexibility. You can gain these benefits in as little as 30 minutes a day, and you can watch television or listen to music at the same time.

For older people, one special alert is chest pain. *Angina* (also called *angina pectoris*) is a characteristic kind of chest pain that usually occurs when exercising and is suggestive of heart trouble. It is usually described as heaviness, squeezing, or tightness that occurs beneath the breastbone and may go into the back, jaw, or left arm, stopping within a minute or so after you stop exercising. If you have any sort of chest pain, be sure to stop exercising right away and have it checked out by your doctor.

Exercising to Lose Weight

Exercise helps you lose weight because it burns calories. But it's hard to exercise enough to lose much weight unless you also make some changes in your eating habits. You would probably have to exercise an hour every single day to lose a pound a week through exercise alone. That would mean walking or running 6 miles or swimming for an hour, every day. There is some evidence that exercise can help you keep off weight you have lost. That's because exercise can help prevent the slowdown in your metabolism that often follows substantial weight loss.

Take Home Messages

- Types of beneficial exercise include aerobic activity, strength training, and flexibility training.
- Aerobic activity and strength training can help improve blood glucose, blood pressure, and cholesterol control, reduce your risk of injury, and improve both your quality of life and your chances for a longer life.
- The American Diabetes Association recommends at least 150 minutes of moderate-intensity aerobic activity a week and strength training at least twice a week.
- Plan for success by picking activities you like and by deciding where and when exercise works best for you.
- Address barriers to exercise by integrating your workouts into your daily schedule and by finding ways to maintain your motivation.
- Learn how exercise affects *your* blood glucose control and make any necessary adjustments.
- If you have any long-term diabetes complications, take these into account when planning your exercise.
- Older adults benefit from both aerobic activity and strength training.

Treating Type 2 Diabetes with Non-insulin Medications

with Shabina Ahmed, M.D.

- "I want to take pills for my diabetes, I don't want to take insulin."
- "The pills used to work perfectly well for me, but now they aren't as effective. What am I doing wrong?"
- "Whenever a doctor says I should take a pill, I want to know what side effects it could cause. I read the insert that comes with the bottle, and then I get upset. How should I interpret what's written in the insert?"
- "I'm always hearing about new pills for diabetes. What's really new? What's proven? What's good for me?"

During World War II, a French army doctor wrote a letter from the front to tell a colleague about a strange observation he had made. When he treated soldiers' combat wounds with the new sulfa antibiotics, some of the soldiers acted as if they had taken too much insulin. His colleague tried to duplicate the finding in dogs and found that their blood glucose levels did indeed go down when they were given sulfa pills. He then removed the pancreas from some dogs and found that in these animals, the sulfa drugs had no effect on blood glucose levels.

That discovery marked a change in the treatment of diabetes. Other medications and herbs had been shown to have small effects on blood glucose levels, but the sulfa derivatives, called *sulfonylureas*, have a major effect in lowering blood glucose, and these became the first of many pills to be used in the treatment of Type 2 diabetes.

In over 60 years of use, pills for treating diabetes—the *oral antihyperglycemic agents*—have undergone some changes, and new agents have come along. Used in the right setting, they are outstanding in their effectiveness. Many people with diabetes are treated successfully with these drugs. But like all medications, they have their limitations and side effects. In this chapter we review the principles for using oral antihyperglycemic agents and take a closer look at the specific drugs.

How the Oral Antihyperglycemic Agents Work

Two fundamental features of oral antihyperglycemic agents are that *they are not insulin* and *they cannot take the place of insulin.* The French researchers first demonstrated this when they removed the pancreas of the dogs and discovered that the sulfa drug no longer lowered blood glucose levels. This meant that the drug needed an intact, insulin-producing pancreas. This is true of all pills that are used to treat diabetes: the person has to be making at least some insulin from his or her own pancreas. So far there has been very little success in giving insulin itself by mouth. Insulin is a fragile chemical that is immediately destroyed by the stomach acids if taken orally, so it must be given by injection.

The practical implication is that oral antihyperglycemic agents will not work for people who have Type 1 diabetes. The pills often do not work well even for Type 2 diabetes if it has progressed to the point where the person is producing very little insulin from the pancreas.

How do the oral antihyperglycemic agents work? One class of these agents, which includes metformin, acts by assisting the action of insulin on the body's tissues (see Figure 15). As discussed in Chapter 2, insulin resistance (a lessened effect of insulin) is a major problem in Type 2 diabetes. There's still some uncertainty about metformin's mechanism of action, but we know that it primarily works to decrease glucose production in the liver. In persons with Type 2 diabetes, the liver makes about twice as much glucose as usual, so the blood glucose level can rise even when they are not eating. Metformin also helps the body's tissues take up and use glucose properly by improving the effects of insulin. Reviews of many studies of metformin have also discovered reduced rates of cancer and death from cancer in persons using metformin.

The sulfonylurea and meglitinide classes of antihyperglycemic agents act primarily by stimulating insulin production by the pancreas (see Figure 16). They act like a booster, giving the pancreas an additional push. They are effective because they not only help the pancreas put out more insulin throughout the day and night but also help it make more insulin at mealtimes.

A third type of pill, the alpha-glucosidase inhibitors (acarbose and miglitol), slows the breakdown and absorption of carbohydrates (starches) in

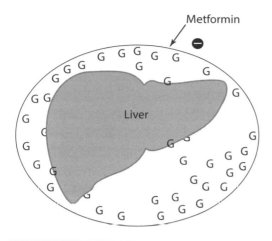

Figure 15. Metformin lowers the blood glucose level indirectly by decreasing the amount of glucose (G) released from the liver.

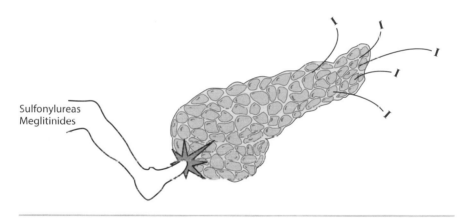

Figure 16. Sulfonylureas and meglitinides lower the blood glucose by causing the pancreas to make more insulin (I). In effect, they give the pancreas a kick to work harder.

the small intestine (see Figure 17). The effect is to reduce the rise in blood glucose after a meal.

A fourth class of pills for diabetes includes the drugs pioglitazone and rosiglitazone. They act by enhancing the action of insulin. Since insulin resistance is a basic problem in Type 2 diabetes, these drugs were initially welcomed as a useful addition to its treatment. However, since they first be-

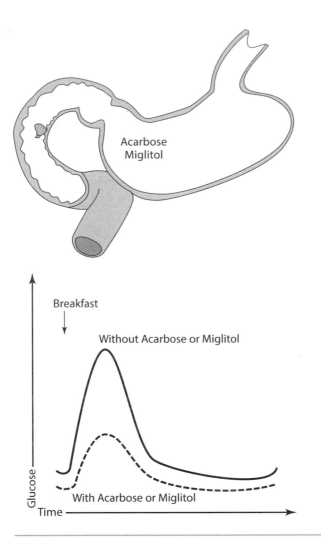

Figure 17. Acarbose and miglitol work in the intestinal tract to slow the absorption of glucose into the bloodstream. This helps to keep the after-meal blood glucose level from going too high.

came available for use, drugs in this class have been shown to have potential adverse side effects, discussed in greater detail below.

Another class of oral antihyperglycemic drugs is the dipeptidyl peptidase 4 (DPP-4) inhibitors. There are currently three drugs in this class: sitagliptin, saxagliptin, and linagliptin. These are medications that help stimulate insulin release in response to a meal, but only when the blood glucose is high, so they do not lead to hypoglycemia when used alone. DPP-4 inhibitors slow the rate at which the stomach empties (stomach emptying), giving the pancreas more time to produce insulin. They also lower the amount of glucose produced by the liver by reducing the release of the hormone glucagon.

Canagliflozin is a medication in the newest class of oral antihyperglycemic agents, the SGLT2 inhibitors, which prevent absorption of glucose by the kidneys. This leads to glucose loss in the urine, a fall in blood glucose, and some weight loss.

Two other classes of drugs that act as antihyperglycemics are glucagon-like peptide 1 (GLP-1) agonists and amylin analogs; these drugs are given by subcutaneous injection rather than taken by mouth. The two GLP-1 agonists, exenatide and liraglutide, work to slow stomach emptying, promote insulin production in response to a meal, reduce appetite, and decrease the secretion of glucagon. The amylin analog pramlintide also slows stomach emptying and decreases appetite and glucagon secretion. It differs from the GLP-1 agonists in that it can be used in Type 1 diabetes, though some studies suggest that GLP-1 drugs may also be useful for people with Type 1 diabetes.

How to Use Oral Antihyperglycemic Agents

As we've noted, the oral antihyperglycemic agents are useful for treating Type 2 diabetes but not for Type 1 diabetes, though metformin can be used for persons with Type 1 diabetes who also have insulin resistance. With the exception of metformin and glyburide, oral agents are also not used for treating gestational diabetes mellitus (GDM), given the possibility of causing injury to the developing fetus. Sometimes when it is not clear whether the correct diagnosis is Type 1 or Type 2 diabetes, the oral agents may be given a trial use.

For best effect, the oral antihyperglycemic agents should be taken regularly every day, not taken irregularly or started and stopped according to blood glucose levels. A wide range of doses are available for several of these drugs, so if the blood glucose is running too high or too low, the dose can be changed. So, to emphasize: these medications are not meant to be used just when you are feeling bad or just when your blood glucose is running high. They can be stopped and restarted later, but this should be done in consultation with your health care professional, not on a whim.

Of course, you should not use a medication if you have an allergic reaction to it. An allergic reaction is typically characterized by a rash all over the body, hives, or difficulty breathing. A true allergy to other sulfa drugs, such as the antibiotics often used to treat urinary tract infections, may signal an allergy to the sulfonylureas also. If you are allergic to sulfas in general, discuss this with your health care provider before beginning to take a sulfonylurea for diabetes. Also, if you have significant stomach symptoms such as nausea, vomiting, or heartburn while taking a medication, stop the medication until you can talk it over with your provider.

Perhaps the most important thing to know about using oral antihyperglycemic agents is that *they are not a substitute for diet and exercise*. People who think they can give up efforts to follow a healthy diet and get regular exercise when they take their pills will be sorely disappointed. Type 2 diabetes is fundamentally a condition treated with diet and exercise, whether or not oral agents or insulin are also necessary.

When the Non-insulin Agents Don't Work

As has been known since the introduction of these drugs in the 1950s, for some people with Type 2 diabetes, the pills work for a while and then lose their effectiveness. Other individuals may continue to respond to pills indefinitely, especially if they follow a good diet, exercise regularly, and control their weight. Needing pills to control your diabetes does not mean you'll end up needing insulin. (Chapter 3 describes how to tell when your treatment is and is not working.)

The general understanding is that the oral antihyperglycemic agents no longer work if the pancreas becomes progressively less able to produce insulin. This natural deterioration of pancreatic function with age occurs in everyone and is the reason diabetes is more common as people grow older. For persons with diabetes, loss of insulin production means other medications become less effective. Therefore, many people with diabetes may end up needing to have insulin added to their other diabetes medications to keep their blood glucose level under good control. Most people prefer to try using the pills rather than moving directly from diet to insulin, even if their response to oral agents lasts only a few years. However, your health care provider may advise you to take insulin early on, even when the diabetes is first diagnosed, if your blood glucose levels are very high—a situation in which pills are often not effective. With time, insulin can sometimes be tapered off as diet, exercise, and pills take their effect.

Adding a different class of oral antihyperglycemic agent, such as adding a sulfonylurea to the treatment regimen of a person who is slipping out of control on metformin alone, may be effective. Individuals often take two or more agents to achieve control of their blood glucose. Another approach that can be very effective is *combined therapy*—that is, the use of insulin and oral agents. This can be tried when the morning (fasting) blood glucose is elevated but blood glucose levels during the day are in a better range. An injection of intermediate-acting or long-acting insulin at bedtime works to lower the liver's glucose production overnight, leading to a better fasting glucose level. Oral agents can then more effectively control blood glucose levels during the day.

Eventually, in many cases, after years of diabetes and when oral antihyperglycemics are no longer effective, both long and short-acting insulin may be needed to keep blood glucose levels under control. If this is the case, your doctor may discontinue some of your oral agents.

Specific Oral Antihyperglycemic Agents

We describe in more detail here the oral antihyperglycemic agents now available (see Table 13), so that you can learn more about the one you take or might be taking and get a good idea of what to expect. We are not trying to provide comprehensive descriptions or to replace the printed material you get with each prescription, but just trying to sort out the most significant differences between medications and to distinguish the more common and the rarer side effects.

Metformin

Metformin became available in the United States in 1995, although it had been used elsewhere for more than 30 years. In the 1960s and 1970s, a large clinical trial was carried out comparing the sulfonylurea tolbutamide (Orinase) and the metformin-like drug phenformin with the use of insulin or diet alone. The study was called the University Group Diabetes Program (UGDP). There were slightly more deaths among participants taking the two oral agents than in the other study groups. Much commentary has been published discussing the UGDP and whether its findings were "real." The FDA could not agree on whether the sulfonylurea used in the study (tolbutamide) was safe. In the end, tolbutamide and other sulfonylureas were not banned but were made available only with a frightening warning on the

Table 13 Oral and Non-insulin Injectable Diabetes Medications

Generic Name	Brand Name(s)	Maximum Daily Dose	Comments
Metformin	Glucophage	2,550 mg	Diarrhea and bloating can occur; better with time and will improve with dose reduction. Improves cholesterol panel, mild weight loss; seems to lessen heart disease and reduce the risk of several cancers. Does not cause hypoglycemia.
Sulfonylureas			Work by stimulating the pancreas to make more insulin. Hypoglycemia is their main potential side effect.
Glipizide	Glucotrol	20 mg	To be taken on an empty stomach; food delays absorption.
Glipizide–extended release	Glucotrol XL	20 mg	Do not break tablet; may be taken once a day.
Glyburide	DiaBeta, Micronase	20 mg	
Glyburide–micronized	Glynase	12 mg	Not equivalent in action to glyburide.
Glimepiride	Amaryl	8 mg	
Meglitinides			Take before each carb-containing meal. Hypoglycemia is main potential side effect for both drugs.
Repaglinide	Prandin	4 mg	
Nateglinide	Starlix	120 mg	
Alpha-glucosidase inhibitors			Take before each carb-containing meal. Gas, bloating, and diarrhea are common side effects. Do not cause hypoglycemia.
Acarbose	Precose	100 mg	
Miglitol	Glyset	100 mg	
Thiazolidinediones			Both drugs can cause weight gain and swelling, worsen heart failure, increase fractures in postmenopausal women. Rosiglitazone seems to increase the risk of heart attacks. Pioglitazone seems to increase the risk of bladder cancer.
Rosiglitazone	Avandia	8 mg	
Pioglitazone	Actos	45 mg	
DPP-4 inhibitors			Work by stimulating insulin, also reduce liver production of glucose. Rarely, seem to cause pancreatitis.
Sitagliptin	Januvia	100 mg	
Saxagliptin	Onglyza	5 mg	
Linagliptin	Tradjenta	5 mg	

Generic Name	Brand Name(s)	Maximum Daily Dose	Comments
GLP-1 agonists			Injectable. Work by stimulating insulin, also reduce liver production of glucose. Rarely, seem to cause pancreatitis.
Exenatide	Byetta Bydureon	20 mcg* 2 mg weekly	
Liraglutide	Victoza	1.8 mg	
Amylin analogs			Injectable. Taken before meals. Works by slowing stomach emptying, reducing liver production of glucose, and inducing satiety (fullness). Nausea is common. Can cause low blood glucose reactions in combination with insulin.
Pramlintide	Symlin	120 mcg*	
SGLT2 inhibitors			Works by blocking glucose absorption in the kidneys, leading to increased glucose in the urine. Causes mild weight loss. Increases risk of genital yeast infections and causes increased urination.
Canagliflozin	Invokana	300 mg	

*mcg = microgram (one-thousandth of a milligram, mg).

package insert. Tolbutamide is no longer used to treat diabetes, and the currently used sulfonylureas seem to be safe.

The case against phenformin was considered stronger. It clearly (though rarely) caused a very dangerous and sometimes fatal complication called lactic acidosis. The FDA therefore decided to ban phenformin and metformin (a related drug), although metformin does not seem to cause lactic acidosis in otherwise healthy persons. Not until 1995, after more than 20 years of additional experience worldwide and after completion of careful trials in the United States, was metformin deemed to be safe and made available in this country.

Many large studies have since emerged that demonstrate the safety and effectiveness of metformin and the sulfonylureas, including the United Kingdom Prospective Diabetes Study Group (UKPDS), the Veterans Affairs Diabetes Trial (VADT), the Action to Control Cardiovascular Risk in Diabetes (ACCORD) trial, and the Action in Diabetes and Vascular Disease: Preterax and Diamicron Modified Release Controlled Evaluation (ADVANCE) trial.

Metformin is usually taken in a total daily dose of about 1–2.5 grams divided into two or three doses, preferably taken with meals. It is available in 500 mg, 750 mg, 850 mg, and 1,000 mg tablets. An extended-release form of metformin may be taken once daily.

Metformin's mechanism of action is not fully understood. The one area of agreement is that it does *not* cause the pancreas to secrete more insulin. Instead, it seems to act at two sites: it primarily helps insulin suppress new glucose production by the liver, and it increases insulin's effect in tissues throughout the body (especially muscle), promoting more effective use of glucose by the tissues. In these ways metformin acts to lower blood glucose, and it definitely needs to have insulin around to have an effect. Metformin also lowers triglycerides and LDL cholesterol by a small amount, and it reduces the levels of abnormal clotting factors that promote blood vessel disease. In the UKPDS, overweight participants taking metformin were shown to have fewer heart attacks, strokes, and diabetes-related deaths than participants taking other medications for their diabetes.

Metformin should be one of the first drugs considered for the treatment of Type 2 diabetes. As we've mentioned, it can be used with insulin (even by people who have Type 1 diabetes with insulin resistance) or with other oral antihyperglycemics. It is safe for use by pregnant women. Recent studies also show that metformin may be protective against pancreatic and other cancers because of its effects on cell growth. More studies need to be done to confirm its anticancer effects.

Side effects of metformin. For many people, one consequence of metformin use is weight loss—or at least, less weight gain. This effect is useful in treating people with Type 2 diabetes, given that most are overweight. Some people taking metformin find that their food has less taste, which may be why they eat less and lose weight. The weight-reducing effect of metformin is inconsistent and needs further study.

The most common side effects of metformin are gastrointestinal (GI) distress, consisting of diarrhea, bloating, abdominal discomfort, or nausea. GI side effects occur in as many as 30% of people taking the drug, but they are less of a problem when starting with a low dose and gradually building it up. Usually, the GI side effects gradually go away with time or if the metformin dose is reduced, and they do not generally cause people to stop taking the medication.

We noted above that metformin does not usually cause lactic acidosis, and this seems to be true *unless* you have certain conditions that predispose you to building up lactic acid in your blood. These conditions include congestive heart failure, severe vascular (circulatory) disease, and advanced kidney or liver disease. In these cases, metformin should be used with caution or not at all. Also, if you are undergoing an X-ray dye study or surgery, you should not take metformin that day and for 48 hours afterward, until tests show that your kidney function has not declined.

Sulfonylureas and Meglitinides

The sulfonylureas have been used for more than 40 years and are effective in treating many people with Type 2 diabetes who do not respond adequately to diet and exercise alone. Indeed, these were the only pills available from the 1970s to 1995 (when metformin and acarbose were approved by the FDA). They act by stimulating the pancreas to make more of its own insulin. If the pancreas is too weak to make much insulin, the sulfonylureas are not effective. And even if they work for a while, these agents may not be effective permanently because everyone's pancreas tends to weaken over the years.

The meglitinides are a subclass of drugs that work like the sulfonylureas but are shorter acting, promoting pancreatic insulin secretion only for several hours after a meal. The two available meglitinides are repaglinide (Prandin) and nateglinide (Starlix). They are taken before each meal. Their side effects are similar to those of the sulfonylureas (described below).

Five sulfonylurea drugs are available in the United States (see Table 13). There are some differences among them, but the similarities are much greater than the differences. They all act by the same basic mechanisms and share some of the same side effects, and there is little evidence that if you fail to respond to one sulfonylurea, you will respond to another.

Chlorpropamide and tolbutamide, the so-called first-generation sulfonylureas, have been in used since the 1950s. They are now used only rarely in clinical practice as second-generation sulfonylureas have come into wider use.

The second-generation sulfonylureas—glyburide (DiaBeta, Micronase), glipizide (Glucotrol, Glucotrol XL), and glimepiride (Amaryl)—became available in the mid-1980s. They are taken at much lower doses than the first-generation sulfonylureas (1–40 *mg* rather than 0.1–3 *grams*), but they act in very much the same way. Glyburide (also called glibenclamide) has an intermediate duration of action and is taken once or twice daily; glipizide has a shorter action, requiring twice-daily doses. Glucotrol XL is a form of glipizide with a long (24-hour) duration of action. Glimepiride also has long-acting properties and can be taken once a day.

There are some relatively minor advantages to the newer, second-generation sulfonylureas, such as fewer side effects and less frequent or less serious interactions with other medications a person may be taking. Glyburide is also safe for use by pregnant women. Because glyburide has a longer duration of action and its breakdown products are active, it carries a slightly higher risk of low blood glucose reactions than the other second-generation sulfonylureas.

Side effects of sulfonylureas. The most common side effect of the sulfonylureas and meglitinides is hypoglycemia. In a sense, this is not a side effect at all but just an extreme of the intended purpose of the pill. Most people who start taking sulfonylureas have significant hyperglycemia (high blood glucose), and it is not common for them to overrespond to the pills and have their glucose levels go too low. But this can happen, especially if the diabetes is mild, meals are delayed, or food intake is markedly reduced, and especially among older and lower-weight individuals.

If you think you may have hypoglycemia due to sulfonylureas, it is important to document it. Check your blood glucose at the time you are having symptoms (see Chapter 5 for a description of symptoms). Remember that fatigue, hunger, sweating, and nervousness are not always due to hypoglycemia. That's why we want you to prove to yourself that your glucose is actually low (for example, less than 60–70 mg/dl) when you are having symptoms, not to automatically assume that you are hypoglycemic.

If hypoglycemia does occur, the treatment is to eat some carbohydrate right away. If it happens with any regularity, your dosage needs to be reduced or the medication stopped altogether.

Other side effects are much less common. Gastrointestinal side effects such as nausea, heartburn, or a full feeling in the stomach occur in less than 2% of people taking these drugs, and these symptoms may go away spontaneously. If they persist, a lower dose may help. Liver function tests may show abnormal results, and rarely, the liver abnormalities are severe enough to cause jaundice, in which case the drug should be stopped right away. Significant anemia is even rarer but has been reported, as have other rare side effects. For individuals with evidence of liver problems or anemia, the condition must be evaluated carefully because it may or may not be due to the sulfonylurea.

True allergy to sulfonylureas occurs in less than 2% of users and usually results in a faint red skin rash on the torso or over the entire body. As noted earlier, people who are allergic to other sulfa-containing drugs such as the sulfa antibiotics are more likely to be allergic to sulfonylureas. But you should be sure to distinguish a true drug allergy from other side effects or unrelated problems. Drug allergies, like food allergies, usually start with a widespread skin rash, which may progress to hives, swelling around the eyes or in the joints, or even wheezing and severe difficulty breathing. This is very different from milder problems such as a full feeling in the stomach, headache, or diarrhea, which are usually better described as an *intolerance* than as an *allergy*. As with most drugs, a serious overdose of a sulfonylurea can be very dangerous. The effect would be to cause severe hypoglycemia, possibly with lethargy, changes in speech, inability to think clearly, or even seizures and coma. This is not likely to occur if someone takes a relatively mild overdose (such as double the usual dose in one day), but it could certainly happen, for example, if a child were to take a handful of pills.

Alpha-glucosidase Inhibitors

Acarbose (Precose) and miglitol (Glyset), alpha-glucosidase inhibitors, act by blocking the enzymes in the small intestine that break down the long chains of sugars in complex carbohydrates into their sugar building blocks, which are absorbed into the bloodstream. The effect of blocking this breakdown is to slow the absorption of carbohydrate, as glucose, into the blood. In this way, these drugs reduce the after-meal rise in blood glucose. They do not depend on insulin for their effect. In fact, they are barely absorbed into the blood; their real action takes place locally, in the intestine. You should take them as soon as you begin a meal.

The downside of acarbose and miglitol is that they cause increased gas production in the intestine in as many as three-fourths of users and produce diarrhea and abdominal pain in a smaller percentage of individuals. These side effects can be reduced by starting with a low dose and building up the dose gradually, but they do reduce the acceptability of these drugs as a medication for everyone. Elevations in liver function tests are uncommon with their use.

Thiazolidinediones

Rosiglitazone and pioglitazone are drugs that work by decreasing insulin resistance. They also improve cholesterol levels by lowering triglycerides and LDL cholesterol and by raising HDL ("good") cholesterol. A single study showed a reduced combined risk of death from all causes, from nonfatal heart attacks, and from stroke with the use of pioglitazone.

An older drug of this class, troglitazone, was pulled from the market because it was found to cause liver injury. Rosiglitazone use was severely restricted in 2011 following studies that showed an increased risk of heart attacks. The FDA has restricted the use of rosiglitazone to persons who are already taking the drug and who cannot take other medications to control their diabetes. Both rosiglitazone and pioglitazone have also been shown to increase the risk of heart failure, mostly in individuals with preexisting heart disease, and to increase the risk of fractures in postmenopausal women. Lastly, a slightly increased risk of bladder cancer has been found with pioglitazone. For now, pioglitazone should be used only after discussing the pros and cons with your health care provider.

DPP-4 Inhibitors

The DPP-4 inhibitors include sitagliptin, saxagliptin, and linagliptin. They work by blocking the breakdown of GLP-1, a hormone released by the small intestine after a meal. GLP-1 helps slow stomach emptying, increase insulin production, and decrease the release of glucagon from the pancreas, lowering the production of glucose by the liver. The advantages of this class of drugs are that they may be used by people with kidney problems (even those who undergo dialysis) and that hypoglycemia is very uncommon. A combination pill with metformin and sitagliptin is available but may not be used by individuals with kidney or liver disease. Side effects of DPP-4 inhibitors include pancreatitis (rarely) and infrequent nausea, diarrhea, and upper respiratory infections.

SGLT2 Inhibitors

Canagliflozin (Invokana) is an SGLT2 inhibitor, a new class of antihyperglycemic agent that prevents glucose from being absorbed into the bloodstream when blood is filtered by the kidneys. In people with diabetes, glucose ordinarily appears in the urine when their blood glucose rises above about 180 mg/dl. With canagliflozin, glucose appears in the urine in greater amounts, even when the blood glucose is below 180 mg/dl. This leads to lower blood glucose and hemoglobin A1c levels. Because of glucose loss in the urine, some weight loss is seen with this drug. A fall in blood pressure and a small increase in total and LDL cholesterol levels have been found in some studies. The most common side effects are genital yeast infections, mostly in women, frequent urination, dizziness, and less frequently, urinary tract infections. Canagliflozin has been shown to be effective when used in combination with diet and exercise or with other antihyperglycemic medications. The dosage range is 100–300 mg once daily. The lower dose may need to be used for individuals with kidney disease, or the drug should be stopped altogether. Canagliflozin can increase blood levels of digoxin, so digoxin levels need to be closely monitored, or the canagliflozin shouldn't be started.

GLP-1 Agonists and Pramlintide

As mentioned above, the GLP-1 agonists and pramlintide are given by subcutaneous injection and can be added to a regimen of oral antihyperglycemic agents to improve blood glucose control. The GLP-1 agonists act like GLP-1—glucagon-like peptide 1—but their structure has been changed so that they last much longer. The agents currently on the market include exenatide (Byetta, Bydureon) and liraglutide (Victoza). Exenatide is taken twice daily as Byetta or once weekly as Bydureon; liraglutide is a once-daily injection. These drugs work by the "incretin" effect—that is, they stimulate insulin production in response to a meal, decrease glucagon production, and slow stomach emptying. They also stimulate areas in the brain that suppress appetite, especially after the person starts eating a meal. They can therefore aid in weight loss, which can further improve blood glucose control. Side effects include nausea and, very rarely, pancreatitis.

Pramlintide is an amylin analog. Amylin is a naturally occurring protein that is produced by the pancreas along with insulin; its role is to slow stomach emptying and promote early satiety (a feeling of fullness after a meal). Pramlintide can be used in either Type 1 or 2 diabetes, but the starting doses are much lower in treating Type 1 diabetes. Its side effects include nausea and hypoglycemia. Persons taking pramlintide who also use insulin should have their insulin dose lowered to avoid hypoglycemia, and you should avoid this drug if you do not have hypoglycemia awareness. Both classes of drugs should be avoided if you have diabetic gastroparesis (delayed stomach emptying) because they may worsen this condition.

Take Home Messages

- Many kinds of oral antihyperglycemic agents are now available in the United States: metformin, sulfonylureas, meglitinides, alpha-glucosidase inhibitors, thiazolidinediones, DPP-4 inhibitors, and SGLT2 inhibitors. All are mainly used to treat Type 2 diabetes, but metformin is increasingly being used in addition to insulin for persons who have both Type 1 diabetes and evidence of insulin resistance.

- The subcutaneous antihyperglycemics—GLP-1 agonists and pramlintide—can be used in combination with oral antihyperglycemic agents in certain cases.

- Many people lose the ability to control their blood glucose levels over time, despite the use of these medications and even with a healthy diet and regular exercise, because the pancreas stops producing enough insulin on its own. This signals the need to start taking insulin.

11

Treating Diabetes with Insulin

- "I'll do anything except take that needle."
- "I don't think of insulin as a drug. I think of it as a little replacement hormone—perfectly natural."
- "I don't want to take insulin. My grandmother took it, and went on dialysis right afterwards."
- "I feel so much better since I've been on the insulin, I can't believe it. My golf game is even better. I wish I had started taking it sooner."

Like most scientific advances, the "discovery" of insulin involved a series of steps, beginning in the 1890s with the demonstration by the German physiologist Oskar Minkowski that an antidiabetic chemical is present in the pancreas. In 1901 a Johns Hopkins pathologist, Eugene Opie, showed that this chemical came specifically from the beta cells in the islets of Langerhans, clusters of cells in the pancreas. Then the race was on to see who would isolate this antidiabetic material in a form that could be used to treat diabetes. Frederick G. Banting, Charles A. Best, James B. Collip, and John J. R. MacLeod are credited with the discovery of insulin in 1921 in Toronto. They worked with tenacity, repeating their experiments and purifying the extract to the point that, in less than a year, it could be used to treat dying children. We highly recommend Michael Bliss's book *The Discovery of Insulin* (University of Chicago Press, 1982); the following events surrounding this dramatic episode in medical history are based on that account.

Before the availability of insulin, treatments for people with Type 1 diabetes were unpleasant and ineffective. Exercise and a low-carbohydrate, semi-starvation diet were all that could be offered. As doctors and families stood helplessly by, patients would lose more and more weight, dying within a year of the diagnosis. One of the first people to be given "Banting's extract" (as it was called), in the winter of 1921, was a terminally ill girl named Elizabeth Hughes, who was 14 years old and weighed just 52 pounds. She received the new extract over several months on a ward of the Toronto General Hospital, and those around her witnessed a "miraculous" transformation: Elizabeth blossomed into a healthy, 109-pound young woman. (She lived into her 70s.)

Scientific egos and jealousies flared within the researchers' little circle, as the world learned about the miracles happening at Toronto General. A Nobel Prize was certain to be given to two of the four researchers, and full-blown battles ensued about who deserved it most. If the truth be told, at least four other investigators, working independently, had also prepared pancreatic extracts that lowered blood glucose levels in animals or humans. But Banting, Best, Collip, and MacLeod pushed their discovery to the point of practical therapy, an achievement that has been called no less than the beginning of modern medicine. For perhaps the first time, health care providers could treat people who would otherwise certainly have died. The 1923 Nobel Prize in Physiology or Medicine was awarded to Banting and MacLeod, who promptly split their cash awards with their allies, Best and Collip.

How Insulin Works

Harold is a professional athlete. For him, getting diabetes was a huge pain. He counts on physical fitness for a living and wants to concentrate on his sport, not his blood glucose. For several years, his blood glucose was adequately controlled with oral diabetes medications, but over the past 18 months, the hemoglobin A1c results had been going up, and although he did not test as often as we would like (no doubt fearing the high numbers), his symptoms were unmistakable. He could not complete a day's workout without a few bathroom breaks, was always thirsty, and often felt excessively tired. Finally, we convinced Harold to take a shot of insulin at night, while continuing his pills during the day. The result, Harold told us, was spectacular. All of a sudden, he felt like himself again. He gained back some needed weight, improved his strength, and felt altogether better. He is the source of the final quotation at the start of this chapter—another therapeutic success with insulin.

No one can live without insulin. If your own pancreas doesn't make enough, you have to take extra. Elizabeth Hughes described insulin as "unspeakably wonderful." She could not have understood exactly how it works, but the evidence was there even with that early use: insulin relieved her of her insatiable thirst and constant urination (by lowering blood glucose); it gave her back her body strength (by promoting muscle development); and it allowed her to gain her normal adolescent fat stores (by promoting the storage of calories as fat). Let's look at these actions of insulin individually.

Many people think of the glucose (sugar) in their blood as coming only from their diet. In fact, it comes from two sources—the diet and the liver. The carbohydrate you eat raises your blood glucose directly, and the liver makes "new glucose" from storage forms (glycogen) or from protein. The liver action is why, if you don't have enough of your own insulin, the blood glucose tends to rise overnight, even when you aren't eating.

Insulin lowers the blood glucose level by both increasing the removal of glucose from the blood and reducing the production of glucose by the liver. To dispose of the carbohydrate you eat, insulin opens the body cells' doors to glucose that is circulating in the blood. The glucose enters the cells and is used as fuel for energy. Insulin shuts down the liver's production of glucose, especially overnight. This is why we sometimes start our patients with Type 2 diabetes on one shot of insulin at night, while continuing the pills during the day.

Insulin also builds muscle. It actually delivers the building blocks of muscle protein, the amino acids, to the muscles. Without insulin, muscles melt away as the amino acids are drained into the liver and inappropriately used for glucose formation. With insulin, the amino acids are put back in the muscles where they belong, and muscle strength increases noticeably.

Finally, insulin signals the body to store extra calories as glycogen and fat, two efficient storage forms to be used by the body during unanticipated fasts. Lack of insulin explains ketoacidosis (see Chapter 21) as well as uncontrolled weight loss. Restoring insulin causes the body to rebuild fat.

Since insulin is at the center of so many of the body's chemical reactions, it is no wonder that it's required for life itself. Various other body functions, such as the complicated hormone changes involved in women's menstrual cycles, are also dependent on the presence of adequate levels of insulin. Insulin is present in some of the most primitive and ancient of living organisms and is the most finely tuned of all the body's hormones. It is, in truth, a miracle of nature, a central regulator of all the body's complex chemical pathways.

Given all these wonderful effects of insulin, why does just hearing the simple words, "You need insulin," elicit such a flood of emotions, all negative? The reason, of course, is that it has to be given by injection.

What People Think about Taking Insulin

The thought of taking several injections every day is not a happy one. People worry about needles, syringes, and pain. They wonder whether the need for insulin means that their diabetes is worse. They ask whether they will have to stay on insulin for the rest of their lives. If you have these thoughts, keep in mind that you are not the first person to wonder, to resist, to be afraid, and to ask hard questions. Any question that you have about insulin use deserves an answer. Consider how the following people with diabetes responded to their need to use insulin.

When 6-year-old Amanda was diagnosed with Type 1 diabetes, her parents thought her life was going to be ruined by endless pain from countless injections. They were amazed when, no more than two months later, Amanda was drawing up the syringe and plunging it right into herself, as proud as she could be and without a whimper.

When Elmer, a man with Type 2 diabetes, was told it was time for him to start using insulin, his first thought was of a relative who took insulin and developed complications of diabetes. He mistakenly blamed the complications on insulin rather than on poorly controlled diabetes.

Jesse thought that taking insulin meant his diabetes was "worse" and would therefore cause more complications. No one told him that insulin was being prescribed to help him avoid complications.

Bernice was afraid that she would go into coma with insulin, because she didn't know that severe hypoglycemia is preventable.

Steve associated the needles and syringes with drug abuse. He was terrified that someone would see him taking an injection and assume that he was a junkie.

All these people hated the idea of taking insulin. What's remarkable to those of us who care for literally thousands of people with diabetes is that we find very, very few who do not accommodate themselves successfully to insulin injections. Like teenage boys learning to shave, after an initial struggle, taking insulin just folds itself into the daily routine. Virtually everyone ends up taking the situation in stride.

Is the diabetes "worse" if you need insulin? It's actually the pancreas that's worse, since the need for insulin by injection means that the pancreas is not able to do the job of making enough insulin, despite whatever diet, exercise, and pills you have been using. In a truer sense, diabetes is "worse" only to the extent that blood glucose levels are higher or diabetes *complications* are worse. Think of how you'll feel and how well you'll live if you take insulin, eat a healthy diet, exercise regularly, and check your glucose levels at home, finding them mostly in a very good range. Then think about how well you'd live if you were suffering severe complications because of having uncontrolled diabetes for a long time. We know you'll conclude that it is having the complications, not taking the treatment, that is "worse."

Is insulin treatment forever? Most often it is, but not always. In Type 2 diabetes, weight loss and increased activity improve the body's response to insulin. For some people, this may mean being able to reduce the insulin dose, even to the point of stopping it altogether. Sometimes loss of as little as 10 pounds makes a big difference. But if your pancreas has stopped making enough insulin, insulin therapy is the only effective way to keep your diabetes under control. In persons with Type 1 diabetes, the immune system has destroyed the insulin-producing beta cells, so insulin replacement is the only option.

Deciding to Take Insulin

When your health care professional recommends insulin, it is only reasonable to expect that she or he will explain the whys and wherefores. If the two of you agree on some definite improvements you can make in your self-care before committing to insulin use, it's certainly worthwhile to give those changes a try and see how they affect your blood glucose levels. But even when you are armed with a plan, it is essential to set a target date by which you'll get your blood glucose down. One month is reasonable. Twelve months is too long to have out-of-control diabetes.

If you need insulin, don't prolong the negotiations with your doctor: "I'll start the insulin after I get done with this work assignment (or this wedding, or the visit from my mother-in-law)." "I'm not sure I want to do it right now, but definitely by next winter." "How about if I cut my calories down to 900 a day and run a mile after every meal?" We've heard them all! When insulin is needed, don't kid yourself by making unreasonable promises, and stop procrastinating.

Principles of Insulin Use

The exact insulin regimen and insulin doses that will work for you depend on lots of different factors:

—How old are you?

—What do you weigh?

—How closely do you follow your diabetes?

—What are the goals you are trying to achieve?

—Perhaps most important of all, what kind of diabetes do you have?

These and many other considerations will be worked out between you and your health care professional. But the fundamental differences between Type 1 and Type 2 diabetes are especially important when it comes to insulin treatment.

As you'll recall, with Type 1 diabetes you have virtually no insulin left in your pancreas, whereas with Type 2 your pancreas still does make some insulin. This means that for Type 1 diabetes, the insulin injections have to "do it all." The doses tend to be more complicated and need to be more fine-tuned. For Type 2 diabetes, insulin injections are just giving the pancreas a helping hand, and while more insulin may be needed than for Type 1, the doses usually aren't so complex. Let's consider each of these situations.

Type 1 Diabetes

With Type 1 diabetes, insulin treatment is always required. Usually, it should be started as soon as the diagnosis is made. There is even some evidence that controlling the blood glucose very well and very quickly may have later benefits by "protecting" beta cells in the pancreas, although this is not proven.

As we noted in Chapter 2, many people with Type 1 diabetes have a "honeymoon period" during which their pancreas seems to recover after insulin treatment begins. The honeymoon may start within a month or so of the diagnosis and last a few months to a year. During this period, the need for insulin drops dramatically or even disappears. This is because the remaining beta cells that haven't yet been destroyed can work better when glucose levels aren't in the 300s or higher anymore. Commonly, the diabetes is very stable, and blood glucose levels are relatively easily controlled. You can be tricked into thinking that the diabetes is going away, but it is more accurate to think of the honeymoon as a final burst of activity from the remaining beta cells in the pancreas. Research is focusing on how to prolong the honeymoon period, with the hope of preventing damage to the remaining beta cells. In the future, Type 1 diabetes might be prevented by learning what the body is trying to tell us with the honeymoon period. In the meantime, for our patients, we look on it as an opportunity to learn good diabetes self-care while things are a little easier.

In treating Type 1 diabetes, replacing the function of the pancreatic beta cells is no easy task. You need *some* insulin all the time, much more at mealtimes, and never too much. Getting this right requires a complicated schedule of injections, preventing gaps in insulin levels and matching the input of carbohydrate taken with meals. Most people with Type 1 diabetes learn by necessity to fine-tune their diet, insulin, and exercise patterns. They learn that inattention to details may have consequences, such as hypoglycemia, that they very much want to avoid.

Principles of "Physiological" Insulin Therapy in Type 1 Diabetes

The goal of replacing insulin for people with Type 1 diabetes, whose beta cells no longer produce insulin, is to give insulin as close as possible to the way the beta cells would release insulin if they were still functioning normally—so-called physiological insulin replacement.

Controlling fasting blood glucose levels. In someone without diabetes, beta cells make a small amount of insulin continuously while the person is not eating, thus preventing the liver from dumping too much glucose into the bloodstream and preventing the production of ketoacids. Diabetologists call this insulin long-acting or "basal" insulin. This type of insulin can be taken by persons with Type 1 diabetes as a once- or twice-daily dose of insulin glargine (Lantus) or insulin detemir (Levemir). The action of these insulins is spread out gradually over a 24-hour period. Some people, especially those taking higher doses of basal insulin, take the insulin twice daily to get more consistent blood glucose control throughout the day.

The job of these long-acting, basal insulins is to keep the blood glucose steady when people aren't eating. The best way to see whether the dose is correct is to track your blood glucose levels during the longest time of fasting, usually overnight. Check your glucose level at least four hours after any food is eaten and, if you take mealtime insulin, after your last rapid-acting mealtime insulin injection of the day (see the section below on mealtime insulin). If your morning blood glucose is within 30 mg/dl or so of the bedtime reading, the basal insulin is doing its job. If your blood glucose consistently rises (or falls) more than 30 mg/dl overnight, the basal insulin should be increased (or decreased), usually by 1 unit at a time until the blood glucose stays fairly stable overnight. If you miss the basal insulin and take no other insulin for eight or more hours, there's a chance of ketoacids developing.

Controlling blood glucose levels when eating. In persons who do not have diabetes, the beta cells make a larger amount of insulin when they eat meals containing carbohydrates, as the carbohydrates are rapidly broken down to sugars. When you have diabetes, the amount of mealtime insulin you take to mimic this natural insulin surge is called "bolus" insulin. For persons with Type 1 diabetes, the best way to prevent glucose levels from rising too high or dropping too low after a meal is to carefully match the amount of bolus insulin to the amount of carbohydrate eaten. One way to do so is to inject the same amount of insulin each day at a certain mealtime and to eat the same amount of carbohydrate at that meal each day. Some people who eat very similar meals each day, especially for breakfast and lunch, find this is an easy way to keep glucose levels stable after eating. If the total amount of carbohydrate and sugar eaten at a meal varies from day to day, the mealtime insulin dose will need to be adjusted each day. Many people will "ballpark" the amount of insulin they take, based on a general sense of how much more or how much less carbohydrate than usual they are eating for that meal. This commonly leads to blood glucose levels rising very high when the carbohydrate estimate is way too low or dropping low if the carbohydrate estimate is much too high.

The best way to match insulin with the amount of carbohydrate eaten is to count the number of carbohydrate calories that foods contain. Based on how much total insulin someone takes each day, we can usually estimate how much carbohydrate is covered by 1 unit of insulin. The calculation we usually use is 500 divided by the total daily insulin dose. So if you take about 50 units of insulin each day, this means 500/50 = 10 grams of carbohydrate covered by each unit of insulin, or an insulin-to-carb ratio of 1:10. This dose can then be fine-tuned until the peak glucose (usually one to two hours after the meal) falls in the desirable 100–160 mg/dl range, the next meal's glucose falls in the 80–130 mg/dl range, and the bedtime glucose falls mostly in the 90–140 mg/dl range.

The rapid-acting insulins lispro (Humalog), aspart (NovoLog), and glulisine (Apidra) act much more quickly than Regular (R) insulin. They begin entering the bloodstream 15–20 minutes after being injected in the skin, much more quickly than Regular insulin, which takes 30–60 minutes. These rapid-acting insulins peak at about 1 hour after injection, rather than closer to two hours as is required for Regular insulin. Since they work more quickly, they also prevent the blood glucose from rising as high after a meal as it does with Regular insulin.

Blood glucose levels begin to rise immediately after you eat a meal containing carbohydrates or simple sugars. Since it takes even rapid-acting insulins 15–20 minutes to start working, we advise our patients to inject their mealtime insulin 15–20 minutes before the meal. Doing so, rather than in the more "convenient" way of immediately before the meal, will lower the after-meal glucose even without increasing the insulin dose.

Correcting high blood glucose readings. It's difficult to account for all the things that can cause glucose levels to rise (the total amount of carbohydrates and fats, the amount of physical or psychological stress, and decreased physical activity), and high numbers will sometimes occur. Fortunately, you can use extra, "correction," rapid-acting insulin dosages to help bring these numbers down relatively quickly. Our patients usually begin with a correction insulin dose of 1,800 divided by their total daily insulin dose. So, if you're taking 60 units of insulin each day, we'd expect 1 unit of insulin to drop your blood glucose by 1,800/60 = 30 mg/dl. This is called a "correction factor" or "sensitivity factor." This can be fine-tuned based on your response to using that amount of correction insulin. We usually target a blood glucose of 100 mg/dl before meals and 120 mg/dl at bedtime to correct down to. Be careful not to use correction insulin more than about once every four hours—unless your health care provider advises you to do otherwise—because it takes that long to see the full effect of a rapid-acting insulin

Type 2 Diabetes

Why is insulin sometimes used to treat people with Type 2 diabetes, when Type 2 is also called non-insulin-dependent diabetes? The answer (discussed more fully in Chapter 2) is that the pancreas of some people with Type 2 diabetes does not produce enough insulin to control the blood glucose, so insulin injections are needed. The old name, non-insulin-dependent diabetes, is misleading.

If you were to ask a room full of diabetes professionals *when* insulin should be used in treating Type 2 diabetes, you'd find some differences in opinion. Some think insulin should be used soon after diagnosis; others, only when other options have failed. Our own practice, simply put, is for our patients to start using insulin when their pancreas cannot make enough. You will know this by the following signs:

—Your blood glucose levels are too high.

—You are losing weight without trying to.

—You are thirsty and urinating too much.

—Other treatments, including diet, exercise, and pills, are no longer working.

People often ask for one last chance. They want to exercise even more or eat even less. Sometimes this is reasonable, especially when blood glucose levels are only mildly high and more attention to self-care will work. But often the insulin-producing beta cells of the pancreas just wear out, and no amount of diet, exercise, or pills will be enough. Insulin is what you need.

Because people with Type 2 diabetes continue to make some insulin in their pancreas, achieving good control of blood glucose levels with injections is usually easier than in Type 1 diabetes. Just one or two injections a day often work fine. Insulin often can be used together with pills. A long-acting (basal) insulin is given usually once, sometimes twice, daily. This helps get the fasting blood glucose under better control and allows the pills to work better to control after-meal blood glucose levels. Usually, the total amount of insulin needed is much greater than in Type 1 diabetes (perhaps 50–150 units per day, especially for heavier individuals). This high insulin requirement has nothing to do with how "bad" the diabetes is; it has to do with how well—or poorly—your body responds to insulin (how "sensitive" it is to insulin).

Pregnancy

If you develop diabetes during pregnancy (gestational diabetes mellitus, GDM; see Chapter 29) and diet alone is not normalizing your blood glucose, you must start using insulin for the well-being of the developing fetus. Oral medications for diabetes generally should not be used when a woman is pregnant or trying to become pregnant. Glyburide and metformin have been studied and seem to be safe in pregnancy, but they are not approved for use because no long-term data are yet available on their safety during pregnancy. Insulin use is usually temporary in GDM. After delivery, most women return to a nondiabetic state and can stop taking insulin, although they have a much higher chance of developing Type 2 diabetes later in life, about a 50% increased risk after 10 years. Of course, if you have Type 1 diabetes before pregnancy, you must continue taking insulin during your pregnancy. Insulin requirements rise and may even double for women with Type 1 diabetes during pregnancy because of the effects of placental hormones. These effects go away right after the baby is delivered, and your insulin requirement will probably go back quickly to the doses you used before pregnancy. For a small number of women, Type 1 diabetes starts during pregnancy. In this case, the diabetes will continue after pregnancy and will continue to require insulin.

Surgery and Other Stressful Situations

People who maintain well-controlled blood glucose levels with their diet or diet and oral medication may find they need insulin to control their blood glucose during periods of stress, such as undergoing surgery. This is another case, though, in which insulin treatment may be temporary. When the stress is over, the person often no longer needs insulin.

Adverse Reactions to Insulin

Like Elizabeth Hughes—and contrary to what you might have anticipated—you too may describe insulin as "unspeakably wonderful." With the right dose of insulin, the bothersome symptoms of high blood glucose disappear, and your overall sense of well-being improves. But for all its wonderful qualities, insulin use has some unpleasant aspects beyond the needle stick. We'll consider some of the adverse reactions to insulin and give suggestions for dealing with them.

Hypoglycemia

Blood glucose that falls too low, or hypoglycemia, is by far the most common downside of insulin therapy. It happens when the amount of insulin taken is too much for the amount of food ingested, the exercise undertaken, or the starting level of blood glucose. There is a smaller risk of hypoglycemia due to insulin in Type 2 diabetes than in Type 1, in part because persons with Type 2 are less sensitive to the blood glucose-lowering effects of insulin. However, when glucose levels fall low, you should notify your prescribing care provider so the dose can be reduced, especially if hypoglycemic symptoms (shakiness, palpitations, sweating, nervousness, vision changes, or confusion) develop. The risk of hypoglycemia is usually low in Type 2 diabetes, can be quickly treated, and can be prevented by following medication and dietary guidelines. Concern over hypoglycemia should not delay your starting insulin treatment when your diabetes is out of control.

Even with generally good blood glucose control, you will miss the mark periodically and have hypoglycemia; usually it can easily be treated by drinking fruit juice or eating glucose tablets or other sugar-containing food. If you are having frequent hypoglycemia—several times a week or more often—you may need to adjust your insulin dose downward. You definitely want to avoid insulin reactions that are severe enough to cause confusion or loss of consciousness. Telephone or visit your health care provider if you are concerned about frequent lows.

Weight Gain

Achieving better blood glucose control while taking insulin means that your body is now working more like the body of a person without diabetes and is properly using the foods you eat. When your blood glucose was high, some of the calories you ate were spilled into your urine as glucose. This drain of calories made losing weight relatively easy. With good blood glucose control, that isn't happening anymore. Instead, any excess calories you consume (that is, beyond what you burn by just living, breathing, and exercising) are stored away as fat. That's right, *fat*. So with good blood glucose control, you become like most people who don't have diabetes: you have to watch your calories closely or your waistline grows. But there are some things you can consider doing to avoid the weight gain that can come with insulin treatment.

Be sure that your insulin dose is not causing frequent hypoglycemia, driving you to eat snacks continuously. If you have to eat to prevent hypoglycemia, you're taking too much insulin. To control weight, you may need to limit your calories (this is best done with the assistance of a dietitian) or increase your activity. Keep in mind that if you diet strenuously, you may have to cut down how much insulin you take.

Needle Phobia

Insulin needles are vastly improved over those that were used in the past. The point of the needle is beveled so that it is very sharp, the needle is shorter, and the gauge or diameter of the needle is "ultra" fine. The needle is coated with a slippery layer of silicone. Sharp, fine, short, slippery needles pierce the skin and slide through the tissue easily, with little or no pain. We find that many patients who learn how to inject insulin during an office visit can overcome their fear right then and there, when they realize how easy and painless the injection is.

Of course, knowing this and being able to inject yourself at home without getting nervous are two different things. As we said, almost everyone eventually gets used to it. But in the beginning, some people have to push themselves. Try thinking ahead ("If I just get it done, I can go on with breakfast"). You may have to make a concerted effort to visualize a relaxing place, such as a beach at sunset, to prevent that cold sweat. If you continue to suffer with the injections and are unable to get the needle in quickly, with a dartlike motion, you might consider purchasing a device designed to do that step for you. A nurse educator can explain the options. But almost without exception, people who take insulin find that injections become easier with time.

Insulin Allergy

Fortunately, as a direct result of using human rather than earlier sources of insulin (see Chapter 12), allergy is a much rarer problem than it used to be. It is so rare nowadays that we are surprised when we see it. Being uncomfortable taking insulin, being sensitive to it, or even getting a bruise at the injection site do *not* mean you have an insulin allergy. With an insulin allergy, there is either redness around the site of insulin injection, often with some itching (this is called *local allergy*), or a reaction involving several body systems (a *systemic allergy*).

A local allergy is rarely severe and is not a reason to stop insulin use. A systemic allergy is much rarer and more severe. It includes hives, rashes on areas of the skin away from the injection site, and sometimes facial swelling or wheezing. Since there are many causes of such allergies, when you have reactions of this type, don't assume that just because you take insulin, insulin is the cause of your allergic reaction. You may be allergic to pollen, a specific kind of soap, nuts, shellfish, or any number of other things. Check the situation out with your care provider, who may want to change the type of insulin you take before setting up a visit to a good allergist.

Insulin Edema

Swelling, or edema, is an infrequent response with the initiation of insulin therapy. This occurs more frequently when blood glucose levels were very poorly controlled before the insulin was started. It goes away in a matter of weeks with a low-sodium diet and short-term use of a diuretic (fluid pill) such as furosemide.

· · ·

Living with insulin therapy makes your life different. There are routines to follow, supplies to juggle, and monitoring to carry out to make sure everything is in balance. But it can also make your life a lot better when symptoms of diabetes disappear and your risk of long-term problems is reduced. As one of our patients said, "Insulin is good stuff when you need it."

Take Home Messages

- No one can live without insulin. If you have diabetes and your pancreas is not making enough insulin, you have to take extra.
- Taking insulin does not mean your diabetes is getting worse. Your diabetes is getting worse only if your blood glucose levels are consistently too high (which increases your risk of developing complications). Insulin is the most effective glucose-lowering medication.
- Basal (long-acting) insulin, taken once or twice a day, can help keep your blood glucose levels under control when you are not eating (overnight and between meals).
- Mealtime (rapid-acting) insulin can help cover the food you eat and keep your blood glucose levels under control after meals.
- People with Type 1 diabetes need both basal and mealtime insulin.
- People with Type 2 diabetes often need insulin. Some take only basal insulin, and some take both basal and mealtime insulin.

12

Types of Insulin

with Nestoras Mathioudakis, M.D.

- "I'm on Humulin insulin. Is that the same as Humalog?"
- "What's the truth about how to store and handle insulin? Where should you keep it—in a refrigerator? an ice pack? on a shelf?"
- "I don't understand the insulin peak. Is it always the same? Does it mean that my sugar goes up or down?"
- "How do I know if my insulin needs to be adjusted, how do I do it, and should I talk with my doctor every time I change it?"

In the last chapter we described the exciting events surrounding the discovery of insulin. But diabetes was far from cured when insulin became available. In fact, early insulin preparations were crude at best, entirely inactive at worst. The insulin was extracted from cow and pig pancreases, was impure, and often caused allergic reactions. Furthermore, because it was originally a weak form of what we now call Regular insulin, the person with diabetes had to inject large volumes three to four times a day, and pits often appeared at the injection sites.

The manufacturing of insulin has come a long way. Today, insulin is well standardized, pure, and of uniform potency. Worldwide, most of the insulin now used is genetically engineered synthetic "human" insulin. Because of this, allergies and other reactions to insulin are much less common than they were in the past. But along with these enormous improvements in insulin has come increased complexity in what's available. Add to this the current focus on improved blood glucose control and you can see that there's more opportunity for confusion than ever before.

In this chapter we explain the characteristics that distinguish different insulin preparations. We discuss the specifics of insulin storage and handling, insulin injection technique, factors that affect insulin absorption, and how to adjust your regimen safely and rationally.

Key Characteristics of Different Insulin Preparations

There are several characteristics of insulin that you should be aware of:

—The timing of the onset and duration of action of the insulin (lispro, aspart, Regular, NPH, glargine, mixed insulins, etc.)

—The concentration of insulin (U-500, U-100, U-80, U-40)

—The different brand names put on each kind of insulin by different companies

Several companies produce and market insulin, and each uses a different brand name. The most widely used insulins in the United States are listed in Table 14. Generally, within a given class of insulin, the pricing is comparable among the different manufacturers. In this chapter we refer to the insulins by their generic names.

Insulin Amounts

Insulin is measured in *units* (U). In manufacturing, insulin is calibrated so that a unit has a particular "biological effect"—it lowers the blood glucose by a certain amount. Many people ask us exactly how much a unit of insulin will lower *their* blood glucose. Unfortunately, for someone who has never taken insulin, we can only guess. The figure will vary enormously from person to person (see the discussion of insulin resistance in Chapters 2 and 7), and of course, any insulin effect on lowering blood glucose will be counteracted by eating carbohydrate. On the other hand, *you* can probably get a pretty good feel for how much a unit (or 5 units or 10 units) lowers your blood glucose, if you pay close attention and test your glucose levels. For patients with Type 1 diabetes, we estimate how much 1 unit of insulin will lower their blood glucose by dividing 1,800 by total daily insulin dose. So, if someone is taking a total of about 60 units of insulin each day, we'd expect 1 unit of insulin to lower the blood glucose by about 1,800/60 = 30 points.

Insulin Concentration

The *concentration* of insulin available in the United States is almost always 100 units in one milliliter (ml), called U-100 insulin. In other countries, U-40 insulin is often available, meaning that the insulin has 40 units in 1 ml. Think of a teaspoon of blue dye put in a half-glass of water—it will make a certain shade of blue. The same teaspoon of blue dye in a *whole* glass

Table 14 Types of Insulin

Generic Name	Brand Name	Manufacturer	Cost*
Rapid-acting insulin analogs			
Aspart	NovoLog	Novo Nordisk	$112 for 1,000 U (vials) $219 for 1,500 U (FlexPen)
Lispro	Humalog	Eli Lilly	$104 for 1,000 U (vials) $198 for 1,500 U (KwikPen)
Glulisine	Apidra	Sanofi-Aventis US	$102 for 1,000 U (vials) $207 for 1,500 U (SoloSTAR Pen)
Short-acting insulin			
Regular	Humulin R	Eli Lilly	$57 for 1,000 U (vials)
	Novolin R	Novo Nordisk	$58 for 1,000 U (vials)
Intermediate-acting insulin			
NPH	Humulin N	Eli Lilly	$57 for 1,000 U (vials)
	Novolin N	Novo Nordisk	$58 for 1,000 U (vials)
Premixed insulins			
NPH (70%) with Regular (30%)	Humulin 70/30	Eli Lilly	$56 for 1,000 U (vials) $291 for 3,000 U (pre-filled pen)
	Novolin 70/30	Novo Nordisk	$58 for 1,000 U (vials)
Aspart protamine (70%) with aspart (30%)	NovoLog Mix 70/30	Novo Nordisk	$110 for 1,000 U (vials) $206 for 1,500 U (FlexPen)
Lispro protamine (75%) with lispro (25%)	Humalog Mix 75/25	Eli Lilly	$111 for 1,000 U (vials) $200 for 1,500 U (KwikPen)
Lispro protamine (50%) with lispro (50%)	Humalog Mix 50/50	Eli Lilly	$107 for 1,000 U (vials) $200 for 1,500 U (KwikPen)
Long-acting insulins			
Glargine	Lantus	Sanofi-Aventis US	$104 for 1,000 U (vials) $188 for 1,500 U (SoloSTAR Pen)
Detemir	Levemir	Novo Nordisk	$103 for 1,000 U (vials) $191 for 1,500 U (FlexPen)

*Listed prices as of late 2012.

of water will make a fainter blue. Likewise, U-40 insulin is more dilute than U-100. One unit of insulin is still 1 unit of insulin; it is just more dilute in U-40 preparations. The easiest thing to do when you travel outside the United States is to take along U-100 insulin. One friend of ours accidentally lost his bottle of insulin down the toilet on a flight to France. In Paris, he couldn't find a pharmacy with U-100 insulin. So you never know when an understanding of insulin concentration will come in handy! Remember this: inject U-40 insulin with a U-40 syringe; then take your usual number of units. As long as you use the correct syringe for the concentration of insulin, you will receive the same amount of insulin. U-500 is a type of insulin that is five times more concentrated than U-100. In other words, 10 units of U-500 insulin are equivalent to 50 units of U-100 insulin. This more concentrated insulin is often used by people who have very large insulin requirements to decrease the amount required at an injection. Although U-500 is a type of Regular insulin, its action is more similar to that of NPH than Regular U-100 insulin, so it is often used twice daily.

Insulin Syringes

Syringes come in several sizes. If you take relatively large doses, say 75 units in a shot, you will use a syringe that can hold a full milliliter, or 100 units of U-100 insulin. Filling the syringe to the 75-unit mark, it is three-quarters full. For lower doses, such as 15 units, there are smaller syringes, holding a maximum of 30 or 50 units. The numbers printed on the side of the syringe are bigger when the full syringe holds only 30 or 50 units, so you can be more accurate. With these half-milliliter or third-milliliter syringes, you still draw up insulin to the mark that corresponds to 15 units, if that is the dose you want. So don't get mixed up by the size of the syringe—always pull up the insulin to the mark that represents your own desired dose.

Insulin Durations of Action

You will almost certainly be using different kinds of insulin—Regular, glargine, aspart, or even mixes of insulins. Each insulin has a different duration of action, and for mixes of insulins, there are two different durations of action to think about. We explain below the differences between rapid-acting, short-acting (Regular), intermediate-acting (NPH), premixed, and long-acting insulins. But first, let's consider some key terms: onset, peak, and duration of action.

When you inject insulin beneath the skin, it is not effective at that very instant, any more than your blood glucose jumps up the very moment you put a piece of bread in your mouth. It takes some time for insulin to be absorbed into the bloodstream and to reach the cells where it acts. The step that takes the longest is the absorption of insulin from beneath the skin into the blood. This time between the injection of insulin and the start of its action to lower the blood glucose is called the *time of onset*. With the rapid-acting insulins, the time of onset is 5–15 minutes, compared with 30 minutes to 1 hour for Regular insulin.

The *peak* of insulin action comes when, after injection, the insulin reaches its maximum activity. If we measure insulin levels in the blood, the peak for an insulin would be the highest level of insulin measured after the injection, a time when glucose is being moved from the blood into cells the most quickly.

The insulin's *duration of action* refers to the time between the start of the effect of the insulin injection and the end of the effect, when the insulin is no longer driving the blood glucose down.

A word of caution is needed here. Everyone talks about these features of insulin—the onset, peak, and duration—as though they were true for everyone. We even present representative curves (see Figures 18–21). But in real life, the duration of action varies substantially from person to person and from injection to injection. The action curves presented here represent only one typical curve for each type of insulin. Action curves may be somewhat different for you. NPH and Regular insulins tend to be more rapidly absorbed when injected into the abdomen, when compared with the arm or leg or upper hip. You can reduce the injection-to-injection variation by always injecting into your abdomen or by trying to inject to the same depth each time. The newer, rapid-acting insulins are absorbed at a similar rate regardless of where they are injected. However, you can't eliminate the variation in action of an insulin entirely.

Types of Insulin

To categorize insulins in terms of their time and action characteristics, we consider four types: rapid-acting, short-acting, intermediate-acting, and long-acting.

Rapid-acting. The rapid-acting insulins include lispro (Humalog), aspart (NovoLog), and glulisine (Apidra). The first of these drugs, lispro (Eli Lilly), became available in 1996 and made use of recombinant DNA technology to change the insulin molecule so that it is absorbed more quickly even than

Regular insulin. Because these insulins enter the bloodstream quickly, they are best taken 10–20 minutes before a meal rather than 30–45 minutes before (as was the case with Regular insulin) (see Figure 18). In addition to being given as injections, the rapid-acting insulins are used in insulin pumps because they better mimic the natural bursts of insulin released from the pancreas both at mealtimes and when fasting.

Regular insulin (short-acting). Regular, or R, insulin has a typical onset within about 45 minutes, its peak action is at about 2 hours, and its duration of action is about 5–8 hours (see Figure 19). For decades, Regular insulin was used to "cover" meals—that is, to prevent glucose levels from rising high after meals. However, Regular insulin has now largely been replaced by the rapid-acting insulins, which act more precisely to lessen the peaking of blood glucose after a meal. Studies have shown that because of its delayed and longer duration of action, Regular insulin allows the blood glucose to rise higher after meals and leads to more hypoglycemia many hours after it's given when compared with the rapid-acting insulins. Regular insulin is now less commonly used, either alone or in mixed combinations with NPH insulin.

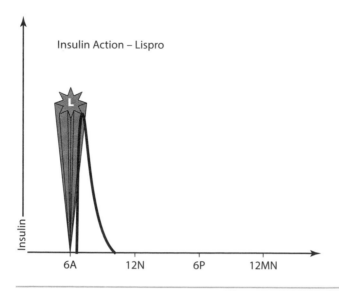

Figure 18. Action curve for lispro, an insulin analog. Lispro has a rapid onset of action—about 15 minutes. Its action peaks in one hour and lasts for about four hours.

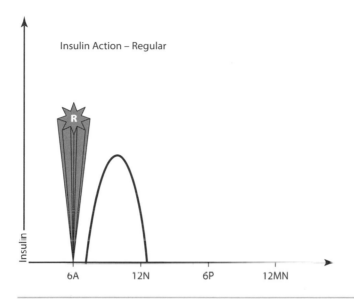

Figure 19. Action curve for Regular insulin, referred to as a short-acting (clear) insulin because it lasts only about five to six hours. It starts working about 45 minutes to an hour after injection and peaks in about two hours.

Intermediate-acting. There are several intermediate-acting insulins: Neutral Protamine Hagedorn (NPH or N), lispro protamine, and aspart protamine. The absorption of NPH from the injection site is slowed down by the addition of a protein called protamine. Similarly, lispro and aspart are usually rapid-acting insulins, but the addition of protamine gives them an intermediate length of action. NPH insulin usually starts working about 1 hour after injection, peaks on average at 6–8 hours, and lasts a total of about 10–16 hours (see Figure 20). NPH is identifiable not only by the "N" on the bottle but also by the cloudiness of the solution. The insulin is actually in the cloudiness, which settles to the bottom when the bottle is allowed to stand. Therefore, you must invert or roll these bottles before use in order to mix the insulin into the solution. NPH is typically taken in the morning to provide some insulin effect through midday and afternoon, covering lunch, or at bedtime to control the blood glucose through the night.

Long-acting. There are two long-acting insulins: glargine (Lantus) and detemir (Levemir). These are considered basal insulins because they mimic the normal baseline insulin released by the pancreas throughout the day,

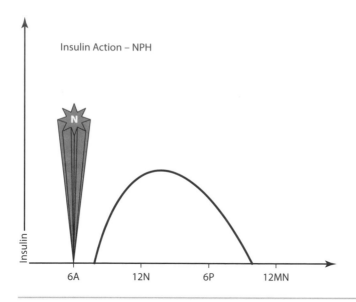

Figure 20. Action curve for NPH insulin, an intermediate-acting (clear) insulin. It generally starts working about 1–3 hours after injection, peaks at about 8 hours, and lasts about 20 hours.

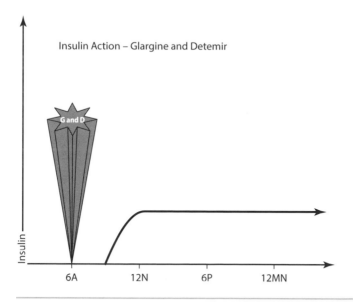

Figure 21. Action curve for glargine and detemir, the longest-lasting insulins available. They start working about 2–4 hours after injection, have almost no peak, and last about 20–24 hours.

whether or not the person eats. Glargine has a duration of action of 20–24 hours. Detemir lasts for 16–24 hours, so sometimes detemir requires more than one injection a day. These drugs are considered "peakless" because they result in relatively steady levels of insulin action throughout the day (see Figure 21). Therefore, they are less likely to cause hypoglycemia than NPH or the rapid-acting insulin analogs.

Insulin Mixes

Several mixed insulins are currently available on the market. These include premixes of the intermediate-acting NPH with short-acting Regular insulin or of a rapid-acting insulin analog with a protamine-modified intermediate-acting preparation of the same insulin. One commonly used mix is called 70/30, containing 70% NPH and 30% Regular. We find these mixes useful for pre-meal dosing when people cannot mix their own insulin reliably. The purpose of these mixes is to cover both mealtime and between-meal blood glucose levels with the combination of the two insulins. Because the 70/30 mix contains so much Regular insulin, it is not a good idea to use it if you are not planning on eating shortly afterward. Mixes containing aspart and lispro (NovoLog Mix 70/30, Humalog Mix 75/25, and Humalog Mix 50/50) are usually taken shortly before the two largest meals of the day. NPH/Regular mixes are usually taken 30 minutes before breakfast and dinner.

Handling Insulin

Insulin is a special medication that needs and deserves to be treated with care. How, exactly, should you handle it? Opinions and even official recommendations have flip-flopped over the years. The fact is that insulin is a fragile protein. It can be damaged by very vigorous shaking or by extremes of temperature. You need to keep several cautions in mind.

Insulin lasts for one month at room temperature and until the expiration date at refrigeration temperature. There is no reason to worry, then, if a bottle has been kept at room temperature rather than cooled, even for days. Since cold insulin can sometimes make an injection more painful, we typically recommend that you keep the bottle of insulin you are currently using at room temperature. Keep your spare, unopened bottles in the refrigerator for long-term storage. For trips to the beach or a cold ski slope, temperature-regulated cases are protective options. Desert-dwelling Bedouins are taught to bury their insulin deep in the sand to keep it cool.

Travel can present special challenges in caring for your insulin. If you fly, keep it (and the rest of your diabetes supplies) in your carry-on luggage, for two reasons. First, the cargo holds of aircraft (and boats, trains, and cars, for that matter) may be subjected to extremes of temperature that can ruin the insulin. Second, it has happened that the traveler goes to London while the checked luggage goes to Hong Kong. Don't get stuck without your insulin. Keep it close at hand.

Insulin Pens

Many of our patients tell us they are uncomfortable giving their insulin injections in public. So they often take their bedtime glargine dose and their breakfast aspart insulin but may skip covering lunch or dinner until well after the meal, depending on their work or social schedule. This leads to glucose levels running high after the missed dose. With the advent of insulin pens, we have mostly been able to get around this problem. No longer do you need to excuse yourself to go draw up insulin from a vial. Now, you can simply dial the dose you need on a portable insulin pen. In other parts of the world, most insulin-treated patients use insulin pens. The pens are becoming much more widely used in the United States as well, and most people say pens are more convenient than syringes and that they make it easier to take all prescribed insulin doses.

There are two types of insulin pen systems: durable and pre-filled. The durable pen uses a replaceable insulin cartridge, so that once the insulin runs out, a new cartridge is loaded and the same pen is used. The pre-filled pen is entirely disposable; once the cartridge is empty, the pen is discarded and a new one is used. Short, thin, insulin pen needles are placed onto the end of the pen and then discarded after the injection. Most types of insulin are now available for use as pens, including the rapid-acting and long-acting insulins, as well as NPH and mixed insulin preparations.

Literally about the size of a pen (though obviously thicker), these devices are discrete and easier to transport than a vial and syringe. Another advantage to the pen is improved accuracy. The insulin dose is determined by dialing a knob, so there is less human error than when drawing up insulin using numbered unit markers on the side of a syringe. This can be important for people who have impaired near vision or limited fine motor skills. Also, since the needle does not have to be inserted into an insulin vial before injecting, the pen needles tend to stay sharper and cause less injection pain. The main disadvantage to the insulin pens is their cost. Generally, compared with insulin vials, insulin pens are $30–$120 more expensive per refill. Since insurance coverage and co-pays for insulin pens are variable in the United States, many individuals still favor the less expensive traditional vial and syringe. Another disadvantage to insulin pens is that different insulins cannot be mixed by the user. If you are taking a combination of NPH and Regular insulin that isn't at a fixed ratio of 70/30 or 50/50, for which pens are available, you'll need to use the traditional syringe method.

Can Insulin Go Bad, and How Do I Know?

Yes, insulin can go bad—due to mishandling or for unknown reasons. The best indication is when it isn't acting normally: when your blood glucose level stays high for no good reason. As we've noted, most insulins available today, whether in a vial or pen, can be kept at room temperature for one month.

Some low-dose insulin users notice that their insulin seems less effective when they get close to the end of the bottle. Around these times, their blood glucose levels trend higher. This could be related to how many times the stopper of the insulin vial has been pierced. If it is happening to you, start a new vial of insulin when the current one gets down to about one-third full, and throw away the ineffective insulin.

Another clue that your insulin has gone bad is that it looks different. If supposed to be clear, it gets cloudy; if normally cloudy, you notice clumps, even after you have rolled it between your palms. Don't take chances with bad insulin: replace the bottle right away, and save yourself the aggravation of uncontrolled blood glucose levels. If there is any question, especially if your vial or pen has been used for more than a month, play it safe and throw the insulin away.

Drawing Up and Injecting Insulin

First, you have to get the insulin into the syringe, then you have to inject it through the skin into the fatty tissue (*subcutaneously*, abbreviated *SC* or *SQ*). Let's consider six easy steps to filling the syringe:

1. To get started, it's just as well to wash your hands and check that the spot you are going to inject is clean. Frankly, infections from insulin injections are very rare, but if your skin is dirty, wash up before injecting.
2. Swab the rubber stopper of the vial (bottle) with alcohol.
3. If you are using NPH, mix it up by rolling or rotating the bottle (see Fig-

ure 22a). Do not shake the insulin bottle, since that could damage the insulin and introduce air bubbles into the solution. (Injecting air bubbles will not cause you any harm, but you will not be getting your full dose of insulin.)

4. It is easier to withdraw insulin from the vial if you first inject air to replace the insulin you plan to take out. Otherwise, a slight vacuum gradually builds up in the vial that can draw the plunger of your syringe back toward the vial. So open the syringe, say, to the 10-unit mark if you are going to draw up 10 units, and inject the air into the vial just before you withdraw the insulin (see Figure 22b).

5. Turn the bottle upside down with the needle still through the rubber septum, so that the tip of the needle is covered with insulin (or you will be drawing up air).

6. Pull down on the plunger, drawing insulin into the syringe—more than you plan to use (see Figure 22c). Give the syringe a few taps with your finger to get air bubbles to go to the top, and push the bubbles back into the bottle. Also, push the extra insulin out of the syringe and back into the vial, until the syringe is full (without bubbles) to the right marker on the syringe (say, the 10-unit mark). Then pull the syringe out of the vial.

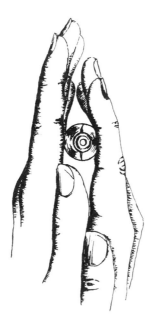

Figure 22a. If the insulin to be injected is a cloudy solution (NPH), roll the bottle between your palms to get the white stuff evenly distributed.

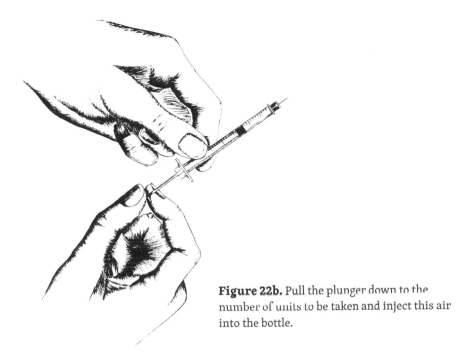

Figure 22b. Pull the plunger down to the number of units to be taken and inject this air into the bottle.

Figure 22c. Turn the bottle upside down and withdraw the insulin by pulling down on the plunger. You may need to push the insulin back into the bottle to eliminate any air bubbles that may have gotten into the syringe. Then pull the plunger down to the number of units to be taken.

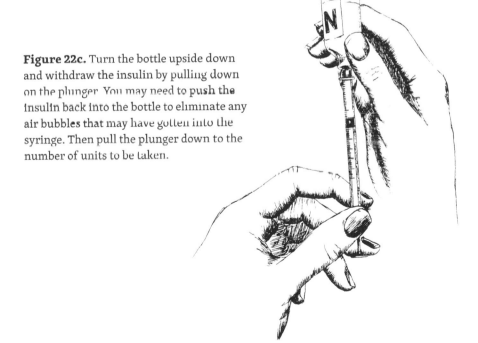

Now for the injection:

1. Pinch up the skin in the chosen area (the choice of a site is discussed below), and poke the needle in at right angles (perpendicularly; see Figure 22d). Some people have the mistaken notion that if they put the needle in slowly, it won't hurt. In fact, the trick is to get the needle in fast, past the nerve endings, before they have a chance to know what hit them.

2. Push down the plunger and withdraw the needle. It's done. Some people recommend pulling back the needle a bit before pushing the plunger, to see that you aren't injecting directly into a vein, but in our experience this is not a real problem. If you see a spot of bleeding, you'll avoid a small bruise if you keep some pressure on the spot for a minute or so.

So there, you've done it! It really isn't that hard, and you don't need to memorize the steps because, after two or three tries, they will become second nature. But there are a few more fine points people often ask about.

Mixing insulins. A rapid-acting or short-acting insulin can be mixed with a longer-acting insulin in the same syringe—for example, 10 units of NPH plus 5 units of Regular—to cut down on the number of injections. In our example, inject 10 units of air into the NPH vial first, and then 5 units of air into the Regular insulin vial. Draw up 5 units of Regular insulin, and then

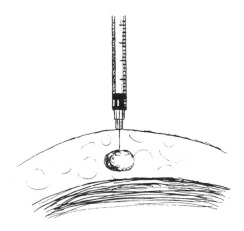

Figure 22d. After pulling the needle out of the bottle, inject the insulin by inserting the needle quickly into pinched-up fatty tissue, at a right angle (perpendicular) to the skin. Push down on the plunger to expel the insulin into the tissue.

the 10 units of NPH (filling the syringe to a total of 15 units). This keeps the additive (protamine) in the NPH from contaminating the Regular insulin. And when you mix insulin, it makes sense not to draw up too much and then reinject the excess into the bottle, since you will be reinjecting the mixture.

Reusing syringes. Studies and anecdotes from our patients suggest that syringes can be reused safely in most cases, but recognizing that the duller they get, the more they will hurt. Be sure to keep the needle capped when not being used, and throw it away if it has touched anything other than your clean skin or the insulin vial. Avoid wiping the needle with alcohol to clean it, as this will remove a coating that allows the needle to pass through the skin more easily. Reusing needles is not safe, however, for people with skin infections or compromised immune systems: those who are HIV-positive or who are taking immune-suppressive drugs for a transplant or an illness such as lupus. Never even think about sharing a syringe with others.

Disposing of syringes. We recommend that used syringes be placed in an opaque container that is thick or hard enough to prevent needles from piercing through. (Why opaque? So that no one sees a supply of syringes and takes them.) Ask your local health department how to dispose of the full containers. There may be local regulations. The Centers for Disease Control website (www.cdc.gov/needledisposal) has links to needle disposal programs available in your state. You can also check with your local health clinic, hospital, or drug store to see whether they have needle disposal containers that you can use.

Dispose of lancets used for blood glucose testing in the same way. It's best not to put syringes and lancets in your trash. You must be especially cautious not to put trash collectors and other people at risk; follow "universal precautions." Everyone should consider their used syringes and lancets potentially infectious.

We recommend *against* breaking off the tip or cutting off used needles, unless you have a device that cuts off the tip and contains the needle inside. Don't place yourself or someone close by at risk from a flying needle or one that accidentally ends up on the floor.

Using Insulin Pens

Compared with the traditional syringe method, there is much less to think about when using an insulin pen. To use a pre-filled disposable pen:

1. Remove the cap from the pen.

2. Screw on or click on a pen needle. Today, pen needles come in a standard size and can be used interchangeably with any type of insulin pen.

3. When using a new insulin pen, prime the pen to remove any air. To do this, dial the knob to 2 units and press the button at the top of the pen (discard 2 units). At this point, the air should be gone and only insulin should remain in the pen.

4. Dial the knob to the number of insulin units you need.

5. Clean off the area of skin to be injected. You do not need to pinch the skin—the needle goes in only a tiny amount. Poke the needle in, perpendicular to the skin. Press the push button on the top of the pen (you will hear clicks) until you can't push any further and the dial reads 0. Keep the needle flush with the skin for a count of 6 seconds. Removing the pen sooner can result in the last bit of insulin dripping from the end of the pen.

6. Put the outer needle cap back on the needle. Twist the needle off, and dispose of it safely.

7. Put the pen cap back on, and you are all done!

Sites for Insulin Injection

Insulin, as we noted, is injected into fatty tissue beneath the skin (subcutaneously). Ideally, it is injected at exactly the same depth each time and near little blood vessels that can absorb it. This ideal cannot be achieved to perfection, but you should try to maintain a technique that holds variation to a minimum. What you want is consistent, reliable absorption of insulin.

Standard spots for the injection of insulin include the outside or front of the thighs, the upper-outer part of the buttocks, the outside of the upper arms, and the abdomen (an inch and a half or more away from the belly button).

But all sites are not created equal. Insulin absorption is fastest from the abdomen, slower from the arms and legs, and slowest from the buttocks. This is more true for Regular insulin than for the rapid-acting insulins, for which there is much less difference in insulin absorption speeds.

It is a good idea to "rotate" injection sites, but you need to think about how this should be done. The best way, if you feel up to it, may be to always inject in the abdomen, rotating around to different parts (upper right to upper left to lower left to lower right, farther from and closer to the belly button, and so on). Many people, however, don't want to inject only into the abdomen.

If you rotate from limb to limb, with or without the abdomen, work out a schedule in which you *inject in the same area at the same time of day*. Maybe you can take your morning shot in the abdomen, suppertime shot in the arm or leg, and bedtime shot in the buttocks.

If you are light in weight, there is likely to be little fatty tissue over your thighs. You are more likely to inject into muscle there, which can be more painful and lead to more bruising. Should this be the case, you should probably avoid your thighs as an injection site.

Factors That Affect Insulin Absorption

The site of injection is not the only thing that affects insulin absorption and its time of action. Be aware that other factors determine how fast insulin action takes place. For instance, exercise can increase insulin absorption, especially if the insulin was injected into a limb being exercised and you exercise within 45 minutes of the injection. So, avoid the leg if you're about to go running, and avoid the arm if you're pitching a ball game.

Overuse of an injection site can also affect absorption. Repeated injections can toughen the tissue with scar tissue over time, which can slow down absorption. That's why, in moving your injection sites around, you should not only change from one large area to another but also keep injections within any one area (like the front of the thigh) at least an inch and a half apart.

Insulin Regimens

Your *insulin regimen* is the plan you have for the types of insulin you take and for the timing and doses of each injection. It is based on your type of diabetes, physical needs, blood glucose goals, and lifestyle (especially eating patterns and activity). Because it involves so many variables, your regimen should, without question, be initiated and fine-tuned in regular consultation with a health care professional knowledgeable in the use of insulin. We want you to be able to modify your regimen from day to day (see below), but you need to start by discussing it with your care provider.

There are as many insulin regimens as there are people using insulin. We'll introduce some of the concepts involved and give some examples.

Insulin Added onto Oral Medications

Sonya has Type 2 diabetes. She was taking maximal doses of oral medica-
tions for her diabetes, but her blood glucose levels were high and she was
bothered by fatigue, blurry vision, thirst, and frequent urination. She found
that her morning blood glucose levels were high (in the 200–250 mg/dl range).
Sonya agreed to try some bedtime insulin while continuing her oral diabetes
medications.

This "combination therapy" is worth a try, especially if the goal is to reduce the morning blood glucose so as to give the pills a better chance to
work during the day. Research has shown that the more normal the glucose
level is in the morning, the more effective oral diabetes medications are at
lowering after-meal glucose levels during the day. Insulin is best given at
bedtime. A long-acting insulin at bedtime helps control the morning glucose by holding the liver's output of glucose in check. In other words, when
there is too little insulin action on the liver overnight, the liver dumps glucose into the bloodstream. This is why people often find that their glucose
level is higher in the morning than when they went to bed, even though
they didn't have anything to eat after dinner.

Twice-a-Day Insulin

Ted is a large man with Type 2 diabetes. He did fine for quite some time on
one shot of insulin before breakfast: 15 units of NPH and 5 units of Regular
insulin. But he began to notice that he was getting up frequently at night to
urinate large amounts. When he tried monitoring his blood glucose four times
a day for a while, he made an amazing discovery: his morning glucose was a
bit high at 140–160 mg/dl, the lunchtime figure was fine at 85–110 mg/dl, and
the figure before supper was okay at 100–140 mg/dl. Ted's bedtime glucose,
however, was 190–260 mg/dl! His doctor suggested switching to a regimen of
70/30 insulin twice a day.

Ted's problem was that he ate a large supper and had no insulin to cover
it. Switching to 70/30 insulin did the job because it contained Regular insulin to cover the supper well and some NPH to last into the night.

Three Shots a Day, Three Opportunities to Adjust Insulin

Maggie is a 29-year-old woman with Type 1 diabetes. She wanted to intensify
her insulin regimen to control her blood glucose levels tightly before attempt-

ing to become pregnant. She had been taking two shots a day of a fixed dose of NPH and lispro insulin: before breakfast at 7 a.m. and before supper at 6 p.m. Her blood glucose control was somewhat erratic, and she was most bothered by middle-of-the-night insulin reactions. With the help of her diabetes nurse educator, Maggie decided to take only lispro insulin before supper and move the NPH to bedtime (11 p.m.). She also learned to adjust her doses further, according to her needs at the time.

The three-shot regimen provided several advantages for Maggie. First, it eliminated the middle-of-the-night low blood glucose because the bedtime NPH was peaking closer to morning; taking it at 6 p.m. had caused a peak action at 2 a.m. Second, the pre-supper lispro covered her evening meal nicely and was pretty much worn out before the NPH kicked in overnight. Finally, three injections provided Maggie with three opportunities to adjust her insulin for variations in control. She learned to take a bit more lispro if her supper was going to be bigger, a bit less if her glucose was low going into supper.

An Intensive Insulin Regimen: Long-Acting Insulin with Rapid-Acting Insulin at Every Meal

William has Type 1 diabetes. He was doing all right with his three-times-daily insulin regimen, but he found that he had to time his meals carefully by the clock. Every day at noon, he knew he had to eat something or his glucose would go low; late in the afternoon, he felt the same way. So William decided he would like to try a regimen that is more intensive but offers the best flexibility while maintaining excellent control. We suggested that he use glargine instead of NPH and take it at bedtime, with a dose of aspart before each meal or snack. With four shots a day, varying the amount of aspart according to his estimated need for each meal, the regimen worked well for William.

The regimen we suggested for William is now the preferred one for persons with Type 1 diabetes: it is the multiple-injection regimen that most closely matches how the normally functioning pancreas makes insulin. Glargine, like detemir, is a "basal" insulin used to provide a relatively stable background level—although it does not provide a truly constant "basal rate" of insulin. But by using a basal insulin with shots of Regular or rapid-acting insulin before each meal, it is possible to mimic fairly well the action of a normal pancreas, which produces a low level of insulin between meals and a much higher level each time the person eats carbohydrate. The intensive regimen that William adopted requires considerable attention on his part and a good knowledge of how much carbohydrate he eats at each meal and how much rapid-acting insulin is needed to cover that amount of carbohydrate.

Matching the amount of carbohydrate eaten with the correct amount of rapid-acting insulin can be challenging, especially if you are eating a large quantity of starches at one sitting, or if you are eating out and are less sure about how much carbohydrate is in the food you're eating. However, taking the time to learn the number of grams of carbohydrate in the most common foods that you're eating will allow you to more accurately dose your rapid-acting mealtime insulin. For our patients with diabetes, we assign insulin-to-carb ratios based on the amount of total insulin they are taking during the day, using the formula 500 divided by total daily insulin dose. So, for someone taking a total of 50 units of insulin daily, the insulin-to-carb ratio is 1:10, or 1 unit of insulin for each 10 grams of carbohydrate eaten. Based on this ratio, the dose of rapid-acting insulin for a meal can be accurately estimated, leading to less glucose variability after meals. For more information on carbohydrate counting, see Chapter 6.

When people are sufficiently interested and committed to take three or four injections a day, to vary their dose of insulin, and to be aware of their carbohydrate counts, we think they should also be introduced to the option of external insulin pump therapy (see Chapter 13).

High-Dose Insulin in Type 2 Diabetes

Ethan's Type 2 diabetes was controlled with pills, but he is now on the maximum doses and his glucose levels are in the 200s. He and his doctor have agreed that insulin treatment should be started, and he is given a prescription for a fairly average starting dose: 15 units of glargine insulin at bedtime. It doesn't work. His glucose levels even increase to the 200–300 mg/dl range. The insulin dose is gradually increased, but only when he gets to 65 units of insulin every morning do his glucose levels come under control. Before long, Ethan needs an additional 30 units of glargine in the morning.

One of the cardinal characteristics of Type 2 diabetes is insulin resistance, meaning that dose requirements are usually high (see Chapters 2 and 7). It is not really surprising, then, that Ethan needs such a large dose of insulin to establish control.

. . .

The following points summarize our overall guidelines concerning insulin regimens:

—We do not think of one regimen as intensive and another as not intensive. We prefer to start with a fairly basic regimen and then "intensify" it until we have reached the number and kinds of insulin injections needed to control a patient's diabetes well. The bottom line is how well your diabetes is controlled, not how many shots you take.

—A basic principle is to use Regular or rapid-acting insulin to cover meals (to hold the blood glucose in control as food is absorbed) and longer-acting insulin to cover between meals and overnight. Regular insulin should be taken at least 30 minutes before a meal so that it is active as the meal is absorbed; rapid-acting insulin is best taken 15–20 minutes before the meal. Many people find that simply dosing the insulin earlier before the meal rather than immediately before the meal will lower their after-meal glucose levels.

Insulin Adjustment

Insulin doses need to be adjusted often, even daily, since very few people have a lifestyle that remains exactly the same, day in and day out. We believe that people with diabetes should understand enough to modify their own doses, safely and reasonably, on a daily basis if necessary. You can't call your health care professional for every larger or smaller meal you eat, every cold you catch, or every period of stress you undergo. Furthermore, with the availability of self-monitoring of blood glucose, people can now keep better track of their own management than ever before.

Here are some suggestions for how you can modify your own insulin regimen:

—*Look for trends.* Don't worry excessively about a single surprising blood glucose. For instance, if a glucose reading is low before lunch one day, it probably doesn't mean much, but if you check it three or four times and find that it is *usually* low before lunch, this is a trend. Act on it. In this case, your morning short- or rapid-acting insulin probably needs to be reduced.

—*Be aware of changes in your diet and in your body weight.* If you make a real effort to eat less and lose weight, there is a good chance that your insulin requirement will decrease significantly. If you gain weight, you will probably need more insulin.

—*Find your high and low blood glucose levels.* If you lead a reasonably consistent life, it is likely that your glucose will be at its highest and lowest at particular times of day and that certain situations or meals will have a consistent effect. For instance, your level may be lowest before lunch (sometimes producing hypoglycemia, with or without symptoms), and it may rise after supper. A particular kind of meal, exercise, or alcoholic drink may cause you to have lows or highs. Chinese food, pizza, and hidden sugar in pasta sauces or bagels are common offenders.

When you are looking for these trends, try to keep other factors constant; otherwise, the trend will not be easy to spot. For example, you won't notice the before-lunch trend if you eat a different kind of breakfast every day.

If your first morning (fasting) blood glucose is high, find out why. Consistently high blood glucose before breakfast can be caused by a variety of factors. The most common is a lack of insulin coverage overnight: whatever doses you are taking are not lasting through the night. A second possibility is the "dawn phenomenon," referring to a period around dawn when blood glucose has a natural tendency to rise due to high levels of cortisol and growth hormone (stress hormones) that occur in the early morning hours. Eating a snack near bedtime that is not covered by or is undertreated with insulin will also cause higher morning glucose levels. The best way to see whether this is the cause is to skip the late-night snack and follow your blood glucose overnight. If it stays at a good overnight level until the next morning when you've skipped the snack, you've got the answer as to why your morning glucose levels have been running high.

Travel Tips

Insulin adjustments are sure to be necessary when you travel across more than three time zones (either across the United States or across the ocean). Look at the length of day and the duration of your insulin. Traveling from west to east, the day is shorter, so you should reduce your long-acting insulin shot (NPH, glargine, or detemir) on your travel day. This prevents an excessive amount of overlapping long-acting insulin as you start living in the new time zone, having lost some hours of the day. The mealtime or high-glucose insulin doses do not change. Traveling from east to west makes a longer day. In that case, on your travel day, you do not need to eliminate the long-acting insulin but will probably need to supplement it with an extra injection of short- or rapid-acting insulin if you have any extra meals or your blood glucose rises too high between injections. You can obtain pamphlets from the American Diabetes Association that provide many additional travel tips.

Self-adjusting Your Insulin Doses

Self-adjustment is a tricky subject because its success varies so much from person to person. As a rule, we encourage thoughtful, safe self-adjustments of insulin dose. But we recognize that it all depends on how sensitive you are to insulin, how much you've been taught, and, frankly, whether you know what you're doing.

A reasonable rule of thumb is to change your basic insulin regimen by no more than about 10%–20% at a time and to change no more often than every three or four days. Of course, this should be done only with the approval of your diabetes health care provider. If you're taking 12 units of glargine at bedtime and it isn't enough (your fasting blood glucose stays high), you can increase the dose by 1 or 2 units, depending on how high the glucose is running. If your blood glucose is going low at lunch with 8 units of lispro in the morning, try 6 or 7 units and see what happens. However, if you've had an alarming problem such as severe hypoglycemia in the middle of the night, you may need to cut back on your overnight, long-acting insulin dose right away—and call your health care professional.

> *Juanita was on an insulin regimen that consisted of 25 units of detemir at bedtime and 8 units of aspart before meals. There was only one problem: she often forgot to take the bedtime insulin and sometimes, when she "felt high" all day, she would increase the detemir to 40 units that night. Juanita couldn't understand why her fasting blood glucose was so unpredictable. And when she started the day with highly variable blood glucose levels, they tended to stay variable all day. That meant she would have to increase her aspart dose from 8 units to up to 13 units with each meal.*

Juanita's problem, of course, was that her bedtime dose was varying way too much, from none to 40 units. Without the basal insulin, she would certainly wake up with high blood glucose levels the following day. She incorrectly reasoned that she could make up for this by taking larger amounts of aspart insulin and doubling the detemir dose the following night. Using rapid-acting insulins to make up for the lack of long-acting insulins can be dangerous—the rapid-acting insulins have more potential to drop the blood glucose quickly. After learning the concept of a basal insulin, Juanita now concentrates on always taking the bedtime detemir and varying it by only 1 or 2 units at a time, based on trends in her fasting blood glucose.

Correctional Insulin

The term "sliding scale" was commonly used to describe the concept of adjusting the amount of insulin to be injected based on the blood glucose level at the time of the shot. We prefer to use the term "correctional" insulin, to emphasize the idea that when the pre-meal glucose level is high, a certain amount of insulin in that dose will be acting simply to "correct down" the glucose into the normal range. In essence, the concept of correctional insulin recognizes that you need more insulin when you go into a meal with a blood glucose of 220 mg/dl than with a blood glucose of 80 mg/dl. Your health care professional will work out the correctional scale. It commonly is calculated by dividing 1,800 by total daily insulin dose, which gives the amount by which 1 unit of insulin will lower the glucose. For example, if you are taking 36 units of insulin for the day, then 1 unit of insulin will drop your blood glucose by 1,800/ 36 = 50 points—a correction factor (or "sensitivity factor") of 1:50. Your care provider will often write down what dose to take for each pre-meal blood glucose range, such as 4 units for 60–100, 5 units for 101–150, 6 units for 151–200, and so on. Alternatively, you may be instructed to add to the mealtime short- or rapid-acting insulin dose that will be covering the meal: 1 unit for a pre-meal glucose of 151–200, 2 units for 201–250, 3 units for 251–300, and so on. This scale depends on how sensitive you are to a unit of insulin—in other words, how much a given unit of insulin is likely to change your blood glucose.

The best way to adjust your insulin dose is to consider both your blood glucose at the time of the meal and what you are going to eat. Today, many applications are available on the Internet and on smartphones that can automatically calculate your insulin dose based on your pre-meal blood glucose and the amount of carbohydrate you are about to eat. This type of technology is standard on insulin pumps.

From experience with our patients, we find that correctional scales are effective. And we believe that, in many ways, they represent the best approach to diabetic control because they strive to match the insulin dose to the actual requirement at the time. But there are some pitfalls to avoid when using a correctional scale:

—It depends on consistent glucose monitoring before meals. Otherwise, you don't know how to adjust the insulin dose.

—Your blood glucose level going into a meal is not the only thing that determines your insulin requirement. Other factors include the size of the meal, recent or planned exercise, and stress or illness. Discuss with your health care professional how much to cut back on your mealtime insulin if you plan to exercise soon after eating, and how much to increase your mealtime insulin when you are ill and your glucose levels are consistently running much higher than usual.

—A correctional scale used before meals may target a lower glucose level than is targeted at bedtime. We commonly target a blood glucose of 100 mg/dl before meals and 120 mg/dl at bedtime, to reduce the risk of a nighttime hypoglycemic reaction.

—The correctional scale is *not* carved in stone. It may be too much or too little, and it may be wrong at only one end of the glucose spectrum. For instance, your scale may say to take 7 units for a blood glucose over 350, but each time you do this you end up with hypoglycemia later; in this case, your correctional insulin needs to be reduced at the high end, say to 5 units maximum. Or perhaps your scale says to take 2 extra units before a meal if your glucose is over 150, but when you do this you find your next reading is always over 200; in this case, your correctional insulin is too low at the low end, and you should take 3 or 4 units instead. With some thought, you'll find that you can make these small adjustments in your correctional scale.

—Be patient when counteracting high glucose levels with correctional insulin. Make sure that you let that correctional dose bring the glucose level down—it can take several hours. Rapid-acting insulin has a duration of action of about 4 hours. Some people repeat a correctional insulin dose once or twice more if their blood glucose level is still high 30–60 minutes after a correctional dose. Doing so can lead to "stacking" of insulin and a high risk for a low-glucose reaction 1–2 hours later.

. . .

Insulin types, doses, and regimens can be the most confusing aspect of diabetes self-care. Still, if you put your mind to it, this is no more complicated than driving a car or setting a digital watch, much less programming your DVD player. In this chapter we have broken down insulin use into its several elements: the kinds of insulin, the various dosing regimens, and the possibilities for self-adjustments.

When dealing with insulin, there is no substitute for a good relationship with a knowledgeable health care professional. Experienced professionals may disagree with some of the guidelines we've presented here, and they may be right to do so in your case. There may also be more than one way to reach the goal of good blood glucose control. So it is essential that you and your treating team work together. We firmly believe that the key to using insulin correctly (and to most other aspects of diabetes care) is a good relationship between you and your health care professional.

Take Home Messages

- Insulin is the most effective medication for lowering blood glucose levels.
- Insulins differ in how quickly they start lowering blood glucose levels and how long they keep working.
- From fastest to longest acting, insulins are classified as rapid-, short-, intermediate-, or long-acting.
- Rapid- and short-acting insulins keep your blood glucose levels from going too high right after meals.
- Intermediate- and long-acting insulins keep your blood glucose levels from going too high between meals and at night.
- Most people in the United States take insulin using a vial and syringe, but insulin pens are becoming more popular.

13

Insulin Pumps

- "I've heard that some people get better control by using the pump. I want to try it."
- "I lead a stressful and unpredictable life. People tell me that I should try an insulin pump. Why?"
- "I've got a good hemoglobin A1c, but it's because I balance my highs with awful lows. Is there a way to even things out? I want to feel better."
- "What are disposable 'patch pumps'?"
- "Can you tell me about something called 'sensor-augmented pump therapy'?"

Insulin pumps have been around for more than 40 years. Today, in the United States, about 25% of people with Type 1 diabetes use insulin pumps.

Over the years pumps have improved a lot. The earliest models, introduced in the late 1970s, were the size of a backpack, so they weren't practically useful. When Richard Rubin's son began pumping in 1983 at the age of 11, he was among a very small number of children using an insulin pump. His first pump was the size and weight of a brick. The pump continually pulled down his pants, and he jokingly takes credit for the current fashion trend among young people of wearing pants way lower than most adults find appropriate.

Pump use has now spread to groups that never used pumps before, including people with Type 2 diabetes, women who develop diabetes when they are pregnant (gestational diabetes), and children—even very young children.

A few summers ago, Rubin spoke at a conference organized by the Children with Diabetes Foundation, which was attended by over 1,000 youngsters with diabetes and their parents. After one of his sessions, a very cute 2-year-old came up to him and said, "Dr. Rubin, would you like to see my pump?" Without waiting for a reply, the little boy whipped up his shirt and there was his pump, attached to his diaper. Rubin was duly impressed. When his son got his first pump, he was one of the youngest kids in the country to have one. No longer.

How Pumps Work

Most insulin pumps are now the size of a cellphone (see Figure 23). The pump includes:

—A reservoir that holds rapid-acting insulin

—A battery-operated pump that pushes insulin out of the reservoir

—A computer chip that lets you choose how much insulin the pump will deliver throughout the day

—A plastic tube (called a cannula) that carries insulin from the pump. The tube has a needle at the end that you stick under your skin. The tubing should be changed every few days.

The pump delivers very small amounts of insulin all day long (see Figure 24). The pump is programmable: it lets you vary the rate of continuous delivery (called the basal rate) so that you can automatically get different

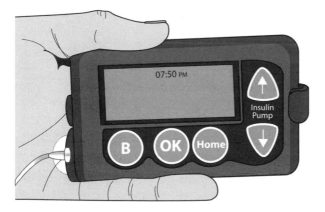

Figure 23. An external insulin pump is about the size of a cellphone. It has an internal reservoir of insulin and a computerized mechanism to deliver insulin through the tubing to the insertion site in precise quantities.

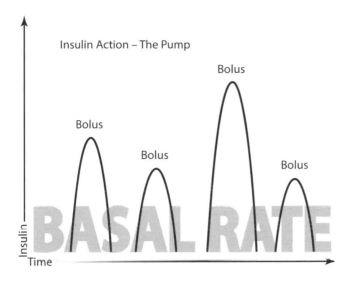

Figure 24. An insulin pump delivers insulin in two ways. The first is in the form of a continuous trickle (the *basal rate*) to meet the body's background need for insulin. The second is as a *bolus*, a larger amount of insulin delivered all at once to meet the body's need for more insulin at mealtimes.

amounts of insulin at different times of day, to keep your blood glucose close to normal between meals and overnight. The pump also lets you take extra insulin (called a bolus) when you eat, to cover the carbohydrates you have just consumed. You can also take a bolus to bring down a high glucose level.

The newer pumps are easier to program, so they can administer insulin with personalized profiles. You can choose bolus profiles based on how much insulin is still active in your body, your insulin-to-carbohydrate (insulin-to-carb) ratio, and your insulin sensitivity factor, and to match the composition of your meal. Pumps contain "food libraries" that help you count carbs, and they suggest bolus sizes based on your personal insulin-to-carb ratio, your insulin sensitivity ratio, and the number of carbs you plan to consume. These pumps also allow wireless transmission of blood glucose readings from a glucose meter to the pump, and you can download pump data to create graphs and reports on your computer. One pump integrates with a continuous glucose monitor (CGM), so the CGM data appear on the screen of the pump.

Advantages of Insulin Pumps

Jeanine is a successful young lawyer. She has had diabetes since childhood, but she'd never found the timing of her day unmanageable until she became a litigator. Now, lunchtime break is up to the judge, the jury, the opposing lawyers, and innumerable other factors she can't control. An insulin pump turned out to be a good answer. She just continues on basal rate until lunchtime comes along, whether it is 11 a.m. or 2 p.m.

Flexibility and Quality of Life

People who switch to pumps generally say that their lives are more flexible and that they feel freer. They say they worry less about when they eat (because their basal rates keep their glucose level stable when they aren't eating). They also worry less about what they eat because they can "bolus" more or less to cover the size of their meal. They can sleep late without running out of insulin and waking up with a high blood glucose. They can exercise without having to eat large amounts of carbohydrate. People say their lives—and their families' lives—feel more normal. All this adds up to a better quality of life. Studies have found that pump users are happier with their diabetes treatment regimen and have higher levels of well-being than people taking insulin injections.

Improved Control

Theoretically, using a pump should give you better glucose control, because the way it delivers basal and bolus insulin is closer to the way a normally functioning pancreas works—though, of course, nothing works as well as a normally functioning pancreas when it comes to blood glucose control. Research shows that pump therapy does have advantages over injections. In many studies, people who used pumps had a greater reduction in their A1c levels than study participants who were taking injections. Though the A1c-lowering advantage was not huge (usually about 0.5%), the difference is considered big enough to reduce the risk of developing diabetes complications.

Research also shows that people using pumps have a reduced risk of severe hypoglycemia compared with those taking insulin by injection. So it seems that pump therapy has the potential to improve long-term glucose control and to reduce the risk of the most serious immediate concern for most people with diabetes: severe hypoglycemia.

Disadvantages of Insulin Pumps

Weight Gain

We have mentioned this one before: if your glucose control improves you will gain weight, unless you either consume fewer calories or burn more calories through exercise. Pumps can lower your A1c, so pump therapy can lead to weight gain unless you make some adjustments. On the other hand, if using a pump leads to fewer glucose lows and less extra eating to bring your glucose back up, that could help with weight control.

Skin Complications

One evening Martin noticed that the area around his infusion set was uncomfortable, but since it was not red he assumed he was okay. The next morning the pain was worse. Martin had a pretty serious infection. A week's treatment with antibiotics got rid of the infection, but Martin learned his lesson—always check immediately when you have discomfort at your infusion site. Infections are much easier to treat when they are caught quickly.

The risk of skin infection is greater with the pump than with injection therapy. With an injection, you stick the needle in and then remove it right away. Bacteria don't have much chance to get into the opening. But with the pump, disposable parts (the needle or cannula, tubing, and reservoir) stay in place much longer (two to five days), giving bacteria more opportunity to infect the site. Some people are more susceptible to infection than others, so they need to do more elaborate skin preparation and change the needle insertion site more frequently. A man with hair on his belly is especially at risk. But almost everyone gets a local infection (something between a pimple and a boil) at one time or another. These infections usually go away on their own once you change the site of needle insertion. Infrequently, an oral antibiotic or even drainage by a doctor is needed.

Diabetic Ketoacidosis

Sheila woke up with a 350 blood glucose. She was surprised it was so high, but as an experienced pumper she was confident that adding a correction bolus to her breakfast bolus would solve the problem. In the middle of the day she started to feel sick to her stomach, and her blood glucose was still around 300. Sheila was puzzled, decided to skip lunch, and took another correction bolus. A couple of hours later she was feeling really sick, got up to go to the bathroom,

started vomiting, and passed out. When the medics arrived she was breath-
ing heavily. Sheila was in ketoacidosis. Her infusion had partially pulled out
of her skin the night before, and for hours she had been getting virtually no
insulin. Now Sheila checks her ketones every time her glucose is high and she
can't explain why.

People using insulin pumps must understand that there is a risk of ketoacidosis (see Chapter 21) if the delivery of insulin stops for any reason. In all
cases, this should be preventable if you are involved in good self-care. The
most frequent cause of flow interruption is a pump that has been allowed
to run dry—and that is totally preventable! Other causes may be that the
needle falls out of the skin, the reservoir is improperly placed in the pump,
or insulin clogs up the line. Whatever the reason, since only short-acting
insulin is being delivered and at a very slow rate, if it stops, the body will
become completely insulin-deficient within a few hours. This is one step
away from ketoacidosis. For pump users, regular monitoring of blood glucose and attentiveness to symptoms should allow you to become aware of
an infusion problem before it gets out of hand.

Cost

A drawback of pump therapy can be the cost of the pump and supplies. The
total cost is probably about twice that of taking three to four injections a
day, but the cost to you depends on your insurance coverage. If you are interested in pumping, look into what your insurance will cover.

Feeling Tethered

Some people say that being attached to the pump at all (or almost all) times
bothers them. For most but not all people, this feeling passes pretty quickly.
One woman did say jokingly that it took her a while to get used to making
love with a pump in place.

Disposable Patch Pumps

Many people see disposable patch pumps as the future of insulin pumping.
One company has a patch pump on the market, several other companies
are applying for FDA approval, and many other companies are close behind.
These pumps are creating lots of buzz because they are much smaller and
lighter than standard durable pumps and because the upfront cost for these
pumps is lower. The patch pump now on the market has two parts. One part

contains the insulin; it is discarded when the insulin has been used. The other part, into which the disposable part fits, contains the computer chip and the mechanism that controls the insulin delivery.

Disposable pumps are sometimes called patch pumps because they attach (patch) directly to your body (usually the upper arm or abdomen). When the pump is attached, the needle that delivers insulin goes right into your skin, so patch pumps, unlike standard pumps, don't have tubes or cannulas. The patch pump currently on the market is controlled by a handheld "personal diabetes manager" (PDM). This means carrying something extra compared with using a standard pump, but that's balanced by the convenience of the PDM having a built-in blood glucose meter. Like standard pumps, this disposable pump has several other useful features: a library of common foods to help you count carbs, a bolus calculator to recommend boluses, and software that lets you download and review your blood glucose, insulin, and other data.

Sensor-Augmented Pumps

Technological advances such as pump therapy and the continuous glucose monitor (CGM), used individually, can improve glucose control and quality of life for people with diabetes. Recently, scientists have been looking at the potential benefits of combining these two technologies. A company that makes an integrated pump-CGM device sponsored a 12-month multicenter study in the United States and Canada to see whether "sensor-augmented pump therapy" (SAPT) had benefits for adults, teens, and children with Type 1 diabetes. Participants in the SAPT group had an insulin pump that also received glucose readings from a CGM every five minutes. The CGM provided alarms for glucose levels that ran either too low or too high. The CGM did not change how much insulin the pump gave—the wearer of the pump had to do that. The study was called the STAR 3 trial; one of us (Rubin) was on the STAR 3 steering committee that helped design and oversee the study.

None of the study participants were using either pumps or CGM when they entered the study. On entry, half the participants began SAPT and the other half continued with their previous regimen of multiple daily injections (MDI) and self-monitoring of blood glucose.

The STAR 3 results were pretty impressive. In fact, they were impressive enough to be published in the prestigious *New England Journal of Medi-*

cine. Adults in the SAPT group saw their A1c average drop 1.0% during the 12-month study, compared with 0.4% in the MDI group. Just as impressive was that the teens and children in the SAPT group also saw their A1c levels go down—by 0.4%, compared with a rise of 0.2% among teens and children in the MDI group. Young people face special challenges when it comes to glucose control, so the effects of SAPT for teens and children is striking. In fact, the difference in A1c change between the SAPT and MDI groups during the study was the same for teens and children as it was for adults—0.6%. That represents a 25%–45% reduction in the risk of kidney, nerve, and eye complications of diabetes. Notably, almost all the change in A1c took place quickly, during the first three months of the study.

Despite the advantages of SAPT for A1c reduction, changes in rates of severe hypoglycemia, ketoacidosis, and weight gain were no different in the SAPT group than in the MDI group. Rates of severe hypoglycemia were very low in all STAR 3 participants, ketoacidosis was practically nonexistent, and participants in both groups gained weight (about 4.5 pounds during the year). The weight gain was probably the result of improved glucose control, as we have suggested in earlier chapters.

The STAR 3 results also underline the connection between self-care behavior and clinical outcomes. The SAPT group participants who, on average, wore their CGM sensor more than 80% of the time, 61%–80% of the time, 41%–60% of the time, and 21%–40% of the time had an average A1c reduction of 1.2%, 0.8%, 0.6%, and 0.2%, respectively. This reminds us of a statement made by Dr. C. Everett Koop when he was U.S. Surgeon General: "Medications don't work for people who don't take them." Apparently the same is true for advanced diabetes technologies.

The use of a sensor-augmented pump was associated with several benefits when compared with multiple daily injections. Adults and caregivers in the SAPT group had a greater reduction in fears about hypoglycemia, and adults, caregivers, and children in the SAPT group had greater improvements in key satisfaction measures: treatment convenience, treatment effectiveness, and overall preference compared with previous treatments.

So SAPT is a very promising approach to treatment for people with Type 1 diabetes. We don't yet have any studies to show how it works for people with Type 2 diabetes. As a further point of interest, the STAR 3 results provide a foundation for building a "closed loop" artificial pancreas, which we tell you more about in Chapter 31.

Is Pump Therapy for You?

The desire for more flexibility, better blood glucose control, and an improved sense of well-being are usual reasons for starting insulin pump therapy. Perhaps you are tired of never being able to get on track with your irregular work schedule, or you want good control for a healthy pregnancy, or you would just like to smooth out the bumps in your control because feeling poorly all the time is driving you crazy. These are all good reasons for considering an external pump.

The decision to use a pump depends on several factors. Before we recommend the use of a pump for one of our patients, we consider the following issues:

—Does he understand diabetes pretty well? Pump therapy won't work if a person can't distinguish an insulin reaction from the flu or a carbohydrate from a fat. So we want the person to have a good basic education in diabetes.

—Does she test her blood glucose regularly and frequently? Without such monitoring, insulin pumps can be dangerous. We want to see the person testing blood glucose at least four times a day for at least a few months, to confirm that she is serious about diabetes control.

—Can he accept the technology of a pump and the mechanics of dealing with it? Every now and then, a person comes along who talks about using a pump but wouldn't feel comfortable changing a light bulb without someone else's help. Usually, the person is relieved when we suggest that perhaps pump therapy is not for him. These people are rare.

—Are her expectations reasonable? If a person has never even tried to follow a diet, has very late-stage complications, or thinks the pump will solve all her problems, then some reality testing is more valuable than starting this therapy.

If you are considering a pump, the most important thing for you to do is carefully question your own motives. Ask yourself some questions. This is not a decision that your cousin or best friend or a pump salesperson can make for you. Work through the issues by yourself, and then perhaps talk them over with someone close to you (as well as with your doctor). It's important to take an honest look at your state of mind about the whole thing.

Do you really think that pump therapy will work for you? It won't work if you're doing it just to get your mother, husband, or doctor off your back. It won't work if you're skeptical or have too high expectations. And it won't cure all your problems. With the additional flexibility comes a heightened responsibility for the components of your diabetes control. You may be used to your doctor telling you exactly how much insulin to take and when. Although you'll have guidelines and education about the insulin pump, many of the decisions related to your diabetes control will be left up to you.

Are you committed to regular blood glucose monitoring? Generally, we recommend that pump users test before each meal and at bedtime. This is necessary not only to get the feedback needed to properly adjust pump rates but also to avoid ketoacidosis should the pump stop.

Are you worried that the pump will get in the way when you want to play sports, go swimming, or have sex? Some prospective pump users do have concerns about "being hooked up to something all the time." Some adjustments have to be made, but most people find they can do everything they were able to do before the pump. It is even possible to go off the pump for an hour or two, or even longer, if you slip in an injection of rapid-acting insulin.

Are you ready to be connected to a device that lets people know you have diabetes? For some people, this is a real and deep-seated concern about being hooked up to a pump. True, the pump can be hidden under clothing, but you know it's there, and at some point others will also. With the pump, more people may find out that you have diabetes. Is that okay with you? Answering this question may mean exploring your feelings about having diabetes.

Is there a health care provider nearby who can help you? This should not be an issue that stops anyone from using the pump, but in some locales it probably is. More and more endocrinologists are becoming familiar with pump use, however, so seek one out if you are interested.

These are not easy questions to answer, and we certainly don't present them in order to be negative. We think pumps are a terrific advance for many people. There are resources to help you. Talk to health care professionals who are familiar with pump therapy. Other pump users can also be an excellent source of information. Your health care provider may be able to put you in touch with some experienced pump users. Also, many areas have an insulin pump support group led by a diabetes educator. It can really help to talk to people who are already using pumps. We regularly hear the testimonials: "I worried about sleeping with it, too, but in two years the needle has never come out while I was sleeping and has never woken me up." "Even after pregnancy, the pump has been great, and I just can't imagine being without it now."

Finally, in considering whether pump therapy is for you, take a look at the equipment itself. Watch a demonstration and check out the important features. Pump company representatives can show you the operation of their specific pump in detail if you don't have an experienced diabetes educator readily available.

Starting an Insulin Pump

Starting to use an insulin pump can be exciting, but it can also be scary. Some pump users say that starting an insulin pump is "like learning about diabetes all over again." There may be a new angle to food: "How much insulin is that plate of pasta worth?" The pump can give a new slant on interpreting blood glucose levels: "My blood glucose is 164, but I bolused 4 units just two hours ago. Should I bolus some more?" It's a lot easier to take another small bolus by pressing buttons than it was to get out all the equipment to take an injection. And the pump also provides a tool to keep from "bottoming out" with exercise: "How much should I reduce my basal to keep from going low with aerobics?"

Starting an insulin pump requires support, equipment, education, and testing. "Support" refers to the team of professionals who will assist you with getting started and becoming comfortable with pump therapy. Usually this means a diabetologist, a nurse educator, and a pump company trainer. We usually ask our patients to also see a dietitian before beginning to use a pump. This is a good time for you to review what healthy eating means; the dietitian will also help you develop some tools to use in calculating the composition of various foods. As you start pump therapy, keep in frequent contact with the team. The time spent in the short term is worth it in the long term. As your questions are answered, you will gain the confidence you need to take on the responsibility of a new management approach.

Your team will help you take the first step in starting pump therapy: choosing the equipment and being trained in its use. Our advice is to find out from your doctor or educator which pumps they are familiar with and whether they recommend a specific brand or model. Once you have a pump, you need to learn the technical steps for operating it: setting the clock, filling the reservoir and tubing, inserting the needle and taping it into place, changing sites of needle insertion, setting the basal rate, programming a bolus, and so on. For our patients, we recommend learning how to do these things before they get started on actual insulin delivery; that way, learning the mechanics doesn't get in the way of learning how to use the pump for blood glucose control.

Some educators like to have future pump users practice with a saltwater solution (normal saline) in the pump so they can learn how to use it without the pressure of making mistakes with insulin. (Usual insulin injections are continued during this "saltwater training" period.) In our area of the country, the pump company provides a very good initial training in the use of the pump, which is followed by reinforcement and further practice with the educator.

The next step is to get started with insulin in the pump. In the first few days the goal is to estimate beginning basal and bolus rates and, with testing, to make modifications until blood glucose levels are reasonably well controlled. Two essential components in these first few days are frequent blood glucose testing (before and after meals, at bedtime, and at 3 a.m.) and frequent contact with the pump team.

Initially, you determine a safe basal rate (or series of rates). If the basal rate is right, your blood glucose should stay relatively stable when you are not eating and when you are not especially active. If the basal rate is too high, your blood glucose will trend down with long intervals between meals; if the basal rate is too low, your level will trend up. You may need several basal rates. For example, you may need a higher rate in the early morning hours (the "dawn phenomenon"), a lower rate at night, and something in between the rest of the time. Ordinarily, basal rates do not require much adjustment after the first few days. You can just program the pump to deliver the same set of basal rates day after day. You may, for instance, need 0.4 unit per hour all night, 1.0 unit per hour from 4 a.m. to 8 a.m. (dawn hours), and 0.6 unit per hour during the day.

Recall that the bolus dose has two purposes: to correct blood glucose levels when they are higher than your target range and to cover food to be eaten. For correction boluses, you need to know how much your blood glucose will drop in response to 1 unit of insulin. This is your *insulin sensitivity ratio*. For many people this ratio remains consistent throughout a 24-hour period. For some people, however, it may vary throughout the day. For example, 1 unit of insulin may bring your blood glucose down 40 points in the evening but only 25 points in the morning.

We estimate the amount of insulin needed to cover food primarily from the *carbohydrate* content of the food. This is your *insulin-to-carbohydrate ratio*.

In the first few days of pump therapy, you and your pump team will be studying your blood glucose levels closely and making adjustments in both basal and bolus dosing. You'll work together to reach the goal of a predictable blood glucose pattern: starting at a certain level before a meal, elevating somewhat after the meal, and returning to your target level four hours later. Of course, in daily living with a pump, all sorts of factors will come into play that will cause the blood glucose to fluctuate in predictable and unpredictable ways. Your pump team will help you learn how to use the pump in your daily life.

On a trip to New York City early in his pumping days, Jethro was really looking forward to a nice restaurant dinner, including a decadent dessert. Unfortunately, his pre-meal glucose level was 240. Still intent on his dream meal, he calculated his correction dose. Throughout the meal he kept track of the carbs he was consuming and bolused accordingly. When he checked his glucose again before dessert, he was delighted to see his level was coming down. He had a slice of his favorite dessert, coconut custard pie, and two hours after dinner his blood glucose was 130. Jethro said, "With a pump and a plan I can do most anything."

Using the Carbohydrate Counting System

Debbie had been on a pump for almost a year, but she still had occasional lows and highs, particularly after a meal. She decided to see if she was taking the right amount of insulin for meals—and she made two important discoveries. First, she wasn't accurately counting carbs for some foods. And second, her insulin-to-carb ratio was actually 1.0 unit to every 15 grams of carbs, not to every 10 grams as she had thought.

Let's assume that 1 unit of insulin lowers your blood glucose by 50 mg/dl, and 1 unit of insulin covers 15 grams of carbohydrate.

Example 1. Your blood glucose is 198. You plan to have 2 cups of cereal, ½ cup of skim milk, and a 9-inch banana for breakfast. You calculate your bolus as follows:

—The nutrition information on the cereal box shows that there are 48 grams of carbohydrate in the cereal.

—One-half cup of milk contains 6 grams of carbohydrate.

—A 9-inch banana contains 30 grams of carbohydrate.

—Your total insulin requirement *for the food alone,* based on your personal
   breakfast insulin-to-carb ratio, is calculated as follows:

   48 + 6 + 30 = 84 grams of carbohydrate

   84 ÷ 15 = 5.6 units of insulin

—Plus, you have a blood glucose target of 100 mg/dl, and based on your
   insulin sensitivity ratio, you calculate the insulin needed to correct your
   blood glucose:

   198 – 100 = 98 mg/dl of blood glucose

   98 ÷ 50 = 2 units of insulin

—Your total bolus is therefore:

   5.6 + 2 = 7.6 units of insulin

Example 2. You are on the road and decide to stop at a deli for lunch. You
do not have your blood glucose meter with you. You order a sliced turkey
sandwich on rye bread and french fries. You can "eyeball" your insulin requirement by estimating the carbohydrates:

—Two pieces of rye bread contain 30 grams of carbohydrate.

—Ten french fries contain about 45 grams of carbohydrate.

—Because you do not know your blood glucose level and do not have any
   reason to think you are running high or low, you bolus for the food
   alone:

   30 + 45 = 75 grams of carbohydrate

   75 ÷ 15 = 5 units of insulin

If you have a smartphone or some other connection to the Internet, you
can look up the amount of carbohydrate in most foods.

Advanced Use of an Insulin Pump

Changing the Basal Rate

In some situations you may need to change your basal rate temporarily.
During exercise and after exposure to hot outdoor temperatures (such as a

day at the beach), you may want to decrease the basal rate or even stop the infusion of insulin for a while. Ordinarily, we recommend that you *do not stop the infusion of insulin for more than a few hours, unless you plan to supplement with an injection of rapid-acting insulin.* (Remember, insulin deficiency can result in a matter of hours if the infusion of rapid-acting insulin is stopped.)

Stress, whether physical (such as an illness or injury) or emotional, may increase your basal insulin requirement. Some women find that in the days preceding their menstrual period their basal requirement is increased. Steroid medications such as prednisone or cortisone (even if only injected into a joint) will also markedly increase your insulin requirement.

A temporary alternative to increasing the basal rate is to take larger boluses based on blood glucose readings. Changing the basal rate is a slow way to change insulin delivery compared with changing a bolus. For example, increasing the basal rate from 0.5 to 0.8 unit per hour for two hours gives only 0.6 unit of extra insulin—an amount more easily given as a bolus.

More about Boluses

Whenever Brenda's glucose went high, she would "over-fix," taking too big a bolus and ending up low. Finally she figured out that if she ate a small snack when she took the large correction bolus, she ended up much closer to a normal glucose level.

Some people are bothered by symptoms of high blood glucose after eating a particularly high-carbohydrate meal: "I know my blood sugar is 250 right now, but I guarantee by lunchtime it will be down to normal." This effect can often be blunted by taking the bolus 15–20 minutes before the meal rather than right before the meal. This will lower the after-meal blood glucose and keep the next pre-meal blood glucose in the same good range, while using the same insulin bolus dose.

Stefan makes regular use of the dual-wave and square-wave bolus features on his pump. He uses the square-wave bolus when he will be eating over a long time. He uses the dual-wave feature (combining a normal bolus and a square-wave bolus) for dealing with previously hard-to-bolus-for meals such as pizza.

High-fat meals may also call for some changes in the bolus. As we've mentioned in earlier chapters, although fat does not affect blood glucose directly, it can slow the absorption of carbohydrate eaten along with it. If too much of the bolus is taken all at once before a high-fat meal, the blood glucose may actually go low before the meal is absorbed. Pump users can compensate for this by using the *square-wave* bolus option, which delivers the bolus over a longer period than the normal bolus.

With boluses, the first rule is to *be safe*, and being safe means not having a severe hypoglycemic episode. For example, it is not advisable to bolus for your supper while you're still at work and assume that the drive home will be the lead time for the insulin. What if you get stuck in traffic? Do you have a glucose source in the car?

Treating Low Blood Glucose

As with any type of insulin therapy, glucose lows should be treated immediately with fast-acting carbohydrate. You may need an additional snack if the low occurs within a few hours after a large bolus, since the bolus may still be acting. Stopping the basal rate will have very little effect. The more important thing is to eat carbohydrate.

Treating High Blood Glucose

If you have unusually high blood glucose, you will need to do some problem solving to find out the cause. The following are common reasons:

—*Missed bolus.* Check the pump to see whether you bolused with your last meal.

—*Insufficient bolus.* This commonly occurs when you eat unfamiliar food and are not sure what's in it.

—*Prolonged use of the needle insertion site.* With extended use, absorption at the needle insertion site may be hampered, and insulin will then become less effective.

—*Pump catheter gets dislodged.* This prevents you from receiving both your basal and your bolus insulins.

—*Illness.* Many people find that their blood glucose levels rise when they are ill.

—*Pump malfunction.* If there seems to be a problem with the device itself—for instance, if the display doesn't respond when you push the button—contact the manufacturer. The company will help you with the problem or send you a new pump.

—*Empty reservoir.* If you're a careful driver, you wouldn't let your car run out of gas. Similarly, you should never allow your pump reservoir to run dry.

If you are not sure why your glucose is high, bolus. If it doesn't come down quite a bit within one hour, change your syringe, tubing, and needle and check to see that the pump is delivering insulin from the needle tip. Then bolus again. Remember, since the pump uses only rapid-acting insulin, you could develop ketoacidosis within several hours if you are not getting any insulin. If you are in doubt or if you have ketones in your urine, take an injection of rapid-acting insulin right away.

Exercise

Darius is the starting goalie on his college lacrosse team, and he enjoys other contact sports as well. The pump never stops him from competing. He keeps his pump in his pocket when he plays. The only adjustments he makes for his diabetes are to check his blood glucose frequently during a game and to make sure he has a glucose source handy. He's also let his coach and a couple of teammates know about his diabetes, "just in case."

Learning your individual response to exercise and to different kinds of exercise is crucial in determining what adjustments to make in your pumped insulin dosing. Pump users have found several strategies helpful in preventing hypoglycemia related to exercise:

—Eat extra carbohydrate before you exercise. If the exercise is prolonged, take additional carbohydrate while exercising.

—Take a reduced bolus for a meal preceding exercise.

—Decrease the basal rate 15–30 minutes before, during, and/or after exercise.

—Eat additional carbohydrate after exercise.

. . .

In the weeks and months after starting to use an insulin pump, you will learn how to handle the many situations that arise while living with a pump: what to do with your pump when showering, how to tell your date what that funny-looking beeper is, where to put the pump during sexual activity, and how to conceal it under a formfitting gown or macho T-shirt. Although you may find solutions to these situations on your own, remember that there are resources out there to help: experienced pump users, your doctor, educators, support groups, counselors, and the insulin pump company. Pump therapy can be a great way to help your self-care.

Take Home Messages

- In the United States, about one-quarter of people with Type 1 diabetes and a growing number of people with Type 2 diabetes use insulin pumps.
- Potential advantages of pump therapy include a more flexible lifestyle, better quality of life, lower A1c levels, and less severe hypoglycemia.
- Potential disadvantages of pump therapy include weight gain (due to improved glucose control), skin irritations and infections, increased risk of ketoacidosis, and higher costs.
- The number, sophistication, and variety of available pumps are growing every year. Today, in addition to standard pumps, there are disposable patch pumps and pumps with an integrated continuous glucose monitor.
- You could benefit from pump therapy if you are willing to check your glucose levels at least four times a day, if you can handle the pump technology, and if you have realistic expectations about what the pump can do.
- When starting pump therapy, it is best to have the active support of your health care provider, a diabetes educator, and a pump trainer who works for the company that supplies your pump.

PART III

Living with Diabetes

We once had three tough individuals in our diabetes self-management program at Johns Hopkins: a retired CIA agent, an ex-Marine, and a New York City cop. Not one of them was thrilled when our psychologist came in to talk about living with diabetes. One of them had never even told his family, much less his friends or coworkers, that he had diabetes; another thought there was no way that anything emotional could affect him; and the third just didn't "believe in" psychology.

Rather than give up, the psychologist used his own skills to make a dent in these men's strong defenses. Gradually, he convinced them that there is a link—as Alan Alda once put it in a commencement address to the Columbia University College of Physicians and Surgeons—between the head bone and the heart bone. Emotions *do* play a role in the success of your self-care. In fact, emotions play a *huge* role.

In Part III we discuss these links between how you feel about diabetes and what you do about it. We even go further, considering how the world around you may react: your family, friends, employer, health care professional, and "the system" (meaning the organization that provides care and pays for it). Your interaction with the world around you, how you get help and support, is a key to successful self-care.

You can't do it without recognizing that emotions play a role, and you can't do it all by yourself—even if you're a CIA agent, an ex-Marine, or a New York City cop.

14

The Emotional Side of Diabetes

- "Even when I do everything I'm supposed to do, I get blood glucose readings that make no sense at all. It drives me crazy!"
- "I've had diabetes for 20 years. The tools for managing my diabetes have improved so much. I feel thankful and hopeful the tools will continue to get better."
- "Every once in a while something about my diabetes makes me laugh. It's amazing how good that feels."

People often tell us that the biggest barrier to taking the best possible care of their diabetes is feeling overwhelmed—overwhelmed by having to deal with diabetes on top of everything else they have to manage in their lives. So if you feel this way, you are not alone. Most people who have diabetes feel overwhelmed at least some of the time. They suffer from a condition variously known as *diabetes distress, diabetes burnout,* or *diabetes overwhelmus.*

And it's no surprise why. There are no vacations from diabetes; it's with you 24 hours a day, every day of the year. Not only that, but few of the things you're supposed to do to manage your diabetes are what you could honestly call pleasant. Like sticking yourself to test your blood or give yourself insulin. How about exercising regularly? It's true that some people actually like being physically active, but it's perfectly clear that most people don't feel this way. The same applies to eating right. Most of us would agree that the tastiest, most satisfying foods aren't usually the healthiest choices. Yet, if you have diabetes, you're supposed to do all these things and more, regularly, for the rest of your life.

And of course that's not all. Even if you did everything exactly by the book every moment of your life with diabetes—an impossibility, naturally—this would not guarantee that your blood glucose control would be perfect or that you would never develop any of the possible long-term complications of diabetes. People with diabetes and their health care providers all wish there was some nice, neat formula for calculating exactly the mix of exercise, food, and medication required to keep blood glucose levels normal all the time. Unfortunately, a few health care providers even act as if this *were* possible. But everybody should know and acknowledge that it's not.

That's what makes diabetes so demanding: you are supposed to make big changes in your life, and you are supposed to maintain those changes every day, forever, even though they are continuous, are unpleasant, can have a serious downside (more frequent hypoglycemia and possible weight gain), and can't absolutely guarantee that you won't develop complications.

So what are you supposed to do? The people who cope best with the emotional side of diabetes, not coincidentally, are also the most successful at sticking with their diabetes treatment plan and maintaining good blood glucose control. We have learned from these good copers that there are two ways to deal with the emotions that trigger diabetes distress. The first is to *change the situation* that causes your distress. The second is to *change the way you think about the situation* that causes the distress.

Sources of Diabetes Distress and How to Change Situations That Cause Distress

Although the emotional side of diabetes is different for everyone, some responses are common. To cope effectively with your feelings, you have to know what they are. Here are some feelings we hear about often—and some ways to cope with them.

Denial and Obsession

- "I just take my diabetes pills and leave everything else to my doctor."
- "No matter what else is going on, diabetes is on my mind. It's the first thing I think about in the morning and the last thing I think about at night. Actually, I never stop thinking about it."

Many people who have diabetes do not acknowledge that they must live as if they have diabetes. Other people go to the opposite extreme and act as if diabetes is the only thing in their lives. Accepting the seriousness of your diabetes without becoming obsessed by it is a tough balancing act. If you slide to either extreme, you'll suffer. If you don't treat your diabetes with respect, your risk of short-term and long-term complications goes way up.

But if you are preoccupied with your diabetes, the concern may take over your life. Either way, you won't do all you can to take care of yourself.

Are you in denial? Do you have symptoms that you prefer not to admit, even to yourself, are caused by diabetes, such as frequent urination, chronic exhaustion, infections, blurry vision, or pains in your feet? Do you avoid getting medical care for fear of what you will be told? Do you believe you can take care of your diabetes by medication alone? Do you tell yourself that your diabetes isn't serious? If so, dealing directly with your denial will help you feel happier and healthier, both today and in the years to come. The information in this book, your health care provider, a diabetes educator, and good websites like the one run by the American Diabetes Association (diabetes.org) can help.

People become obsessed with their diabetes regimen because they desperately want to believe that if they do everything perfectly, diabetes and its consequences can be perfectly controlled. Unfortunately, diabetes management is *not* a precise science, so a compulsive approach to diabetes can't provide the desired benefits. (Compulsive *behavior* is the result of obsessive *thinking*.) Leonard Pray, author of *The Journey of a Diabetic*, once wrote, "Don't try to be perfect. Try for good control, to be sure, but perfection lasts for a moment, and diabetes lasts a lifetime." These are words to live by.

Anger

- "Nobody else has to eat like I do. It's not fair!"
- "My doctor has no clue what it's like to live with diabetes. All he does is get on my case about the high glucose levels in my log and about my weight."
- "Just once I'd like to get a word of support from my husband when it comes to my efforts to manage my diabetes. Instead, all I hear is 'You should get more exercise.'"
- "When my blood glucose is really low I feel like screaming at anyone who is anywhere near me."

Anger is another emotion all too familiar to people with diabetes. Many people tell us they feel angry because diabetes is such an *imposition*: they are angry because of all the things they *have to do*. Others say they are angry because diabetes *deprives* them of so much: they are angry because of all the things they *can't do*. People are also angry because diabetes is forever. They are angry because *they*—rather than their parents, siblings, spouses, neighbors, friends, or strangers—developed diabetes. They are angry because they can't eat what they want, because they have to schedule and plan in ways no one else has to, because they feel like pincushions as a result of all the shots and blood tests. Surely, there is no lack of things to be angry about.

A common target for the anger is health care professionals. Health care providers don't appreciate how difficult it is to live with diabetes, people say. "They don't care how I feel." "The nutritionist gave me a meal plan that has nothing to do with real life." "The nurse acted as though I were lying when I told her what I actually do." "The doctor was offended by my questions." "The doctor was too rushed to listen to me." We've already touched on the issue of your relationship with health care providers, and we go into more detail about this in Chapter 17.

Another trigger for anger is the feeling that family and friends are unsupportive. Sometimes they minimize the demands of diabetes. At other times they may act like police, monitoring your eating, exercise, and blood glucose results, as though you can't do it for yourself. This can make the person with diabetes feel like a prisoner, surrounded by guards rather than loved ones. We discuss diabetes as a family affair in Chapter 15.

Finally, angry feelings are often the result of extremes in blood glucose levels. We've heard countless stories from people who lose control emotionally when their blood glucose levels skyrocket or bottom out.

To deal with diabetes-related anger, start by asking yourself *precisely* what you are angry about. Is it that you can't ever have another treat? Or that you can't have as many treats as you used to? Or perhaps you can't stand seeing your coworkers devouring goodies at work. By specifying in your own mind what bugs you, you may find that solutions present themselves: have a small treat once a week, carry a snack that you can munch on at work when your coworkers pass around the cookies or candies. Even if you don't come up with a solution, at least the true magnitude of the problem will be clear: no, you can't eat everything you used to eat. Whatever the source of your anger, you can choose to deal with it directly rather than stewing about it.

Frustration

- "My doctor put me on a new medication. I was really hopeful it would help, but my blood glucose is even harder to control, I've gained 10 pounds in two months, and it costs a fortune. Very frustrating."

- "I do exactly the same thing every day when it comes to managing my diabetes, but every once in a while I get blood glucose readings that make no sense at all. It drives me up the wall."

Many of the things that make us angry also make us frustrated. People with diabetes feel frustrated that they have to keep diabetes on their minds every waking hour. They feel frustrated by the lack of freedom and flexibility. People are also frustrated by the relatively slow progress of science in its efforts to find a cure for diabetes. Ten years ago one of us gave a talk with the theme "a cure for diabetes in 10 years." Unfortunately, we could probably talk on that same theme today.

For most people the biggest source of frustration is the unpredictable nature of their own bodies. Like those times when you try really hard to lose weight; you change your diet and you exercise much more. But when you step on the scale, your weight hasn't budged. The worst thing about frustration is that it may lead people to give up, to say, "To hell with it, it doesn't matter anyway." While understandable, this reaction initiates a downward spiral. As one of our patients said, "When you take a 'to hell with it' attitude toward your diabetes, that's exactly where you go."

To avoid "chucking it all" when you feel frustrated, try some positive diabetes self-talk. Imagine this scenario: your meter reads 287 (or any number that you would consider high). You might feel like saying, "I never do anything right!" or "That's it. I give up!" But try another approach instead. Try analyzing the situation: "That's really high. I hate it when I'm that high." After considering the likely possibilities, you might decide that there's no good reason for your numbers to be high that day. So you say to yourself, "Something is up, but I haven't a clue what it is. I'll try to get my level down right now, and if I'm still high in a day or so, I'll call my doctor or nurse and see if two heads are better than one." It may take lots of practice before you can talk to yourself this way, accepting some blood glucose results without understanding them and without excessive frustration. But it's worth the effort.

Fear

- "I'd rather die than start taking insulin. I know it means my diabetes is getting much worse."
- "I live in fear of going low. It happened once while I was driving and I

had an accident. Luckily no one was seriously hurt, but it was an awful experience."

- "Both my grandparents and my mother died of diabetes complications before they were 60 years old. I'm 54 now and I can't help thinking I have only a few years to live."

Diabetes is a scary disease, so it's probably inevitable for people with diabetes to feel fearful and to think more about death than the average person does. These worries are even more likely to plague you if you have older relatives with diabetes who did poorly. People tell us about many diabetes-related fears. Among people with Type 2 diabetes, one of the most common is the fear of having to take insulin. We discussed this fear in Chapter 11.

Diabetes fears, which are all understandable, are usually a mix of fact and fiction. Starting insulin is hard for some people: insulin reactions are unpleasant, and there is some risk of long-term complications. On the other hand, going on insulin does not mean that your diabetes will have a worse outcome. On the contrary, the risk of complications goes way up if you need insulin but don't take it. Insulin reactions can be avoided or treated by detecting mild, early symptoms. And many, many people live long, healthy lives despite diabetes. So recognizing and dealing with your own particular fears can be liberating.

Guilt

- "Every time I eat something I shouldn't, I see my doctor standing there shaking her head."
- "My exercise clothes are right by my bed so I can slip into them and do my routine in the morning when I get up. Whenever I don't, I feel guilty the rest of the day."
- "My meter reads 240 and I immediately start beating myself up about whatever I might have done to cause the high number."

Many people with diabetes tell us they feel guilty. No question about it, there are plenty of opportunities to feel guilty when you have diabetes, what with all the things you are supposed to do and all the others you are not supposed to do. One of our patients provided a perfect description of these sentiments:

- "I know I don't go to the doctor as often as I should. I don't go because I always end up feeling so guilty. She asks me if I've been exercising, if

I've been testing my blood, if I've been eating better and lost any weight, if I've stopped smoking. And for every question I have to give the same answer. 'No.' It's not like she's criticizing me on purpose; she's actually really gentle. Then she tells me that there's nothing she can do if I won't make the commitment to helping myself. I know she's right. What's wrong with me?"

Guilt is the one emotion that seems to have no positive side, and yet we see guilt all the time. Many patients come to our office with marginal notes in their diaries: "I cheated!!" "Really pigged out today!" "I was bad!" It might be natural and normal, but guilt is a paralyzing emotion. It gets you down on yourself, and when that happens, you're focused *backward*, on things in the past that you can't ever change.

We recommend looking *forward* rather than backward. Instead of looking backward and feeling guilty, try looking forward and finding ways to be more responsible to your own expectations. Pick anything you feel guilty about—eating more than you should at a restaurant dinner, for example. Instead of beating yourself up for something you can't change (since it's already happened), think of how you will handle the situation differently next time. This takes a lot less energy and is much more likely to help you feel better and take the best possible care of your diabetes.

Embarrassment

- "I was at my future in-laws' for dinner. It was the first time I had met them, and I got hypoglycemic just before we sat down to eat! I told them I had diabetes and ate a glucose tablet. But afterward they all treated me as if they felt sorry for me. I hated it."

- "I used to keep my diabetes a secret as much as I possibly could. After a while I realized that it just took too much energy to hide it, so now I let a few friends and one colleague at work in on 'the secret.' I still don't let everyone at work know, but this is easier."

When you have diabetes, feeling different is inevitable. That's why managing diabetes in social and work settings is a big issue for many people. It is each person's choice whether to tell and how much to say about diabetes. There are some dangers, however, to keeping your diabetes a secret. You could have a diabetes-related emergency and no one would be able to help you. Your friends could present you with all sorts of temptations without even knowing what they are doing.

At least your closest contacts at home and at work (or at school) should know enough about your diabetes—especially about recognizing and treating hypoglycemia—to help you if you are in trouble.

Anthony went canoeing with his friends, to an island in the middle of a lake, where they all planned to enjoy a midday picnic. The canoers got off to a late start, though, and all of a sudden it was 1 p.m. Anthony needed to eat, but the party hadn't even reached the island yet, much less set out the picnic. Luckily, Anthony had anticipated the possibility of a delay and brought some fast-acting sweets along. He just popped some candies and kept paddling.

The key here was that Anthony, like so many others with insulin-requiring diabetes, knew enough never to leave home without a ready source of sugar. You never know when a meal will be delayed. If he hadn't had the sugar on hand, think of the disruption. He might have had a hypoglycemic reaction out on the water, while a bevy of canoes circulated around and his companions panicked, having no notion of how to help. Anthony, at a minimum, would have felt awkward, frustrated, embarrassed, and guilty. So it makes sense to do everything you can to minimize how often your diabetes stops the action, causes you embarrassment, and scares your friends or colleagues.

Reframing: Changing the Way You Think about Situations That Cause Distress

- "Once you replace negative thoughts with positive ones you'll start getting positive results."—Willie Nelson.

Are you aware that you are always talking to yourself? It's true, no matter where you are or what you are doing, your mind is busily at work, filled with thoughts.

Some of these thoughts are *practical*—keeping track of the traffic as you drive to work, for example.

Other thoughts are *judgmental*. Some are positive judgments of the world around you ("What a beautiful day!") or of yourself ("The dinner I prepared was delicious"). Unfortunately, much of our self-talk is negative ("The country is going to hell"; "I'll never be able to control my eating"). It's these self-critical thoughts we'd like to talk about here.

Thoughts are powerful. But how can you follow Willie's wonderful words of wisdom, when it comes to managing your diabetes?

Pay Attention to Your Self-Talk

The first step is to recognize what you are saying to yourself. That's a challenge for many of us because most of our self-talk is unconscious and automatic. For example, most people go unconscious when they eat. Are you one of those people? If you are, and you "tune in" to your thoughts just before you eat something you know you shouldn't, you might find yourself thinking something like this: "I deserve it" or "I've already blown my diet for the day, so what I do now doesn't matter" or "I'll never be able to control my diabetes." Do any of these thoughts sound familiar?

One of the tricky things about these negative thoughts is that they *feel* true. So if you don't stop and think about what you are saying to yourself, you act as if these thoughts *are* true (for example, that you will never be able to control your diabetes), and that leads to feeling discouraged and doing things like eating that extra dessert, or staying in bed instead of getting up to exercise, or skipping a blood glucose check you know you should do.

Challenge Negative Thoughts

Once you recognize thoughts that lead you to do things you shouldn't, you can begin challenging those thoughts. This can be easier than it seems if you use a process we call *reframing*. Reframing means taking something you are struggling with and looking at it from a different perspective, a perspective that helps make the situation less overwhelming and more manageable.

Let's talk about some tried-and-true positive frames that could help you live better with diabetes.

Keep Your Eyes on the Prize

- "I want to be around to see my first grandchild walk across the stage and get her high school diploma."
- "I want to lose 20 pounds in the next year so I'll look my best at my daughter's wedding."
- "If I get my A1c down to 7.0%, I'm going to treat myself to a trip down the Amazon River."

Be very clear about the benefit for *you* in actively managing your diabetes. We mentioned this earlier in the book, but it bears repeating. We are not talking about the reason your doctor or your spouse offers. We are talking about your own personal reason. The reasons people do anything challenging are always personal, and the most powerful reasons are usually positive—like the ones above. What's your reason? Keeping it clearly in mind will help you maintain your motivation for taking the best possible care of yourself, avoiding negative thoughts, and dispelling diabetes distress.

Focus on Your Successes

- "I don't like diabetes. But it has forced me to learn how to take better care of myself, and I wouldn't give that up for anything in the world."
- "Whenever I get down on myself for not doing everything I should to manage my diabetes I make myself think about what I am doing right. That helps me feel better, and it also makes me feel more motivated to do better."
- "My blood glucose log looked terrible when I went for my last doctor's visit, with lots and lots of highs. I expected a lecture, but instead my doctor asked me about the days when my numbers were pretty good. I was so relieved, and looking at the good numbers gave me some idea what I could do to get good numbers more often."

When you have diabetes it's natural to focus on things that you have to correct—like eating more than you should or not exercising regularly. And it's also natural to focus on why you are not doing the right thing. But we'd like to suggest a radically different approach to improving your diabetes self-care: focus on what you are doing *right*.

It really works, for a couple of reasons. First, it can help you feel better right away. It helps you see that you are doing *some* things right, a fact you might lose sight of when you focus on where you are off track. Reminding yourself what you are doing right can help lift your spirits.

And that's not all. Figuring out *why* you did the right thing can help you be successful more often. If you can identify *why* things went better when they did—why you were able to stick to your eating and exercise goals, for instance, or why your blood glucose numbers were closer to your targets—you have tremendously valuable information for getting better results more often.

See "Slips" as Experiments

- "I know how much I should have for my evening snack. When I eat more than that I often just keep eating and eating. I tell myself, 'I've already blown it. Does it really matter by how much?'"

- "I thought I had taken the right amount of insulin for the meal I ate at the restaurant, but when I got home my blood glucose level was really high. I started beating myself up, thinking I should never eat out again."
- "I was doing a great job with my new exercise program, but then I skipped exercise a couple days in a row. I thought to myself, 'Here I go again, I've never been able to stick with exercise.' Then I caught myself and realized I had just skipped a couple days; I hadn't failed, and I wouldn't fail if I just got back on track right away."

When it comes to diabetes, of course, things don't go right all the time, or even most of the time. The people we know who are most successful at avoiding or resolving diabetes distress think about what we might call mistakes or slips as *experiments*. Experiments are designed to provide information for future experiments. You could think of life with diabetes as a very long series of experiments. Let's say you decided to have ice cream and cake at a party, thought you took enough insulin to cover the carbs, but ended up with a very high blood glucose level before bed. You could beat yourself up for eating the sweets or for underdosing your insulin. Or you could see what you did as an experiment. What did you learn from this experiment? What would your next experiment be?

A great example of this kind of thinking is a story about the famous inventor Thomas Edison. We mentioned this in Chapter 7, but it's a good illustration to repeat here. Edison tried approximately 5,000 experiments before he succeeded in creating the first electric light bulb. Just before he finally succeeded, a reporter came to his lab and asked him how he managed to keep going after failing 5,000 times. Edison responded that he hadn't failed a single time; he was moving 5,000 steps closer to the ultimate solution. Edison was right because, though none of his first 5,000 experiments resulted in a light bulb, every experiment provided him with information that brought him closer and closer to ultimate success. In every experiment Edison gained information that took him one step closer to his ultimate success. By the way, Thomas Edison had Type 2 diabetes.

Find the Humor

- "A woman woke up in the throes of a really bad low. She awakened her husband, who staggered groggily down the stairs to fetch her some juice and crackers. The minutes passed as the woman lay in her bed, shaking and waiting. Finally, her husband came staggering back up the stairs, empty-handed. 'Where is my food?' the woman demanded indignantly. 'Oh my gosh! I ate it myself,' her husband blurted."

- "When a colleague asked how his trip to Europe had gone, a man said, 'Well, I learned to say hello in 2 languages and sugar-free in 12.'"
- "A 6-year-old was working on his homework. In response to the question, 'Name one thing in your house you measure with,' he wrote, 'syringe.'"

You might be thinking, "There is nothing humorous about diabetes." And we admit it can sometimes be tough to find anything about diabetes to laugh about. But have you ever heard someone say, "I don't know how I would have made it if it wasn't for my sense of humor"? Maybe you've even said something similar yourself.

Humor is magical. For one of us, it certainly saved the day in lots of diabetes-related interactions with his son. Here's one example. When Richard Rubin's son Stefan was first diagnosed with diabetes in 1979, he took only one shot of insulin a day. About a year later he had to start taking a shot at dinner, as well. For some reason, this second shot felt like the end of the world to the then 9-year-old boy. Every dinnertime became a nightmare, with Stefan screaming and crying and pleading to be spared this second shot. "Why can't I just take one shot a day!?" he would shout.

Several weeks went by this way. Until the day his father stopped responding with factual information about the benefits of that second shot and took a different approach. "I can't think of any reason in the world why you can't have one shot a day," he said. "But why stop there, how about one shot a week?" Stefan's first response was a puzzled look. Then his eyes brightened and he joined right in, "Could we make that one shot a month?" he asked. Not to be outdone, his father said, "Let's go for it, how about one shot a year!"

Stefan frowned for a moment. Then, spreading his arms as far apart as he could, he added, "But think about how big the syringe would be!" Laughing, he quickly calculated the answer: 12,775 units. One very big syringe, he and his father agreed, as Stefan took his dinner shot without protest for the first time ever. What a relief. And Stefan never again fought his dinnertime shot.

We told you humor is magical. Only it just *seems* like magic. What was really going on that night between father and son was something else. The problem was not the second shot; the problem was Stefan feeling overwhelmed. What Stefan needed was lifting up, and laughing together with his father at a problem they had struggled with for weeks was very uplifting. Uplifting enough for Stefan to get right back to taking wonderful care of his diabetes, something he has been doing for more than 30 years now.

That's the magic of humor. It helps us cope with challenges that would otherwise bother or even overwhelm us. These challenges may be diabetes-related or not, including problems at work or at home. Humor feels good too. And it's good for you. Laughing has even been called "internal jogging." In fact, laughing seems to release endorphins just like exercise does. So you may be able to get a "runner's high" by just laughing. And at least one study found that laughing can lower your blood glucose level. Any way you look at it, adding a little laughter to your life is a good thing.

Take Home Messages

- For many people the biggest barrier to optimal self-care is feeling overwhelmed by the demands of life with diabetes.
- Common diabetes-related emotions include denial, obsession, anger, frustration, fear, guilt, and embarrassment.
- These feelings can be managed by changing situations that cause distress.
- These feelings can also be managed by thinking differently about ("reframing") situations that cause distress.
- Positive frames include keeping in mind your personal reason for working hard to manage your diabetes, focusing on your successes, seeing inevitable "slips" as "experiments," and finding humor in your life with diabetes.

15

Lessons for Families Who Live with Diabetes

- "My husband tells me that ever since I got diabetes I'm mean as a junk-yard dog, and I guess maybe he's right."
- "We have six people in the family, but since one of us got diabetes, it's tearing the family apart. We just don't know how to deal with it."
- "My husband will not take care of his diabetes, but when I say anything to him, he jumps right down my throat."
- "I was diagnosed four months ago, and the diabetes has actually brought my wife and me closer. We walk miles every day, and we talk and talk."

Diabetes is a family affair, in more ways than one. First, since diabetes is in part a genetic disease, you are more likely to have it if another member of your family has it already. In addition, the effects of diabetes are so powerful and pervasive that they touch everyone who loves, lives with, or cares for a person who has diabetes.

You want the best for family members who have diabetes. You want them to stay healthy, and that means eating right, staying active, taking their diabetes medication, checking their blood glucose levels, and a whole lot more. You want to help your loved one do the right thing, but without nagging. That can be easier said than done. Sometimes simple caring can be misinterpreted, and tensions can spread throughout the family unit. We hope those of you who have diabetes will read this chapter too, so you can learn more about what your family might be thinking and feeling. Our goal is to help everyone in the family live better with diabetes.

We offer 10 suggestions that we've developed over the years. Each is introduced with a real-life anecdote, some of which you may find familiar. Think about these suggestions when the tension seems to be rising around diabetes-related issues in your family. We think they'll help.

Lesson 1: Learn about Diabetes

When Sara's diabetes was diagnosed, her husband, Leonard, was even more upset than she was. He seemed really down and withdrawn, not at all like his usual warm, sociable self. Sara was hurt. She could handle having diabetes and all the changes it would bring, but she really needed Leonard's support. For weeks Sara felt she was dealing with her diabetes on her own. She went to the doctor's office alone, she took a diabetes class at the local hospital alone, she planned the family's new, healthier meals alone, and she got up early before work to walk alone. Finally, she confronted Leonard. He immediately apologized and started crying. Sara had not seen Leonard cry since their first child was born, 18 years ago. Leonard said, "I know I'm going to lose you in a few years. My grandfather got diabetes and he died just five years later. I don't know what I'm going to do." Sara knew what he was going to do. Leonard went on the American Diabetes Association website, joined Sara for her next doctor's visit, and attended a diabetes education class for family members. He learned that Sara's future was much, much brighter than his grandfather's had been and that there was a lot he could do to help.

Diabetes treatment is improving every day. Understanding diabetes and how it is treated makes it easier to help your loved one. Ask your loved one to explain things to you. Read the rest of this book. Go on the Web for useful information; the American Diabetes Association website (diabetes.org) is a great resource. Attend a diabetes education class together. These classes are available at many hospitals. Knowledge is strength when it comes to diabetes. That's true for those who have diabetes and for those who love someone who has it. Understanding diabetes helps you know what you need to be concerned about and what you don't need to be concerned about.

Lesson 2: Don't Act Like a Police Officer

Tanya was extremely frustrated because her husband, Phil, refused to care for his diabetes. His attitude was, "If I die, I die." Earlier in their marriage, before Phil had diabetes, she had found his devil-may-care attitude attractive, but now all she could think of was that he was killing himself. Tanya refused to accept Phil's fatalism. So she acted like a domestic police force, constantly bugging him to do the right thing: "Don't eat that, get off your duff and exercise, check your blood sugar, keep your appointments." All to no avail. Tanya was beside herself because her love and concern for Phil were turning to anger and frustration. She couldn't control his diabetes, and their relationship was suffering as well.

Attempting to police someone's behavior rarely works. In fact, it usually has the opposite result, and it can ruin your relationship, whether the target is your spouse or your child.

We know that it's hard to follow this guideline. For one thing, the worrying and nagging are done out of love. We talk to many people who are frantic because they see a family member denying his or her diabetes and refusing to take responsibility for it. If they really didn't care what happened to their family member, they wouldn't get so upset.

So let's consider how Tanya could be more successful in dealing with Phil. First, she should recognize that she's frustrated because she *does* care, not because the man she loves is insufferably stubborn. Next, she has to accept that her attempt to police his behavior doesn't work and will never work. The trick is not to give up caring but to change the way that caring is expressed. Maybe Phil sees Tanya's efforts as a challenge to his independence or his masculinity or as accentuating his "differentness." Whatever is going on inside Phil's head, it's obviously enough to keep him fighting every effort on Tanya's part. What a waste of energy for both of them!

So Tanya needs to develop more effective strategies and rebuild their relationship. Following the next several lessons would help.

Retiring from the role of household police officer is hard. It takes conscious effort, time, and patience. But it is the only approach that works.

Lesson 3: Find Out What Your Loved One Really Needs

Jeanette struggled at home every day, all day, with her husband Frank's diabetes. Being a naturally open, talkative person, Jeanette had a habit of mentioning his diabetes to others. She made benign little comments to waiters ("Frank can't have any dessert because he has diabetes") or to friends ("Frank's diabetes is acting up today, so I hope you don't mind if we leave early"). Their friends all knew Frank had diabetes, and it just seemed natural to Jeanette to refer to it. But one night, maybe during a glucose low, Frank blew his stack and roared, "I don't want you ever mentioning my diabetes to anyone, ever again. It's my diabetes, I take care of it, and that's it!" Jeanette was stunned and hurt.

Jeanette loves Frank. She felt she was helping him, but clearly Frank felt otherwise. This makes a very important point: we never know what another person wants unless that person tells us. We might think we know, and we might even be right, but the only way to know for sure is to have the other person tell us.

This is especially important when it comes to a complicated, sensitive matter like diabetes that affects so many aspects of our lives. Try asking the following four questions. Ask them at a time when you are feeling close and comfortable together, and ask your loved one to answer the questions as specifically as possible. Maybe write the questions down, so if your loved one can't answer them right away, he or she can think about the questions and answer them later.

1. What is the hardest thing about living with diabetes?
2. What do I do that makes it easier for you to manage your diabetes?
3. What do I do that makes it harder for you to manage your diabetes?
4. What can I do to help that I am not doing now?

Lesson 4: Offer the Help Your Loved One Asks For

The Crosby family always had snacks around: potato chips, ice cream, choco-lates. When son Saul developed diabetes, it just didn't seem right to make the whole family suffer. So Diane Crosby tried to teach her son not to eat the snacks, but she often found empty potato chip bags, ice cream cartons, and candy wrappers under his bed. And his blood glucose levels frequently re-flected the results of these late-night eating escapades. Diane would yell and Saul would pout, but nothing changed. Diane kept stocking the cupboard and freezer, and Saul kept doing his part in emptying them. Finally, at the end of her rope, Diane sat down with Saul and asked him what he wanted her to do. After a moment Saul replied, "I wish you and Dad and Jessie could just live without that junk. Then I would, too." It turned out that the rest of the family was glad to give up their favorite fatty and sugary treats for an end to the constant battles between Diane and Saul. They all agreed to get one treat a week that everyone could share. Peace and better glucose control returned to the Crosby household.

Take to heart your loved one's answer to the question, "What can I do to be helpful that I am not doing now?" Whether it's limiting the availabili-ty of sweets in the kitchen, running to the drugstore when your husband runs out of glucose-monitoring strips, making healthier eating easier for your son or daughter, or offering encouragement when your wife is feeling down, do your best to make your loved one's wish come true.

Lesson 5: Talk about Your Feelings

Tanya's frustration with her husband, Phil, finally boiled over one night when he "forgot" to take his medication and ended up with a very high blood glucose. This had happened many times before, but for some reason this time was the last straw. "Are you trying to kill yourself?" she screamed. "You're driving me crazy." Phil shot back, "Why should you care? It's not your diabetes. If I kill myself, I kill myself." That stopped Tanya in her tracks. Why did she care? She cared because she loved Phil. She cared because she was afraid of losing him. She cared because she felt helpless to do anything about it.

You don't have diabetes, but as a person close to someone who does, you are living with diabetes. Diabetes affects your life in countless ways, especially if your loved one is struggling in his efforts to manage it. You have your own hopes, frustrations, and fears. Talking about these feelings and not about your loved one's behavior can put you both on the same side of the fence. It's much easier for your loved one to hear that you want to spend many happy, healthy years together, that you are afraid of losing him, and that you feel helpless, than it is to hear you get on his case about all the things he's doing wrong. Sharing your feelings cuts down on nagging and builds closeness and cooperation. And that's a good thing.

Lesson 6: Offer Support and Comfort, Especially When Things Aren't Going Well with the Diabetes

George knew that for his wife, Sue, her diabetes was getting to be more and more of a struggle. What used to be easy—taking one shot in the morning and not worrying about it—had intensified into a multidose daily insulin regimen that seemed to consume her time and energy. Then she went to the ophthalmologist and was told she had "a spot of diabetes in one eye." Sue was devastated.

People with diabetes are especially sensitive when their blood glucose levels are bouncing around or when they get what they interpret as bad news. In Sue's case, the "spot of diabetes" was in fact of very little importance, but to her it was devastating. A little extra thoughtfulness in word and deed can go a long way toward keeping things positive.

Much has been written about the tendency to want to *do something* instead of just offering support. It's much easier sometimes to react by saying, "Well, I'm going to make you an appointment with two other ophthalmologists to see if your doctor is really right, and then I'm going to the library to look up exactly what the diagnosis means and what to do about it." This is not always the most helpful response. What Sue needs is a good hug, maybe a cry, and the feeling that George will always be there. The skill required here is the ability to give one of the world's greatest gifts—genuine, loving support.

Speaking of gifts, everyone loves them, and maybe they should be tangible. What are the gifts your loved one most appreciates? Cards, unexpected phone calls, flowers, a special night out, a back rub? Gifts are great to cheer up someone who is down. Spontaneous thoughtfulness is especially nice. It's bound to help your loved one feel better about himself or herself, and that will undoubtedly provide extra motivation for diabetes care.

Another true story can drive home the importance of simply showing your unconditional love, letting it be known within the family.

> When Stefan was 10 years old, he went through a period when he tried to minimize the pain of his insulin injections by giving his shots as slowly as possible. He would sit with the needle poised, often for minutes at a time, while his dad exhorted him to get it over with, arguing that Stefan was actually prolonging his agony. Needless to say, his father's approach didn't help matters. Finally, one day his dad took a different tack. He said, "I know those shots must really hurt, and I wish I could take some of them for you. You're really brave and I love you." Stefan smiled at his dad and said, "It's not that big a deal." Then he pushed the needle right in.

Stefan needed that extra bit of loving support that goes a long way toward making life with diabetes more manageable. This support may even explain Stefan's attitude toward his diabetes. When he was 11 years old, his father told him that one of his greatest wishes in life was for Stefan to no longer have diabetes. To this Stefan responded, "I don't like having diabetes. In fact, there are times when I hate it. But it has forced me to learn how to take care of myself, and I wouldn't trade that for anything in the world."

We hope that everyone who has diabetes will find a way to grow stronger and closer to those who love them.

Lesson 7: Be Especially Patient When Your Loved One Has a Low Blood Glucose

Herman's mother, Mabel, had come to live with Herman and his family. This was the first time he'd really experienced her life with the disease on a daily basis. She seemed to handle it very well, taking her insulin injections in the morning, checking her blood glucose level several times a day, eating the healthy meals Herman and his wife prepared for the family, and even walking a few blocks with Herman when he came home from work. But one day when Herman asked his mother if she wanted to go for a walk, she lit into him. "Why would I want to walk with you," she yelled. "You are always dragging me out when I don't want to go. And you make me eat that food you call healthy that I can't stand. I've a mind to move out tonight." His mother's behavior was so out of character that he suspected she was having a blood glucose low. He figured that asking her if she was low would only get her angrier, so he went into the kitchen, poured a glass of orange juice, put it on the table next to the chair where his mother was sitting, and then sat down himself without saying a word. His mother gulped down the juice. In a few minutes her blood glucose was rising and her temper was cooling.

Low blood glucose is always uncomfortable for the person with diabetes, and it can even be dangerous. It is also often uncomfortable for anyone witnessing the low, especially if the person with diabetes is acting out, as is often the case. Fortunately Herman did the right thing, and his mother responded positively. Things don't always work out so well, though, even when you do the right thing: people have been known to throw glasses of orange juice instead of drinking them.

When your loved one is having low blood glucose and is acting out, you have to keep reminding yourself that when hypoglycemic, she just isn't the person you know and love. When they are hypoglycemic, people will say things they don't mean, will be violent when it's not in their real nature, and will act in all sorts of ways that seem calculated to make you miserable. What's more, when it is all over, it's possible they will not remember a thing!

When your family member is having a glucose low, you have to keep your wits about you, keep your emotions under control, and offer any practical help you can.

Lesson 8: Look for Opportunities to Help, Especially in Public Situations

After 30 years of living together, Fred knows his wife's diabetes routine, and he has learned many little things he can do, unobtrusively and almost without thinking, that make Frieda's life easier—things she's told him would make life with diabetes easier for her. He buys the glucose test strips and makes sure there's always a supply handy. He orders the food at a restaurant, keeping control over that roving eye that spots the most tempting dessert on the menu. He is also the exercise coordinator and cheerleader. Every Sunday, after a relaxed breakfast, they plan their weekly activities. Fred always has at least one new suggestion, to keep things from getting boring—a new place to walk, for instance, or a new activity, like going to the Saturday night dance at the senior center.

Eating right, testing, and staying active are challenging for anyone. Making these daily responsibilities easier or more fun can make a world of difference for your loved one with diabetes. Be alert for opportunities to make things a little easier. The key to success here is to do things your partner or other family member wants you to do and not to make a big deal of it. It's not something you're doing for praise or thanks, it's just part of your love and support. And it's great for your relationship.

Lesson 9: Get Help

Pam was really worried. Her husband, Jake, who had always been a cheerful person, had been anything but recently. He just looked sad all the time, he wasn't taking his usual good care of his diabetes, and he had stopped playing softball with his friends on Saturdays. These games had always been the highlight of Sam's summertime weeks. When Pam asked what was going on, Sam just said, "Nothing's fun any more."

If your family member seems really sad, encourage him to talk about it. Just getting out his feelings with you can help, but he might also need professional help. If it seems that he does, encourage him to talk to his health care provider to get a referral for a mental health provider, such as a psychiatrist, a psychologist, or a social worker. Depression is common in people who have diabetes, and it's a double whammy for them. When people with diabetes are depressed, they not only feel terrible but usually have more trouble sticking with their diabetes self-care as well. And that means higher blood glucose levels and more health problems. The good news is this: effective treatment for depression—medications and/or counseling— can turn things around, helping people feel better and bringing down blood glucose levels. So if your loved one might be depressed, do everything you can to encourage him to get help.

Lesson 10: Try a Little Humor

Glynda told us about an experience with her husband, Jack. One night, after they had been asleep for several hours, Jack started thrashing around. Glynda woke up and realized he was in the throes of a severe hypoglycemic reaction. She got him to drink some orange juice, and Jack slowly regained full consciousness. Finally, at about 3:30 a.m., he was back to normal. Glynda, exhausted and a little frustrated, tried to go back to sleep. But no, Jack decided it was time to make love. This was the last thing on Glynda's mind, so, thinking quickly, she said, "Honey, we already did that." Jack gave her a puzzled look, started to laugh, and fell asleep.

Stefan developed diabetes when he was 7 years old. To confirm the diagnosis and to begin learning to live with diabetes, Stefan and his mother and father went to the pediatrician's office. There they received instructions about diet, insulin, exercise, and the countless other things they would need to know. All through this process, Stefan's father was feeling more and more discouraged, overwhelmed by the prospect of living with his son's disease. At some point the pediatrician suggested that Stefan's father pull down his pants and stick his leg with a syringe, to show his son that it didn't hurt too much. Spontaneously, Stefan's father blurted out, "At least I'm wearing clean underwear." At this, everyone laughed, and the tension level came down a bit.

Along with clear communication and love, humor can go a long way toward making your family's life with diabetes easier. You've probably heard people describe some difficult situation they've lived through and then add, "I don't know how I could have made it if I hadn't been able to laugh about it." And you surely know people who can make a whole room happy just by their sense of humor. Identifying something humorous in an otherwise difficult diabetes-related situation helps restore the problem to manageable proportions. Our patients have offered us many examples of how this helps keep all members of the family working together. And you don't need to be a comedian to lighten your load through humor. Humor is everywhere, and the more trying your day, the more important it is that you find a light side.

. . .

Staying strong and close as a family is essential when you are living with diabetes. The problems of living are hard enough without adding unnecessary family friction. We find that, very often, the things that create friction in a family are trivial when they are considered in isolation. But they do usually form patterns: specific hot-button issues, as we have described, specific actions and failures to act. We also find that in most cases, these things can be easily remedied. You don't need to be a professional family counselor to become aware of your own family's dynamics. Think over the 10 lessons described above and see what applies to your family. Then do something positive about it.

Take Home Messages

- Diabetes affects everyone who loves or lives with a person who has diabetes.
- You want to help your loved one live well with diabetes, but your efforts can be misinterpreted and lead to tension.
- There are things you can do to be truly helpful without creating tension. Learn about diabetes. Don't be a police person. Find out what your loved one really needs and offer the help he or she asks for. Talk about your feelings. Offer support and comfort, especially when things aren't going well. Be especially patient when your loved one has an episode of low glucose. Get help when your loved one is depressed. Try a little humor.

16

Dealing with Psychological Problems

- "With my diabetes it's just one thing after another. I feel hopeless and everything I used to enjoy seems meaningless."
- "Before diabetes, I used to worry some, but now I worry all day long about everything, even things that make no sense at all."
- "I discovered I could control my weight by taking less insulin than I should. My blood glucose runs really high, but my weight stays down."
- "I felt so down I could hardly drag myself out of bed in the morning. My doctor gave me some medication and sent me to a counselor. It took a while, but now I feel almost back to my old self."

In Chapter 14 we talked about the emotional side of diabetes and about diabetes distress. For some people this distress is very severe, severe enough to qualify as a psychological problem that could require professional help. Among the more common and serious problems for people with diabetes are depression, anxiety disorder, and eating disorders. People with diabetes who suffer from an anxiety disorder or eating disorder often also suffer from depression.

The consequences of a psychological problem are especially severe for a person who has diabetes. Episodes of depression last longer, feel worse, and recur more often. In addition, psychological problems make diabetes management more difficult. For example, depression can make it much harder to do the things you need to do, like sticking to a regimen for eating, exercise, and blood glucose monitoring. And an eating disorder can seriously undermine your efforts to achieve good glucose control. Putting it plainly, having both diabetes and a psychological problem is a bad combination.

How can you tell whether you have a significant psychological problem or are just down in the dumps? And if you do have a serious emotional problem, where can you turn for help? These are the issues we address in this chapter.

It isn't always easy to distinguish between garden-variety distress and true emotional disturbance, but we hope our description of each disorder will give you an idea of where you fall on the spectrum. If you aren't sure, it makes sense to seek professional help in evaluating the seriousness of your problem. Ask your doctor what he or she thinks about referring you to a mental health professional. A single meeting with a mental health specialist, especially one who has experience in treating people who have diabetes, may be enough to determine whether you need treatment for your emotional problem. Of course, you don't need to be suffering from a diagnosable emotional disorder to benefit from a visit to a mental health professional. Counseling from such a person can help you cope with the normal stresses of life with diabetes.

Depression

- "I know I have no energy when my blood glucose levels are high, but when the feeling went on and on, and got worse and worse, I figured something else must be going on."
- "Everything goes to pot when I'm depressed; I stop exercising, I eat anything I feel like, and I even stop monitoring my blood glucose. Needless to say, the results are not pretty."

People with diabetes are twice as likely as people who don't have diabetes to suffer from depression. People with diabetes who have very high A1c levels or who have two or more diabetes complications are the ones most likely to be depressed.

Recent research shows that people with diabetes who are depressed (even those with low levels of depression symptoms) don't manage their diabetes as actively as people with diabetes who have no symptoms of depression. Those who have at least some symptoms of depression exercise, monitor their blood glucose, and take prescribed medication less often, and they are also less likely to stick to a healthy diet.

Given the association between depression and less active self-care, it is no surprise that other researchers have found an association between depression and high blood glucose levels and higher diabetes complications rates in those who are depressed. One study even found that people with diabetes who were depressed died much sooner, on average, than those who were not depressed.

Depression is the pits, whether or not you have diabetes, but if you have diabetes, it is the pit of the pits. The thing that makes us saddest is that so many people with diabetes are suffering needlessly; there are effective treatments for depression. So, if you think you might be depressed, please read on.

When most people say they are depressed, they aren't using the term in the clinical sense. They just mean they are sad and dragged out emotionally. Everyone feels down from time to time. But these normal downs come and go, usually in a couple of hours or a couple of days and usually in response to a fairly clear cause. Clinical depression is different. It takes you down further and keeps you there longer. Often, it has no particular precipitating event, or if there is such an event, your emotional response to it is extreme. To see whether you might be clinically depressed ask yourself these two questions:

1. During the past two weeks have you felt down, depressed, or hopeless all or almost all of the time?

2. During the past two weeks have you lost interest or pleasure in doing things you used to enjoy?

If you answered yes to either question, make an appointment with your doctor for a full assessment and to discuss treatment options. When you talk to your doctor, be sure to mention the specific question or questions we just asked for which you answered yes. This might be hard to believe, but you may have to be very clear about how you are feeling for your physician to recognize that you might be depressed.

Professional Help for Depression

- "I don't believe in mental health treatment, but after feeling down for so long I didn't think I'd ever feel better. I decided I'd better give it a try."
- "It took a while for the antidepressant my doctor prescribed to kick in, but once it did the whole world looked brighter."

Only 30% of people with diabetes who are depressed have their depression diagnosed. That's because many physicians lack the time and training to diagnose and treat depression, and many others believe that depression will go away if a person's blood glucose control improves. Better control can help some people feel less depressed, but not most. Diabetes and depression are two separate diseases, and most people need a separate treatment for each.

There are two types of professional treatment that seem to be effective for relieving depression in people with diabetes. One is counseling or psychotherapy, and the other is antidepressant medication. One or the other of these treatments works for some people, and others get the most relief from a combination of the two.

There are many different types of mental health professionals. They include psychiatrists, psychologists, clinical professional counselors and clinical social workers, and some nurses. One form of therapy, called cognitive behavioral therapy, seems to work particularly well for people with diabetes, so you might want to look for a counselor who specializes in this approach. In cognitive behavioral therapy, the counselor helps you identify the thoughts that trigger your depression and helps you find ways to deal better with stressful situations and to take better care of yourself. Counseling for depression might last three to six months, often with occasional checkups after that. Naturally, it is important to find a counselor you are comfortable with, though it can take a couple of sessions before you can tell.

Antidepressant medication can also relieve depression. These medications can be prescribed by your physician or by a psychiatrist, if you are referred to one. There are many different such medications, all of which seem to have similar benefits when it comes to relieving depression, so the physician who prescribes one for you should take several things into consideration, including your specific symptoms and the medicine's potential side effects. Some antidepressants also relieve anxiety symptoms. That is important because many people suffer from symptoms of both depression and anxiety.

You should know that although antidepressant medications are very effective, finding the right one and the right dose for a given person can take some work. So your physician may have to increase the dosage you take or even prescribe a different medication before you get what you need. Also keep in mind that some people find it can take as long as six weeks before their medication kicks in and they start to really feel better. So try not to get too discouraged if it takes a while for your medication to work. Just pay close attention to your symptoms and report them to your doctor.

Other Steps to Help Relieve Depression

- "Once the counseling started to help me feel less depressed, I got back to exercise. It had always been the one part of my diabetes regimen I actually enjoyed, but when I got depressed I stopped. I'm convinced that the combination of counseling and exercise works for me."

- "Feeling depressed made me always focus on the negative. I saw only the things that were wrong in my life. Once my depression started to lift, I followed my doctor's advice and started making lists of the good things that happened that day. It might sound funny, but that helps."

Professional help in the form of counseling, medication, or both is the most effective depression treatment, but there are some things you can do to help relieve depression symptoms, especially once professional help has started to produce some benefits.

One thing you can do is to be more active. In the Look AHEAD trial, which we talked about in Chapter 7, depression symptoms declined among participants in the lifestyle intervention group, who had a goal of 175 minutes of moderate-intensity exercise a week. Potential mechanisms for these benefits include the effects of exercise on feelings of self-confidence and an increase in endorphins—substances produced by our bodies that improve our feelings of well-being.

You could also try some nonphysical exercises that were part of a study designed to help people feel less depressed and happier. People who participated in the study completed questionnaires that assessed happiness and depression before they began their assigned exercise, after completing the exercise, and one week and one, three, and six months later.

Here are the exercises (each participant did just one of these):

—*Gratitude visit.* During the next week, write and deliver a letter of gratitude to someone you have not properly thanked.

—*Three good things in life.* Each night for a week, write down three things that went well that day and why.

—*You at your best.* Write about a time you were at your best, and reflect each night for the next week on your personal strengths that made that time your best.

—*Identify signature strengths.* Identify your personal signature strengths— that is, things you like to do and are good at.

—*Using signature strengths in new ways.* Identify your personal signature strengths, and use at least one in a new way every day for a week.

—*Early memories.* Write about your earliest memories each night for a week.

The last exercise was included as a "placebo": the researchers did not expect the early memories exercise to have any effect on happiness or depression. Comparing the results in this group with the results in the other groups provided the most accurate estimate of the benefits of the "real" exercises.

The results of the study were very interesting:

—All participants were happier and less depressed right after completing their exercise than they had been before they started it. This included participants in the placebo group.

—Only two of the exercises—three good things and using signature strengths in new ways—led to long-lasting (six-month) improvements in happiness and depression.

—The gratitude letter exercise had the biggest immediate effect on happiness and depression, but these benefits decreased over time and had disappeared six months after the exercise.

—People who kept practicing their exercise on their own (after the week it was assigned) stayed happier and less depressed than those who didn't keep practicing. This was true for all exercises.

It seems that reminding yourself each day of things that went well and why can contribute to lasting happiness (and less depression), and using signature strengths in new ways can have the same benefits. Keep in mind that the people participating in this study were looking for something to help them feel happier and that their scores on the depression questionnaire indicated that they tended to be mildly depressed when they started the study. But it's pretty amazing that people in the study got the benefits they did from nonphysical exercises they did completely on their own, with no professional help. So you could benefit too, if you are only mildly depressed.

Anxiety Disorder

- "I'm anxious all the time, sometimes about my diabetes and sometimes about everything else in my life. Sometimes I'm so anxious I feel I can hardly breathe."
- "I couldn't tell if I was anxious or depressed; maybe I was both. My doctor gave me a drug that works for both and it really helped."

Everyone who has diabetes worries about diabetes-related concerns. Worrying about your blood glucose or about diabetes complications is as normal as worrying about your job, your marriage, and your children. A clinical anxiety disorder, like clinical depression, is different from this kind of normal worry. It makes the worrying so intense, so uncomfortable, and so long-lasting that you may hardly be able to function.

A *clinical anxiety disorder* would probably be diagnosed if you are uncontrollably anxious and if you worry excessively about particular events or activities (such as work or school performance or your diabetes management). The two most common forms of anxiety disorder are *generalized anxiety disorder* (GAD) and *panic disorder*. Anxiety disorders are as common as or more common than depression, and like depression, anxiety disorders are more common in people who have diabetes than in people who don't.

Symptoms of GAD include:

1. Trouble controlling constant worrying
2. Worrying more than you know you should
3. Inability to relax
4. Difficulty concentrating
5. Difficulty falling asleep or staying asleep

Symptoms of panic disorder include:

1. Feeling of intense dread
2. Fear you are losing control or are about to die
3. Pounding heart or chest pain
4. Difficulty breathing
5. Trembling or shaking

Panic disorder symptoms are more severe than the symptoms of GAD, but both are serious problems. You probably also noticed that some of the symptoms of GAD are similar to those of clinical depression. There is an overlap, both because some psychological problems share similar symptoms and because some people suffer from more than one disorder. This again brings up an important point: if you have any signs of a clinical psychological disorder, get help. What particular disorder you are suffering from matters less than that you are suffering.

First, talk to your doctor about your symptoms. Like depression, anxiety disorders are generally treated with counseling or psychotherapy, medication, or both. Again, as with depression, cognitive behavioral counseling can be especially useful to help you think, behave, and react in ways that help you feel less anxious.

Your doctor may also prescribe medication to treat anxiety disorders. Some medications are used specifically for anxiety disorders. Some of these work very quickly, but they generally should not be used for long periods. As we mentioned earlier, some antidepressants are also effective for treating anxiety disorders. These drugs take longer to work. Some people do best with cognitive behavioral therapy, some with drugs, and some with a combination of the two.

There are also helpful things you can do on your own if you have an anxiety disorder. These things are most likely to help if your anxiety is not too intense. First, identify the fears that are triggering your anxiety. Then see whether you can do anything to relieve those fears. If fear of hypoglycemia is disturbing you, for example, read some of the suggestions in Chapter 5 and see whether they provide any relief. If you are afraid you may develop complications, ask your health care provider for the facts about exactly where you stand and what you can do to minimize your risk. If you are anxious about the effect your diabetes may be having on your family life, refer to the discussion in Chapter 15 and try talking out these fears with your loved ones.

Eating Disorders

- "I just can't stop eating, even when I'm full. I know something is wrong with me."
- "When I eat more than I should, I have a magic trick to keep from gaining weight. I just skip an insulin injection, or I take much less than I should."
- "I was so embarrassed by my inability to control my eating. I often waited until my husband went to bed before raiding the refrigerator. One night he caught me in the middle of a binge and I broke down and told him the truth. The next day I called my doctor, who referred me to a counselor who specialized in eating problems."

If you take good care of your diabetes, you probably spend a good deal of time thinking about food and watching what you eat. And you are probably concerned about your weight as well. For some people with diabetes, concerns with eating and weight are extreme enough to qualify as an eating disorder. There are three basic types of eating disorder: *binge eating, bulimia nervosa,* and *anorexia nervosa.*

Binge eating is the most common eating disorder among people with diabetes, as it is in the general population. Key signs of binge eating disorder include:

1. Eating until uncomfortably full
2. Eating large amounts of food when not physically hungry
3. Eating very rapidly
4. Eating alone because of embarrassment with how much you eat
5. Feeling disgusted, depressed, or guilty after overeating

Binge eating by people who have diabetes is most common among those with Type 2 and among those who weigh more and who have psychological problems like depression.

Bulimia, as traditionally defined, is rare among people with diabetes. Key traditional signs of bulimia include:

1. Eating in a discrete amount of time (e.g., within two hours) much more food than most people would consume.
2. Lack of control over eating during such episodes.
3. Compensatory behavior to prevent weight gain from overeating (e.g., laxatives, diuretics, self-induced vomiting).

Bulimia in people with diabetes is much more common among young women who have Type 1 diabetes and who carry out *insulin purging*, sometimes called *diabulimia*, as a "compensatory behavior." Many young women (and some young men) control their weight by skipping or reducing insulin doses. This causes blood glucose levels to rise and results in frequent urination, as the kidneys must work overtime to get rid of the extra glucose. The chronic high blood glucose levels caused by insulin purging can lead to many health problems, including immediate problems such as dehydration and fatigue and an increased risk of long-term diabetes complications. So insulin purging is very dangerous. But health care providers understand why it has a strong appeal for some people, despite the dangers.

Anorexia is very rare among people with diabetes. Signs of anorexia include:

1. Weight that is less than 85% of a normal weight for height, body frame, and age
2. Intense fear of gaining weight, even when underweight

3. Exercising far more than is necessary to stay fit

4. Denying the seriousness of low body weight

If you have an eating disorder or suspect you might be suffering from one, get help. We make this recommendation in full awareness of how difficult it is to admit you have an eating disorder and to ask for help. If you are like most people suffering from these problems, controlling your eating this way feels crucially important, and you feel terrified at the prospect of giving up control. In fact, you are probably even terrified at the prospect of anyone discovering that you have an eating disorder. Besides that, you are probably ashamed.

You may also believe that no one can understand your problems and that no one could possibly help you. But there are people who can help. Tell someone you can trust about your problem and ask for help. If you aren't comfortable talking to your parents or spouse, maybe there is a relative, teacher, religious adviser, or health care provider you could approach. What you need to do, with the help of someone you trust, is to see a mental health professional who treats people with eating disorders; you may be able to find such a person who also knows something about diabetes.

· · ·

As hard as it is to admit you have any of the emotional problems we've discussed in this chapter, it's critically important to do just that and to ask for help. Your life is at stake, and that is precious. So get the help that could save your life. Many of our patients have discovered the relief of living with just one medical condition—diabetes—rather than two.

Take Home Messages

- Psychological problems such as depression, anxiety disorders, and eating disorders are more common among people with diabetes.
- Psychological problems make diabetes management more challenging, and they can lead to higher blood glucose levels and to more diabetes complications.
- There are effective treatments for psychological problems, and getting these treatments can help you feel better and live healthier.
- Effective treatments include counseling and medication. Often a combination of these works best.

17

Interacting with Health Care Professionals

- "I just found out that I have diabetes. Should I see a specialist?"
- "I spend months keeping a detailed record of my blood sugars, diet, and activity, and then my doctor spends less than five minutes looking through it!"
- "Everyone says I need to lose weight to get the diabetes under control, but nobody tells me how to do it."
- "Now that I've learned how to manage the diabetes, my doctor and I can work together as a team."

The relationship between you and your health care professional has tremendous potential for satisfaction—and for frustration. It is, after all, your comfort, your body, your very life at stake. You look to your health care professional to make you well. You have all sorts of reasonable expectations, and maybe some unreasonable ones too. The opportunities for disappointment and disillusionment are great.

Still, according to surveys, most people like their own doctor, regardless of what they think about doctors in general. In this chapter we discuss what you can do to foster a good relationship with your doctor and with other health care providers. We begin by describing the members of the health care team then suggest some keys to building and maintaining a good relationship between you and your health care providers.

The Health Care Team

The *health care team* is a model that has much to recommend it. It involves coordination and communication: multiple players all working together for your benefit. A reality test is occasionally needed for this dream-team concept, however. Sometimes the members of the health care team don't

274

communicate all that well. In this, as in so many other aspects of diabetes management, you may have to take charge yourself.

> Julio, one of our patients, is an extremely well-organized person who is accustomed to being in charge. He comes to office visits well prepared, with his data nicely summarized and his questions lined up. Last year, when he developed a serious orthopedic problem, he not only communicated with each of the people on his health care team but went so far as to arrange a conference call for the whole team—four doctors and a patient. It was an unusual step, but it was a good example of the patient making sure that all the members of his health care team communicated, and it was done in such a friendly and gracious manner that all the doctors enjoyed it.

Even if you are not such a take-charge person as Julio, you can still manage your care very well if you make the best use of available resources and know whom to seek out when. To do this, you have to start with a list of the players who might belong on your diabetes health care team.

You

You are the central person on your health care team. You make the decisions: what to eat, when to eat, how to exercise, how to take medications, when to seek help, and so on. You may be the sort of person who wants everything spelled out for him, who just wants to follow directions, or you may be the kind of person who bridles at the thought of losing control of her own decisions, who wants always to do it her own way. Wherever you are on that spectrum, you are the one who leads the life and experiences the consequences of your actions. Still, we haven't met the person who doesn't need some help at some point. This usually starts with a primary care provider.

The Primary Care Provider

The medical professional who takes responsibility for and coordinates your overall health care is your *primary care provider*. You should know who this person is; you should not have to wonder. You should have his name and telephone number posted near your home phone, noted on a card in your wallet, written out for your friends, and so on. This is the person to call first in an emergency. This is the person who knows you and cares for you on a regular basis.

In this day of shifting health care systems, primary health care providers might change with disturbing frequency. We suggest only that you be aware of any changes. Visit the "new doc" early, get to know him, and let him get to know you.

The training and background of your primary care provider is less important than clear identification of the role. Most often, we recommend a general internist (a physician trained in internal medicine) or family practitioner. Increasingly, it will be a nurse practitioner. Primary care providers have varying levels of expertise in managing diabetes, but they can recognize the problems, provide advice about many parts of treatment, and coordinate whatever specialty care you need. Many are skilled in diabetes management, as a large percentage of their patients probably have this diagnosis.

Remember that a general physician or nurse practitioner probably won't be a specialist in diabetes, and this is not a bad thing. He will be able to deal with the variety of health care problems you have. When the need arises, especially when your diabetes becomes more difficult to manage, the generalist should freely refer you to a specialist.

Endocrinologist or Diabetologist

An *endocrinologist* is a physician who took advanced, specialized training in the field of endocrinology (hormones and glands) after completing training in internal medicine or pediatrics. Diabetology is less well defined as a specialty. A *diabetologist* is generally a physician, usually an endocrinologist, who has special expertise in the treatment of diabetes. Most often, a diabetologist is an endocrinologist who subspecializes in the treatment of diabetes. Health professionals who are not physicians and whose primary training is as a nutritionist, herbal specialist, or "holistic medicine" specialist would not be called diabetologists.

Do you need an endocrinologist or a diabetologist on your team? Our opinion is that not everyone with diabetes does, but quite a few people do. A simple way to decide is to think about how you are doing with your current provider. Are your questions answered reasonably well? Are your examinations reasonably thorough? Most important, is your diabetes under good control? If not, you should consider whether specialty input from an endocrinologist or diabetologist is needed. Sometimes you can see a diabetologist to help get your diabetes back under control, then return to the care of your primary care provider once your glucose levels have remained stable after several visits.

Endocrinologists or diabetologists may be primary care providers or may work on a referral basis, in tandem with primary care providers, in treating persons with diabetes. Let's consider four different patients with different needs.

Edgar is a 72-year-old man with Type 2 diabetes who has several other health problems as well: high blood pressure, arthritis, and a prostate problem. He has a primary care provider who is a general internist, and he also sees a diabetologist about every six months, or whenever the primary care provider would like to get the specialist's opinion on some aspect of Edgar's health.

The variety of Edgar's illnesses makes it important for him to have a generalist coordinating his care. The diabetes is only one of several problems, and the generalist is asking for help as needed.

Sandy is 27 years old, with a 14-year history of Type 1 diabetes. An endocrinologist is her primary care provider. Her blood glucose levels are unstable, she has some developing problems with her diabetes, and the endocrinologist is best suited to give her most of the care she needs. He regularly refers Sandy to a gynecologist and an ophthalmologist.

In this case, Sandy's Type 1 diabetes is her most significant health problem, and it's a difficult problem to manage. It makes sense for her to have a specialist for ongoing care.

Michelle signed up for a managed care option in her health insurance plan that turns out to be quite restrictive. She is having significant insulin reactions and thinks her insulin regimen needs adjustment, but the generalist seems unfamiliar with mixing insulins. Worse, when Michelle asks about the possibility of seeing an endocrinologist, the generalist tells her that it really isn't necessary. Translated, this means that Michelle can consult whomever she wants, but she'll have to pay for it out of pocket.

Often, managed care organizations are perfectly willing to approve needed consultations or ongoing primary care by a specialist. But apparently not in Michelle's case. The roadblocks she hit, such as the generalist's unwillingness to refer, despite clear indications that the current regimen wasn't working, definitely suggest that Michelle needs help. She should get it from her managed care organization, and she should not have to pay out of pocket.

Antoine is 30 years old and has had diabetes since the age of 5. His primary care provider is—well, in fact, Antoine's not quite sure who his care provider is since his company changed health coverage plans a year ago. He liked his old endocrinologist and may return to her for care, but he will now have to pay out of pocket because the new plan doesn't include her as a care provider. As a result of the confusion, Antoine hasn't seen a doctor in 18 months.

Antoine has let inattention get the better of him. Maybe he's in denial about his diabetes. Whatever the cause, all people with diabetes need regular care by a good medical care team.

Diabetes Nurse Educator

A nurse educator may provide a variety of services for the person with diabetes. A primary role is teaching self-management skills. Just what this involves will vary from place to place and person to person. For example, a nurse educator may be associated either with a large hospital or diabetes center or with just one practitioner's office. After assessing your individual needs, the educator may decide to concentrate on certain facets of self-care, such as insulin durations of action and injection technique, foot care, or diet.

Just how much individual patient management a diabetes educator does also varies. Some diabetes nurse educators work with a physician in providing follow-up care. The physician prescribes your initial insulin regimen, and the nurse educator then helps you fine-tune it over time, under the direction of the physician. At our diabetes center, some of our diabetes educators are also nurse practitioners, who can both begin a patient's medications and adjust medication dosages. Only doctors, nurse practitioners, and physician's assistants (with various state regulations applying to each profession) have the right to practice medicine independently, but a nurse educator can often help you a good deal in addition to assisting you with learning good self-management.

To find out if the educator you see has special expertise in diabetes, ask whether she is a *certified diabetes educator*, or CDE. Any health professional can become a CDE, but earning the certification requires having considerable experience in patient education and passing an examination.

Dietitian

A dietitian provides nutritional care, education, and counseling. A *registered dietitian*, or RD, has met the standards of the American Dietetic Association.

Dietitians with a CDE designation have specialized in the dietary aspects of treating diabetes.

It is hard to imagine treating diabetes effectively without a dietitian being involved. Contrary to popular belief, the principles of healthful eating for diabetes are *not* well known and are certainly not the same as they were 20, 10, or even 5 years ago. Individualizing diets requires expert professional knowledge. Matching the requirements of a particular diet with an individual's personal and ethnic preferences takes another level of skill. Don't try to learn what diet to be on by yourself. Talk with a dietitian.

Mental Health Professionals

As we discussed in Chapter 16, depression and other psychiatric illnesses are more common among persons with diabetes than among persons without diabetes. These illnesses make diabetes more difficult to manage, and treatment by mental health professionals has been shown to improve both psychological well-being and diabetes control. The term *mental health professional* encompasses people with a variety of backgrounds, degrees, and skills. Some are trained formally in psychology, some in social work with an emphasis on psychiatric social work, some in sociology and counseling, and some in another area. The level of education is signified by the degree obtained: a bachelor's degree (B.A. or B.S.) means the person has graduated from college; a master's degree (such as an M.S.) usually requires one to two years of postgraduate work; and a Ph.D. requires about four to six years of education after college. A psychiatrist is a medical doctor (M.D.), with four years of education and training after college plus three to four years of training in psychiatry. A psychologist has a Ph.D. Most counselors trained in social work have a master's degree.

In essence, the mental health professional can help you reduce your psychological and emotional response to stresses in life. This may involve helping you learn coping skills to deal with the additional demands of diabetes in an already busy life. It could mean providing counseling and training in coping skills either as part of a larger treatment plan for diabetes or for a specific psychological problem. Only medical doctors and nurse practitioners can prescribe medications such as antidepressants, but other mental health professionals are able to recognize the need for psychiatric care or medications and can refer you to a psychiatrist or another M.D.

The most important point about mental health counseling, in our view, is that you recognize you have the need and take advantage of what's available. Thinking of getting counseling as somehow meaning you are weak or inadequate is a very outdated notion. Working with a counselor is really no different than an athlete working with a coach. Please take advantage of all the help that's available for all your needs.

Ophthalmologist

An *ophthalmologist* is a medical doctor (M.D.) with specialized training in diseases of the eye. Chapter 23 describes the work of ophthalmologists in more detail. Everyone with diabetes needs a regular eye exam by an ophthalmologist. This examination should be arranged by your primary care provider.

Optometrist

Optometrists are not physicians but professionals who have been trained in specific aspects of eye care. Optometrists vary widely in their experience in examining eyes for evidence of the diabetes-related eye condition called diabetic retinopathy. Some are experienced at picking it up with a careful dilated-pupil eye examination, but others are not. How can you evaluate this? First of all, no eye exam for diabetic retinopathy is adequate if the pupils are not dilated, unless performed with a special camera that can take pictures of your retina without pupil dilation. Be sure to look out for yourself by asking the optometrist about her skill in screening for diabetic retinopathy and by checking back with your primary care provider or diabetologist.

Physical Therapist

Physical therapists are professionals with special training in improving physical function. Usually they work with individuals in rehabilitation after injuries or strokes, but they also have a role to play in prevention—for example, in avoiding foot injuries. Physical therapy services are often underutilized. Just as people don't automatically know how to prepare a diabetic diet, they are not born knowing how to safely build strength, endurance, and flexibility. The physical therapist does have this knowledge. He can get you started on a safe exercise program, especially if you have a physical problem, such as a bad back.

Podiatrist or Other Foot Care Specialist

Podiatrists, orthopedists, and even physical therapists may specialize in the foot care of people with diabetes. But the *podiatrist* is the person who deals with feet as the only focus of her professional activity. Podiatrists can provide a variety of services, from trimming the toenails to examining the foot for structural abnormalities that could develop into ulcers without proper treatment and performing some surgical procedures. Chapter 26 describes how to use the services of a foot care specialist.

Other Health Care Specialists

There are other health care specialists involved in caring for people with diabetes. A social worker or case manager may be important, for example. Other medical specialties, such as obstetrics, gastroenterology (for stomach or intestinal problems), dermatology (skin), nephrology (kidney), cardiology (heart disease), and urology (bladder and sexual function), offer their own special focus. Your care team has to be customized to your needs as well as to the resources available where you live. Once you've assembled your team, you have to know how to get along with its members.

Working with Health Care Professionals

How can you best establish a good relationship with your health care professional? First, you need to understand your own expectations, the expectations the health care professional may have, and how to meld the two.

Your Reasonable Expectations

As the person with diabetes, you quite naturally think of your own needs first, especially when it comes to health care. You have a right to expect communication, honesty, competence, professional standards, and high-quality care from your health care professional. You can also expect clear communication between members of your health care team. You have a right to switch doctors (although, as we discuss in Chapter 18, your health plan may have strict regulations about whom you can see under what circumstances). In Chapter 18 you'll also find a "patient's bill of rights," and we urge you to check it out. It is what you deserve.

But it makes sense every now and then to step back and consider the viewpoint of the health care professional. What is she dealing with and thinking about with respect to your best health outcomes—and what is he or she thinking of *you*? Are any of your expectations unreasonable?

Your Encounter with the Treating Professional

It's certainly fair to assume that the treating professional wants what is best for you and that his motives are good ones. If you have any doubt about that, you should definitely move on to someone else. But all health care professionals operate within certain constraints and restrictions. First, the care provider must know what's medically *possible* and what is not. As much as you may want a cure for the circulatory problem in your leg, for instance, an experienced vascular surgeon may know that it is not possible.

The time element. There is always a time limit. These days very few professionals can spend as much time as they might like talking with each patient. To be sure, you deserve whatever time is necessary, and you shouldn't feel pushed out the door. But reality may fall somewhat short of the ideal in this modern world of time management. It's better to expect a specific amount of time, say 15 or 30 minutes, and use it well than to have unlimited expectations and be disappointed.

Specialist or generalist? If you find the doctor who knows everything, please let us know—that would be quite a find! More likely, the specialist will know a good deal about diabetes, insulins, pills, diabetes complications, and so on. The generalist will know something about the general aspects of diabetes and a lot about all aspects of health care for you. Neither one will know your particular diabetes as well as you do. If you've just read something in a diabetes magazine or on the Internet, it's very possible that your treating professional won't know what you're talking about. A good professional is one who will admit, "I don't know." Then, if the issue is potentially important, she will find out or tell you how to find out about it. But good health care is not a quiz show where the smartest doctor or the smoothest talker wins.

The human being behind the white coat. And then, dare we say it, there's the matter of being human. Is a health care professional allowed to feel frustration, disappointment, defensiveness, or even anger? To a degree, there's probably no avoiding it. The care provider must maintain a level of professionalism, but you can't expect, and probably wouldn't want, a person with absolutely no emotion.

Making a list, checking it twice. One of the relatively simple steps you can take to improve your interaction with health care professionals is to make a list of your main points before you go into the office: what's bothering you, what questions you have, what your priorities are. Show your doctor the list early in the visit. If 15 minutes of a 20-minute visit are spent on unimportant chit-chat, the doctor isn't going to be excited about addressing a whole new set of serious issues just when he thought the visit was ending.

Try to have your records, your diaries, and your dates in good order. You may become nervous in the office, so if you have prepared everything neatly and legibly and organized it well, you will save a lot of time. Also, if you make sure beforehand that laboratory results or notes from other physicians have been sent to your doctor's office, time won't be taken away from your visit to track them down.

Turning on the charm. Don't be afraid to use your own charm, your own tact, your own "bedside manner." You should recognize two different interaction styles:

- "You said take 16 units of insulin in the morning. Dr. Jones said take 20 units. What's the deal, don't you two talk, and are you right or is Dr. Jones right?"
- "I saw Dr. Jones after seeing you, and she suggested that maybe 20 units of insulin would help. This is higher than the dose you recommended to me before. Does that dose sound like a good idea to you?"

The first style is brusque, even combative, and is not likely to help your relationship with your health care provider. The second style is not only more tactful but also more cooperative; it is more of a teamwork approach.

Don't take offense too easily. Some doctors may seem abrupt or even gruff: "You're way too heavy." Others say the same thing rather differently: "I believe you would be healthier and your diabetes better controlled if you could lose a few pounds." Some seem to accuse you of "cheating" if the treatment isn't working perfectly. Others don't. But in the end, the words they use may not be as important as the care they give. So if you are truly offended by a professional's approach, find someone else. But our advice is to try to ignore the superficial and concentrate on what really matters.

Communication between professionals. Don't expect instant or perfect communication between professionals. They all have busy days, and even telephone or fax communications may take some time. Furthermore, some communications are simply more important than others. It probably doesn't matter much whether your ophthalmologist knows the exact status of your prostate, but it's important for your primary care doctor to know if you see a cardiologist who changes your medications.

Changing horses. A final word about talking to doctors and changing doctors: try not to worry about speaking out and asking questions. See if you can make the relationship work so that you get what you need out of it. But if you can't, and if you want to change doctors, don't worry about that either. We are amazed at how far some people will go to protect the feelings of a doctor. He will be okay. There will be other patients. If you feel you have to change, just do it. The important thing is for you to get your health care problems solved.

Problem Solving

So far we've put the emphasis on personalities and interpersonal communications. But in the end the issue is not how closely your personalities match but whether you and your health care professional can get the job done. And the job, quite simply, is problem solving. There must be clear communication between the two of you concerning the nature of the problem, from both your point of view and the doctor's. Once you agree on the problem, you can put your heads together and work out a plan.

> Jean comes to her endocrinologist's office with three things on her mind: her ankle is still sore after she sprained it a few days ago while playing tennis; she wants to know whether the advertised herbal product she just bought will make her feel more youthful; and she has had some low blood glucose reactions at night. Her doctor comes into the room with other concerns: Jean has not had an eye exam in two years, and her hemoglobin A1c tested in the office is considerably higher than he would like. In the interview, Jean gets a little nervous and keeps coming back to the ankle and natural alternatives to replace some of her medications. Her doctor gets irritable, not showing much interest in the ankle, and he's not enthusiastic about discussing an herbal product he's never heard of. Jean leaves with a sense, shared by the endocrinologist, that it wasn't a very useful visit.

Jean and her doctor never got to the stage of problem solving. They didn't even begin to work on some changes that might help with three important features of Jean's case: her need for better average blood glucose levels (A1c level), her need to avoid nighttime hypoglycemia, and her need to revisit her ophthalmologist. The reason? Jean and the endocrinologist had different agendas. Her ankle was still bothering her, and she wanted to know whether an advertised natural product would make her feel more youthful. The endocrinologist's agenda was to talk about blood glucose control, but he let himself get sidetracked by an ankle he wasn't going to treat and an herbal product for which he was unable to find any scientific data.

Let's run that scene over again, slightly rescripted:

Jean comes in her endocrinologist's office with three things on her mind: her ankle is still sore after she sprained it a few days ago while playing tennis; she wants to know whether the advertised herbal product she just bought will make her feel more youthful; and she has had some low blood glucose reactions at night. But she thinks, "Wait a minute, he's not going to deal with ankles or herbal supplements. He's a specialist. Let's talk diabetes." Her doctor comes into the room with some other concerns: Jean has not had an eye exam in two years, and her hemoglobin A1c was considerably higher at her last visit than he would like. He's sorry to see her limping on a sprained ankle and says so. In the interview, they immediately agree on the problem: how do they improve the blood glucose average and still avoid the nighttime hypoglycemia? Together, they work on problem solving. Before Jean leaves, the doctor jots down his suggestions for changes in insulin doses and also reminds her, in writing, to have her eyes examined.

This version seems a lot more satisfactory, doesn't it? The key to a better outcome was Jean thinking over what she really wanted out of the visit and making that clear. Of course, the endocrinologist helped by being sympathetic about her ankle, even if he wasn't treating it. But getting to the problem solving was the important thing—plain and simple.

Sometimes during the office visit, too many suggestions are made, too many warnings are given, too much is said. Many people feel overwhelmed as they walk out the door. And don't think that it will all become clearer once you leave the office. It is well known that as soon as people leave the doctor's office, they *forget* most of what was said.

There are several ways to fend off the barrage of information and prevent information overload. Sometimes your doctor can write down or print out the points she is making. You can also take notes yourself as she is talking. It's a way for you to slow your doctor down and to see whether you understand what she is saying.

Another approach to enhancing communication and keeping instructions to a reasonable number is to draw up a contract. Your contract is an agreement between you and the health care professional as to what you will do as a result of the office visit. Any contract involves benefit to two parties: in this case, you get improved health care, and your doctor gets the satisfaction of helping. By "contracting," you end up with a short list of instructions that you understand and agree to try to carry out.

Whatever the interpersonal chemistry and the methods of communication between you and your health care professional, you want to leave that office with some problem-solving suggestions. Then you can work on them yourself, making use of all available resources.

Other Resources

As you leave the health professional's office, especially if it has been a supportive and positive setting, you may well have a sudden sense of being alone. You're the one with diabetes—and no one else out there knows what it feels like. Even if your doctor and nurse are caring people, they have only so much time to interact with you. You may find it helpful to seek out other people with diabetes.

One avenue is a diabetes support group. Affiliates of the American Diabetes Association (ADA) usually sponsor such groups, as do some hospitals and universities. Joining the ADA and the Juvenile Diabetes Research Foundation (JDRF) can bring a lot of information right to your door and provide opportunities to interact with others in educational or fund-raising activities.

One particularly useful service of these organizations is the magazines they publish. The ADA has a monthly magazine called *Diabetes Forecast* that features articles on people with diabetes, recipes, research updates, discussions of specific treatment measures in the management of diabetes, and product information. You can also find the magazine articles on the ADA's website, www.diabetes.org. The magazine of the JDRF, called *Countdown*, focuses on research on Type 1 diabetes and is published quarterly. The JDRF's website is www.jdrf.org.

There are many other resources out there as well. If you have access to a computer, modem, and Internet service provider, you'll be able to locate not only the ADA's and JDRF's websites but also chat pages, bulletin boards, blogs, discussion groups, and a variety of other websites about diabetes. A healthy dose of skepticism is useful, however, when you read nonprofessionals' discussions of diabetes. Remember that when individuals make a statement about *their* diabetes, their situation, their understanding, that doesn't make it true for you. We recently saw a patient, a woman in her late 70s, who had just developed diabetes. Her well-intentioned granddaughter had collected all the information she could find on the Internet and sent a three-inch-thick printout to her grandmother. Unfortunately, the material was haphazard and disorganized, and the older woman was overwhelmed. Information overload can be as dangerous as no information at all.

. . .

You and your health care professionals are a team, working together to control your diabetes and help you lead a healthy life. Maybe your team is a small one, well versed in the intricacies of your diabetes management. Or maybe it involves many specialties. Maybe it's everything you want, and maybe not. But in the end the goal is the same: to figure out how the various team members need to come together to control your diabetes and keep you feeling well. Whatever you can do to make this work, it's worth the effort.

Take Home Messages

- You are the central person on your health care team. You make the decisions: what to eat, when to eat, how to exercise, how to take medications, when to seek help, and so on.
- Your primary care provider is the medical professional who takes responsibility for and coordinates your overall health care.
- Other health care professionals with expertise in treating diabetes include endocrinologists, diabetes nurse educators, dietitians, mental health professionals, eye specialists, physical therapists, and foot care specialists. Each can help make your life with diabetes healthier and easier.
- Effective communication is your key to the best possible diabetes outcomes: effective communication with your health care team and effective communication among your diabetes health care providers.
- Organizations such as the American Diabetes Association can also be part of your health care team when you make use of their publications and Internet resources.

18

Interacting with the Health Care System

- "My insurance covers some things, like pancreas transplantation, that seem so useless to me, but it limits the number of blood glucose testing strips I can get, which are obviously essential. It makes me get special prescriptions with a list of restrictions: only 30 days' worth, no refills, written as a generic, signed by the doctor. Why are they hassling me?"
- "I just don't understand all these plans offered by my employer. HMO, PPO, Indemnity, Network. Some are much cheaper than others, but are they as good?"
- "My daughter has diabetes. She just left school, and all of a sudden I realized that she is no longer covered by my insurance plan. Is this a problem?"

Whatever else you think of the health care system in the United States, you probably recognize that it's not really an organized system at all. It's a complicated set of policies, plans, providers, and insurers that evolved with no apparent overall planning. You may believe that it is the best system in the world, or that it is in serious need of reform, or both. But if you have diabetes in your family, your immediate problem is how to get along in the current system. In the United States, the Affordable Care Act of 2010 was the first major reform to the health care system that guarantees more health care choices.

This chapter provides an overview of the *system*. It doesn't look closely at your personal interactions with individual health care providers (a topic covered in Chapter 17). Instead, we are dealing here with aspects of health care that may be even more frustrating: the forms, the phone calls, the coverage, the payments, and so on. Although we can't discuss all the innumerable existing plans and options or unscramble all the acronyms, we discuss your rights and concerns, what's out there to help you, and ways to make the system work to your advantage. Your primary interest is your own good health.

We start with a brief description of your rights *as we see them* (we're not implying that all insurers see things as we do). We then describe the various kinds of health coverage and summarize the most important considerations when choosing a plan or using a plan to your best advantage. No matter what the advertisements say, there's very little that is simple or obvious or even logical about health insurance. It takes some thought and a lot of persistence to come out on top.

A Patients' Bill of Rights

A bill of rights for patients is not an uncommon document these days. The American Diabetes Association, for example, spells out as a matter of policy what your rights are when it comes to high-quality diabetes care. Many hospitals, too, have a patients' bill of rights framed and prominently displayed. Unfortunately, the Framers of the U.S. Constitution did not write health care, much less glucose monitoring strips, into the Constitution. On the contrary, to this day federal law is nonspecific in regulating what must be provided and what need not be provided as part of health insurance. So you have to be careful in selecting a plan and assertive in claiming your "rights."

We believe that the right to quality diabetes care starts with your own responsibility to do what you can for yourself. No amount of technology, no team of specialists or education program, will be adequate if your own self-management is poor. But assuming that *you* are acting responsibly, what should the system provide? In short, what constitutes quality diabetes care? This is where the debate begins. Let's start by setting out the basic elements of good diabetes care to which we believe everyone is entitled:

—An accurate diagnosis and ongoing care

—Diabetes education

—Provision of necessary supplies and medications, both disposable and permanent

—Access to health care professionals, both for primary care and for any specialized needs

Accurate Diagnosis

A problem that we covered at the start of this book (see Chapter 1) is how often people are unclear about whether they have diabetes or not. You really should know. We recommend that you get tested if you are at high risk (overweight, strong family history, unexplained weight loss, or other typical symptoms) and, most important, that you ask for a straight answer from a health care professional—do I or don't I have diabetes?

Diabetes Education

Nothing is more important in managing your diabetes than understanding it. People are not born knowing about diabetes, and usually the information they pick up from general sources (Aunt Matilda's second cousin, the man down the street, a 30-second news clip) is incomplete at best and often totally inaccurate. It's up to you to learn about diabetes.

The settings for diabetes education vary widely. Some people have several one-on-one visits with a diabetes educator; others may get their diabetes education in a group, along with other people who have diabetes. Sometimes diabetes education consists of a single intensive class, and sometimes it is extended over a longer period of time. It is rarely necessary for someone to be hospitalized for education.

These days the educator should be a certified diabetes educator (CDE), and the program should be well structured and comprehensive. Education does not consist of a few casual comments or a simple handout on diet. In addition to sessions with a CDE, there is no substitute for an individual consultation with a qualified dietitian.

Today, insurance companies will reimburse for the cost of diabetes education, though different plans cover different types and amounts of education.

Necessary Supplies and Pharmaceuticals

The things people have to buy just to manage their diabetes, to fill their prescriptions, can be expensive. These include pills, insulin, syringes, glucose test strips, glucose meters, insulin pumps, and so on.

The supplies and pharmaceuticals that are recommended by your doctor ought to be covered by an insurance plan. You may not be in a position to insist on getting reimbursement for supplies and pharmaceuticals if they are specifically excluded from the coverage in your plan, but you should try.

Access to Health Care Professionals

People with diabetes want, deserve, and need to have continued care by competent professionals. In Chapter 17 we mentioned that although primary care physicians are usually not diabetes specialists, they may be excellent physicians who can care for you very well without knowing all the details about meters, new insulins, and other diabetes-related matters. So for most people with diabetes, their care can be well managed by a primary care physician. However, people with unusually unstable diabetes, complications, or other special problems need to have their care managed by a specialist.

In addition to a primary care physician, many people need to have at least some contact with specialists. For example, all people with diabetes should regularly see an ophthalmologist (specialist in eye diseases). Input from other specialists is often indicated too, such as that provided by a nurse educator, psychologist, cardiologist, podiatrist, or dietitian. Whatever your health plan coverage, you are entitled to both primary care and necessary specialty care.

Types of Health Insurance Plans

A convenient way to consider health insurance options is to divide them into government entitlements, traditional insurance coverage plans, and managed care plans. (A glossary at the end of this chapter includes some of the many terms used in defining insurance coverage and health plans.)

Government Entitlements

Government entitlement programs have fixed criteria for eligibility, which are written into law. The eligibility criteria may be complicated, and to interpret them many people need the assistance of a social worker or benefits manager. In most cases, such as Medicare and Medicaid, the programs represent a commitment by the state or federal government to pay bills; within the military and veterans' health care systems, the programs actually deliver the care. These federal entitlements are probably the largest health care delivery systems in the world.

Medicare, the health insurance program for the elderly (currently, 65 and older) and disabled, is the largest single expenditure of the U.S. federal budget after payment on the national debt. (We recently heard of a woman who complained, "I'm not going to let government get in the way of my Medicare"—a nonsensical comment.) Medicare is not a means-tested program, so age and long-term disability, rather than income, are generally the basic criteria for eligibility. Medicare has significant co-payments and limitations of coverage. Insulin is covered, but newer diabetes pills (DPP-4 inhibitors) or injectable medications (GLP-1 analogs) are not. When Medicare insurance does not cover certain drugs or diabetes services, senior citizens may want to look into paying separately for Medigap policies, also called Medicare supplemental insurance, that specifically fill the gaps in Medicare coverage.

Medicaid is a combined federal and state program that pays for health care for the poor. Unlike Medicare, Medicaid is a means-tested program, meaning that eligibility depends on income and net worth. Income and size of family are the basic criteria for eligibility. Benefits vary considerably from state to state.

There is no doubt that if you qualify, the government entitlements are the most advantageous programs for you. They adhere to insurance principles in that they are supported by a very large base of people paying into the system (taxpayers), and they do not exclude people because of preexisting conditions or high health risk. Increasingly, though, they are being scrutinized as budget items that should be limited. Many Medicaid and Medicare programs, for example, are entering into managed care plans rather than simply paying bills. This often means that people are either forced or induced (by the lure of lower out-of-pocket payments) to join specific health plans. Being enrolled in a government entitlement program does not guarantee any particular level of coverage. Increasingly, benefits are being limited as part of the overall effort to lower government expenditures.

Traditional Insurance Coverage Plans

The idea behind traditional (indemnity) insurance is really very simple: every person in a large group of people pays premiums to an insurance company; then, when a person gets sick, the provider (doctor, hospital, pharmacy) generates a bill, and the insurance company pays it out of the pool of money it has collected as premiums. Interestingly, insurance companies make most of their profits by investing the premiums before they are paid out to providers, rather than by paying out less than they collect. State insurance commissioners regulate how much the insurers are allowed to skim off as administrative expenses and profit. By calculating the likely amount of illness in a given group of insured people, the insurance company tries to anticipate what the payouts will be and to charge adequate premiums to cover these payouts plus expenses and profit. When faced with uncertainty, the traditional response of insurers is to increase premiums to cover potential losses.

Blue Cross and Blue Shield plans across the country are a slightly different type of insurance. They generally operate as nonprofit corporations and thus receive certain tax breaks. Increasingly, though, like the for-profit insurance companies, they are diversifying into managed health care, and in some states they are taking on a for-profit status.

The theory of insurance dictates that the insurer collects a large pool of members (called *covered lives*) so that the risk of illness is spread widely and is therefore relatively predictable. Some members will get sick, but many will remain healthy. You can see that it makes quite a difference for insurers whether the population being covered is elderly or young.

Insurers prefer to cover such large groups, assuming that this will spread the risk among the healthy and the sick. When individuals or very small groups (such as a mom-and-pop store) apply for coverage on their own, the insurer is much more skeptical. Are any of these people already sick? Will they require payouts from the insurance company right away, no questions asked? How much does the insurance company know about these people? What is the insurance company's risk and how can it be minimized? These questions lead to some obvious answers. Faced with a request for individual or small-group coverage, an insurer is very likely to require careful physical exams, to increase the premiums significantly if the person or small group is found to have significant illness or a higher average age, and to try to refuse coverage for preexisting illness. While these are logical reactions in the for-profit insurance business, they do not work to the benefit of individuals or small groups applying for traditional insurance, especially for someone who has diabetes.

Even when covering large groups with actuarially sound premiums and low profit margins, traditional insurance has a tendency to become more and more expensive. This is because these insurers pay all legitimate bills that are submitted. They pay on a fee-for-service basis—the insurance equivalent of piecework. This means that if a doctor does 20 operations in a week, she earns twice as much as if she does 10 operations in a week. If a person goes to the doctor five times in a month, the insurer pays five times as much as if the person goes once a month. The insurance company will probably try to raise premiums the next time around, but as long as the company has little control over the volume of service, costs will tend to escalate. This feature of traditional insurance, as much as anything else, has led to the explosion of health care costs generally. It has also led to new developments in health coverage, typified by the managed care approach, which is rapidly replacing traditional insurance as the most common way Americans pay for and receive health care.

Managed Care Plans

In the broadest sense, *managed care* refers to the management of who goes where for what health care services, and who gets paid how much by whom. Patients' care is "managed," meaning that people are not entirely free to go wherever they want for whatever medical service they want. The providers are tightly managed as well: they, too, are restricted not only in what they may charge for a given service but also in how often the service can be delivered.

As with traditional insurance, managed care plans depend on relatively large groups of covered lives. Typically, the plan receives payment on a capitated (per capita) basis. A large group of people (say, a large company) contracts with the plan to *deliver* all the health care for group members (not just pay for it, as with traditional insurance). The managed care company takes a fixed annual amount—for the sake of this example, let's say $100 per employee per month, or $1,200 per employee per year, for each of the company's 1,000 employees. It guarantees to deliver health care with the $1,200,000 it has collected for the year.

How the managed care company chooses to spend the dollars delivering care is up to the directors of the company. They can hire their own doctors or negotiate deals with independent doctors, own hospitals or negotiate deals with hospitals, even own suppliers of pharmaceuticals or negotiate deals for pharmaceuticals. This diversity of options is what makes the differences among managed care plans so complicated. And as the managed care companies know very well, whatever they do *not* pay out, they keep as profit. This makes the business profitable.

To an even greater extent than with traditional insurance, the amount of illness in a population is crucial to the managed care company's profits. A traditional insurance company can adjust premiums, at least to some extent, and reduce its risk. But managed care plans usually offer one basic capitated rate and make their profit by controlling what they pay out for delivery of care. If the population is relatively healthy, the number of doctor and hospital visits and expenses incurred can easily be controlled by using a gatekeeper. But every sick person who joins the plan eats directly into the company's profits.

Because there is so much profit to be made in collecting generous fees for the care of healthy people, managed care plans have long been accused of "cherry picking," or choosing a healthier-than-average population to enroll. Regulations have been made in an attempt to counteract this tendency of managed care plans, but if the regulations are not successful—if plans collect average fees for healthier-than-average people—the whole concept of managed care is undermined.

There is a science—some call it an art—called risk adjustment that is designed to calculate just how much the care of a given population should cost and to set payments to the insurer accordingly. It is a complex subject, however, filled with such imponderables as how much care is enough, what constitutes quality care, and who deserves what level of care. Ultimately, though, risk adjustments will be necessary if managed care is to have a lasting incentive to deliver excellent care.

Specific Types of Managed Care Plans

All managed care plans control, or manage, the expenses of providing health care. Exactly how they do so varies enormously from plan to plan.

Health maintenance organization (HMO). The classic HMO may be "closed panel" or "open panel." The closed panel HMO hires its own doctors and nurses, owns their office space, pays them a salary, and closely regulates their practices (controlling, for example, how many patients the professionals see in a day, what drugs they prescribe, and how many consultations or lab tests they order).

The medical care provided to members of an HMO usually is coordinated by a single primary care provider. The open panel HMO may hire some providers, but it also negotiates with many outside doctors to deliver care at a reduced rate. While an independent practitioner may normally charge, say, $60 for a visit, an HMO can approach the doctor and offer 500 visits at $40 per visit. The way physicians are hired and how they feel about the organization can have consequences that may affect you. Sometimes the doctors get more personal income if they order less testing and make fewer referrals to specialists, and there have been cases in which physicians were prohibited from revealing such arrangements to their patients. The turnover rate of physicians in a particular plan can give you an idea of how happy they are, which may also be an indication of how free they are to practice as they think best.

Preferred provider organization (PPO). A PPO manages the delivery of care somewhat differently, extending the practice of negotiation with independent providers. The company does not hire a large number of providers, but instead sets up a long list of physicians who have agreed to accept the PPO rates of payment and to play by PPO rules. The providers, for example, may agree not to refer patients to specialists without prior approval, or they may agree to have all lab work done through a particular commercial laboratory with which the PPO has negotiated favorable rates. Under this system, any physician who turns out to be more "expensive" than anticipated (in other words, one who makes too many referrals or orders too many tests) may be taken off the list. This would mean you could no longer receive your care from that doctor.

Indemnity or fee-for-service plans. Indemnity plans allow members to see any doctor and go to whatever hospital they want, but at a price. A moderately large deductible usually has to be paid before the insurance company reimburses members a set percentage of the cost of the service. Because of the greater freedom members have in choosing whom they see, the cost of these plans is usually greater than other plans.

Network plans. These plans also allow patients to direct their own health care, but within a network of providers. Networks usually also require members to pay a co-pay at the time of office visits. How much members pay out of pocket depends on where they see the doctor: visits at the plan's regular office may involve no fee, an approved urgent care center may require the patient to pay 10%–30% of the total bill, a visit to an emergency room may cost the patient 15% of the bill, and a visit to an unapproved specialist may cost the patient a deductible, a co-pay, or 20%–100% of the bill. Many network plans also require members to pay a deductible before medical expenses are covered.

Hospitalization and Managed Care Plans

Hospitalization is a major expense and therefore a prime target of all managed care plans. Most managed care programs, and even traditional health insurers, now require preauthorization before hospitalization. This means that the physician has to call a special phone number, where someone (it is often not clear who this person is or what medical credentials he or she has) takes the information provided and decides whether hospitalization is necessary and, if so, for how many days. Once the patient has been hospitalized, record reviews are a routine procedure; the reviewers decide when the patient should be discharged. This process, called *utilization review*, has resulted in much less hospitalization and the closing of many hospital beds and even whole hospitals.

. . .

We have tried to avoid the temptation to label different insurance plans as good or bad. Naturally, our opinions, like yours, are often based on our own personal experiences. But experiences will vary tremendously; a plan that one person has found to meet her needs perfectly may be terrible for someone else. There is no doubt, though, that systems of payment for health care are changing dramatically. New plans and companies are formed almost daily. Rather than bemoaning this (or wishing for the old days when the friendly local doctor pulled up to your door in his buggy and cared for your sick child in exchange for a plucked chicken), we recommend that you accept this new world and work on bending it to your own needs.

How Do I Get the Best Health Care Coverage for Myself?

There are two times to consider the question of how to get the best health care coverage: when you are choosing a plan and when you are in one. In either case, remember that if you have diabetes, you need to disclose and discuss that fact. Keeping a known health condition secret is a prescription for losing coverage altogether, and you should use every means available to you not to be without insurance. If diabetes is a fact of your health care life, it should be dealt with. There are predictable medical costs in sight, and the last thing you want is to have needed health care unaffordable due to lack of an insurance plan.

Qualifying for an Entitlement Program

As we mentioned above, government entitlements are often the best type of health care program. If you think you might be eligible, you should contact the relevant office of the federal or state government and find out whether you qualify. The federal government's website www.medicaid.gov will let you find out whether you qualify for Medicaid or, for your children, the Children's Health Insurance Program (CHIP).

Choosing a Traditional Insurance Plan through a Large Group

Earlier, when we described what goes on in the traditional insurance sphere, we explained that it is advantageous for people to enroll in large group plans rather than seeking insurance as an individual or in a small group. This is particularly true for someone who has an illness, such as diabetes. Large group plans are most often offered by established, large employers. As few as 20 people may qualify as a group. Unions are another good source, since many unions have negotiated very favorable health plans over the years. But there are other ways to get into a large group. Consider associations, fraternal organizations, and clubs. Simply by bringing together many people, these groups may have developed plans that will allow you to join, despite having diabetes. A spouse's policy may be able to cover you. When you are choosing employment, be sure to consider whether the employer offers a group health insurance plan. It may well be worth sacrificing other elements of a job, such as a higher salary, to get good insurance coverage.

Some states have pooled risk plans, in which so-called uninsurable risks are allowed into a state-run plan. Where available, these plans can provide insurance at a reasonable rate even when you have serious health care expenses coming up.

Choosing a Managed Care Plan

You may very well find that managed care plans of one kind or another are increasingly favorably priced. This can be the deciding factor in the choice of a plan, and there is certainly nothing intrinsically wrong with choosing a plan with a good price as well as good care. But you need to make the effort to understand what you are getting into. Here are some questions to ask about managed care plans. Be sure that you have the answers to these questions *in writing* from someone with the authority to be held responsible for the answers.

—To what extent can I choose my doctor?

—Is my regular doctor able to continue caring for me?

—As a person with diabetes, will I be seeing a board-certified internist? family practitioner? endocrinologist? Can I see a specialist if my care is not going well?

—Are retinal exams, diabetes education, glycated hemoglobin (hemoglobin A1c) tests, and other diabetes-related tests that I may need routinely covered?

—Are there limits to the number of test strips covered?

Our advice is to find out about the plan before you join. Use whatever sources of information are available: your employer's human resources department, people already enrolled in the plan, company brochures or lists of covered services, and/or plan salespeople. No one likes having major coverage surprises.

Working within a Plan

Here are three suggestions to help you "work the system" once you have enrolled in a health insurance plan:

1. *Learn the rules for getting coverage and getting office visits, and play by them.* Sometimes the rules seem almost cruelly complicated, and sometimes you'll get the impression that they are nothing but barriers put up to confuse and discourage you. But if you learn the rules, you can profit by your knowledge. If the plan requires four identical prescriptions, each saying a certain thing, get them. If you have to have a written preauthorization, get it. Whether or not the health plan has good reasons for establishing a set of complex regulations, chances are you will not be successful in going around them, so you may as well go through them.

2. *Be persistent.* If you think you deserve a specific coverage, keep asking. Make it a game, a personal challenge. Write back, call back, talk with a supervisor. Write down the date and time of every phone call you make, and ask for and write down the name of the person you talk to and what is said. You'd be amazed at how many people end up getting positive responses just by coming back at insurers over and over again.

3. *Apply pressure when needed.* If some needed service is not covered, there is always the last resort of trying to force a change in coverage policy. Maybe a letter to the president of the company will work. Perhaps your union or association, your state's insurance commissioner, or a politician can help. There are certain necessary elements of diabetes care that you probably know better than most. Don't be afraid to speak up.

. . .

To our way of thinking, health insurance coverage for high-quality diabetes care is your right. How such a statement actually plays out will vary, but it is worth making anyway. We have to assume that very few traditional insurance plans or managed care plans are oblivious to their responsibility to provide quality health care. We believe that by being smart and aggressive, we can all work our way through the maze that is the U.S. health care system and come out reasonably successful.

How Do I Get the Best Health Care Coverage for My Child with Diabetes after He or She Graduates from School?

In the past, children could no longer be covered by their parents' insurance plan after they finished their education. The Affordable Care Act allows young adults to stay on their parents' health insurance up to age 26, unless the child's employer offers health insurance coverage.

Take Home Messages

- As a person with diabetes, you have the right to an accurate diagnosis and ongoing care by qualified health care professionals, diabetes education, and the supplies and medication you need to take good care of yourself.
- A convenient way to consider health insurance options is to divide them into government entitlements (like Medicare and Medicaid), traditional insurance coverage plans, and managed care plans.
- Government entitlements are often the best type of health care program. If you think you might be eligible, you should contact the relevant office of the federal or state government and find out whether you qualify.
- You may very well find that managed care plans of one kind or another are increasingly favorably priced. Before you enroll, though, be sure to find out what choice you will have in doctors and hospitals, what services (e.g., eye exams) and supplies and medications are covered, and what your out-of-pocket expenses will be.

Glossary of Insurance Terms

Actuary The person who tries to calculate exactly what the amount of illness will be in a given group of people and therefore what the payouts will be for an insurance plan.

Adverse selection The situation when a plan gets more than its share of sick people (the opposite of *cherry picking*).

Capitated payments Payments based on the number of people in a plan, providing the same payment per person. For example, if a provider such as a doctor's office takes on the care of 100 people at a capitated (or per capita) rate of $50 per person, the provider receives $5,000 for delivering that care, regardless of what the care actually costs.

Catastrophic coverage Insurance coverage that starts only when expenses are very high. It is a policy of last resort, not paying for small or even average expenses but only for the very high (catastrophic) ones. Because these catastrophes are relatively rare, catastrophic insurance is relatively cheap.

Cherry picking The practice of picking the predictably healthiest people to join a plan (the opposite of *adverse selection*). This can be done subtly by steering advertising campaigns toward healthy people or overtly by excluding people with known illnesses.

COBRA A federal law requiring many employers to extend health insurance coverage to all laid-off employees for 18 months. Individuals are required to pay 100% of the cost of the insurance.

Co-pay The amount a patient pays out of pocket for a partially covered service. For example, if the insurance plan pays 80% of a given bill, the patient's co-pay is 20%.

Covered benefit A material or service that is paid for. For example, certain drugs or glucose meters or routine outpatient visits may or may not be covered benefits in a given plan.

Deductible The amount that must be paid by the covered individual every year before any insurance coverage kicks in. For example, if you have a $2,000 deductible, you pay the first $2,000 of all expenses each year before your insurance policy pays for anything.

Disposable supplies Supplies that are used and thrown away, such as syringes, glucose test strips, and alcohol wipes.

Durable medical equipment Supplies that last rather than being used then thrown away. Blood glucose meters and insulin pumps are examples.

Entitlement A program such as insurance coverage that a person is entitled to by virtue of his or her situation in life. The term usually refers to government programs. Medicare, for example, is an entitlement for which one qualifies by being age 65 or older. Medicaid is usually based on low income, veterans' benefits are based on having been in active military service, and so on.

Fee-for-service plan See *Indemnity health plan*.

Gatekeeper A person (or system) that directs the flow of people to particular providers. For example, if you have bronchitis, the gatekeeper (perhaps a nurse practitioner or a family practitioner) will probably decide that he or she can treat you and that you do not need to see a specialist. If you have a broken bone, the gatekeeper may decide that you need to see an orthopedist. The gatekeeper is your entrance into the system; you cannot decide for yourself which specialists you see.

Health maintenance organization (HMO) An organization (usually a for-profit company) that collects premiums from insured people or their employers and hires a staff to provide all health care.

Indemnity health plan A plan that allows you to choose which doctor or hospital to go to; also known as a fee-for-service plan.

Means-tested program A program in which eligibility depends on income and net worth. Medicaid is the classic means-tested program, meant to ensure health care for the economically disadvantaged. Medicare and the health insurance plans of the Department of Veterans Affairs are not at present means-tested programs.

Medigap An insurance policy designed to fill in the coverage gaps of Medicare; also called Medicare supplemental insurance. Ideally, for a reasonable cost, these policies cover only what is left uncovered by Medicare. The buyer has to be wary, though, that coverage is not overlapping or duplicated.

Network health plan A plan that allows members to choose from a large number of physicians, other health care providers, and hospitals that are part of the plan's network; also known as a point of service (POS) plan. Different levels of coverage are provided depending on where the patient receives the service. For example, you may be covered 100% if you go to one of the doctors in the plan, but if you choose to go outside the network—see an outside specialist, have surgery at a hospital other than the recommended one, and so on—you may have to pay 50% or more of the bill out of pocket. So, using providers or hospitals outside the network will cost more out of pocket.

Open enrollment period A period of time in which there is open enrollment in an insurance plan. For a month or so, people can sign up for the plan (sometimes still subject to certain limitations). Between open enrollment periods, a plan can decide whether or not to let you in.

Point of service (POS) plan See *Network health plan.*

Pooled risk plan A plan, usually run by a state government, that insures people who are otherwise too ill or too much at risk of illness to be eligible for usual coverage. The pooled risk plan may use government funds to pay some proportion of the high premiums charged by insurers to take on high-risk individuals.

Preauthorization The requirement to get approval before any test, procedure, or hospitalization is done. Typically, criteria are set up at a central computer, so when a physician's office calls for preauthorization, the information provided is put into the computer and the request is then approved or denied. If your plan requires preauthorization and it's not obtained, you may end up paying the entire bill out of pocket.

Preexisting condition *A medical condition (such as diabetes) that exists before a person signs up for a given health plan.* Many plans state that they will not cover preexisting conditions or will cover them only after a certain period of time. Starting in 2014, one of the provisions of the Affordable Care Act mandates that persons with disabilities can no longer be legally denied access to health insurance.

Preferred provider organization (PPO) A network of physicians and other health care professionals who have agreed to accept patients from a specific managed care plan, usually for a reduced fee per visit, to ensure that they have a flow of patients.

Provider The person or entity that delivers a health care service. A provider may be a doctor, a group practice, a nurse, a nutritionist, a hospital, or an entire health care system.

Risk adjustment The science of deciding how much risk (e.g., for illness) there is in a given group of people and adjusting payments accordingly.

For example, for health insurance, the risk is much higher if the average age in a population is 60 than if it is 30; a fair adjustment would be to have greater financial resources within the plan covering the 60-year-olds.

Utilization review The process of reviewing expenses in progress, usually applied to hospitalization, in which teams of chart reviewers check the charts of patients daily to decide whether continued hospitalization is necessary. Utilization review is now also being applied to outpatient care.

19

Employment and Diabetes

with Shereen Arent, J.D., and Katie Hathaway, J.D.

- "I want to be a police officer. Is there anything wrong with that? Why can't I be a police officer, if I want to?"
- "At the job interview today, they asked me if I have diabetes. I said yes, and the tone of the interview changed on the spot. I think I blew it."
- "I have a job in health care, where if I have a bad insulin reaction, it could really hurt someone. Should I get out of the field of health care altogether?"
- "What can I do to show my employer that I can be an excellent employee with diabetes?"

Throughout this book we encourage you to take control of your diabetes, and we provide tools to help you do so. But if diabetes keeps you from getting or keeping a job, it is controlling you, regardless of how well you manage your blood glucose. In this chapter we talk about how to hold your job regardless of diabetes. We describe, first, responsibilities and rights—yours and your employer's. We discuss employment discrimination, how to make it through job interviews, and what to consider in various kinds of employment. Finally, we offer some real-life scenarios and practical advice about performing successfully in the workplace—how to keep diabetes from dominating the situation.

Ideally, every job should be available to every qualified person, every employer should have an enlightened and intelligent approach to diabetes, and every employee should be successful at managing his or her diabetes without any interruption of work. But this is not a perfect world. Since every person and every workplace have unique features, employment problems can arise. Just remember: having diabetes is only one of your individual characteristics. You can work with it.

305

On the Job

Your Responsibilities

You have a responsibility both to yourself and to your employer. You need to take good care of yourself for the long run. If work is interfering with good self-care, you have to modify your regimen, modify the job, or seriously consider changing jobs. The goal is to be able to do your job while managing your diabetes for both long-term health and short-term safety, doing everything you can to avoid the worst-case scenario: having a severe insulin reaction on the job that causes injury to yourself or others. We have heard of a case that went to court for just this reason: the employee, a police officer, had one severe insulin reaction during which he put people in serious danger by crashing his patrol car. The county wanted to fire him from the force without a second chance. This was a case of "one strike and you're out." It was a situation you never want to be in.

You have a responsibility to your employer to perform your job reliably and well. This means, among other things, not taking unnecessary risks that could interfere with your job performance.

It is a good bet that your employer knows little about diabetes—a lot less than you do—and it's also likely that he or she isn't all that interested. So the best option is to make your diabetes self-care compatible with good job performance. If push comes to shove, though, it doesn't hurt to have a working understanding of what constitutes employment discrimination.

The Employer's Responsibilities

The Americans with Disabilities Act, the Rehabilitation Act of 1973, and state antidiscrimination laws form the basis of your legal rights as they relate to employment and diabetes. The laws state that employers cannot discriminate against a person because of disability, if that person can perform the essential functions of the job with or without reasonable accommodations made by the employer. Diabetes fits within the definition of disability covered by these laws. When you are applying for or holding a job and have diabetes, it is not legal for an employer to use your diabetes against you unfairly. It cannot be a factor in your advancement or your continued employment, unless it keeps you from doing your job. There may be more subtle, but also damaging and illegal, limits put on you. For example, restrictions on your areas of work must be based on a realistic assessment of your capabilities and any potential dangers. In one case, a worker was not fired but his activities were so restricted that there was no chance of advancement. The employer must be able to justify such restrictions.

You are also legally entitled to changes or modifications to your workplace, known as "reasonable accommodations," because of your diabetes. Just what is "reasonable," of course, can be a matter of serious contention. You may feel that you need regular work breaks, regular hours, no night work, and the right to have food with you at all times. That would be nice, but the employer may be unable to make these accommodations for all jobs. Some jobs require certain work hours (a teacher or receptionist, for example), and for some jobs it is trickier to find a way to keep food nearby at all times and to take unscheduled breaks (although there is almost always a way to work this out). An employer does not need to provide accommodations that pose an "undue hardship," which typically means great difficulty or expense. And if your diabetes interferes with your job performance and there are no reasonable accommodations that can help you perform the job, or if the accommodations you need cannot reasonably be made, then all bets are off. Such disputes sometimes end up being settled in court. So think carefully about your responsibilities as a good employee.

Finally, one reason that employers worry about hiring people with disabilities is their concern that the company's health insurance premiums will climb if an employee becomes sick and makes more health care claims, or even if the health plan just finds out that an employee has diabetes. The employer may not be happy about keeping a person who has diabetes for this reason, but it is illegal to let an employee go just because his or her health may affect insurance premiums. It is also illegal to deny health insurance coverage to family members (dependents) because they have diabetes. Once the Affordable Care Act is fully implemented in 2014, it will be unlawful for any insurance plan to deny coverage or charge higher premiums because of diabetes.

Looking for a Job

In our transient society, where people frequently change jobs and even locations, at any given moment many people will be in the process of seeking employment. The issue of employment discrimination often comes up at the time of a job interview. A potential employer is permitted to ask you whether you have any health problem that would interfere with your ability to do the work. But he or she *cannot* ask you specifically whether you have diabetes or otherwise seek to obtain information on your health status. Under no circumstances is the potential employer permitted to list a series of diseases and ask if you have any of them—even if, as noted above, the reason is a wish to avoid increases in health insurance premiums.

What do you say, then, when the interviewer begins questioning you about your health status? This is a tough one. We don't recommend lying, but we do suggest that you try to answer only what the potential employer has a right to ask. Consider the following exchange:

Employer. "Well, Ms. Perkins, I like you very much, and I think you'll be a valued employee with Acme, Inc. But I just want to be sure you'll always come to work and won't get sick on us—you know, raise our insurance rates or anything like that. You don't have any health problems I should know about, do you?"

Job Applicant. "Why, no, Mr. Dunning, I am sure I could do the job just fine. I've always been a very reliable worker with a good attendance record, as my recommendations attest." [*True.* And Mr. Dunning does not, in fact, have a right at this point to know that Ms. Perkins has diabetes.]

Employer. "Well, Ms. Perkins, I'm sure that's right. But I mean, you don't have any horrible *disease* or addiction or anything like that, do you?"

Applicant. "Why, no, Mr. Dunning. I take care of myself very well. I'm sure there's nothing horrible about me, Mr. Dunning." [*True.* And this is not the moment to educate Mr. Dunning about diabetes.]

We know it's hard to sit in the hot seat and come up with the right answers, without antagonizing your interviewer or backing yourself into lies. There's no perfect solution. You don't want to be in a position of losing the job or filing suit. So we suggest that if you are interviewing for a job, you do not volunteer information about your diabetes.

There may be a point in the pre-employment process where the diabetes becomes known. Although you cannot be asked about your diabetes before you are offered the job, for some jobs, an offer is contingent upon every potential employee passing a medical exam. Other jobs do not require this, and in that case you have no legal obligation to reveal your diabetes. If you are required to complete a pre-employment medical exam, your having diabetes will inevitably come out, so it is important to understand your rights. *Diabetes is not a disqualifier. The issue is, Can you do the job?*

Where Diabetes May Be a Problem

There used to be many jobs considered off-limits to people who have diabetes, but today many fewer jobs have a blanket ban excluding people who have diabetes. In recent years both the Federal Bureau of Investigation and the State Department were sued to challenge rules that prohibited hiring people with insulin-treated diabetes for jobs as Special Agents and Foreign Service Officers. Today, people with diabetes can hold either of these jobs. People who treat diabetes with insulin must first obtain a waiver from the government to work as interstate commercial truck drivers, and sometimes bus drivers are singled out for restrictions based on diabetes. Hiring rules for police and fire departments vary greatly, but medical standards now exist to allow qualified people with diabetes to work as firefighters and police officers.

But there are still a couple of jobs closed to people who have diabetes. You cannot become a commercial airline pilot if you use insulin. And people with diabetes are not allowed to enlist in active duty military service. People who develop diabetes while in the service, depending on which branch of the military they are in and the job they are doing, may have difficulty staying in the service whether or not the diabetes interferes with their work.

What does this mean? Are these major employers breaking the law? Is it hopeless for a person with diabetes to try for employment in the face of rules that say no one who has diabetes need apply? It's true that changing the rules at the FBI, the State Department, and the Department of Transportation took decades. And it took a lot of advocacy, led by the American Diabetes Association, to break these bans and to develop a framework that police and fire departments could use to make sure they were hiring people who could safely do the job, but today you will find many highly qualified people with diabetes working in these public safety jobs. Yet there are still employers, large and small, who are uninformed about diabetes and believe it's okay not to hire you because of your diabetes. But it is precisely because the management of diabetes has come such a long way since the days when the rules banning people with diabetes from certain jobs were written that, today, many cases of discrimination can be fought—and won—because the law is on your side.

It is important to understand why, in the law, diabetes is defined as a disability. Diabetes is defined this way because it provides a legal tool to protect people against discrimination. As we have pointed out, in recent years the law has changed to make sure people who have diabetes are covered and protected. This means that in more and more situations, the law is on your side.

The Realities of Working with Diabetes

Having discussed some of the legalities, we should consider the question of whether there are, in fact, certain kinds of work that are particularly hard to do if you have diabetes. The answer depends on your own personality and your own condition. Examples abound of people with diabetes succeeding in virtually every kind of work, from the National Football League and National Hockey League to politics, television, jazz, and scuba diving. But your situation is unique. If you can't control your diabetes during vigorous exercise (or if you don't have much athletic ability), you should forgo professional athletics. If you have long-term complications due to diabetes, these have to be put into the equation. If you don't have complications, we suggest that, when considering what job to choose, you don't worry about whether you might develop them at some future date.

We are often asked whether stress on the job makes diabetes worse, and our answer is that there's no set answer. Any adrenaline rush does tend to raise blood glucose, but you can take extra insulin, tighten your diet, or fit in some regular exercise. On the other hand, if your response to high-stress situations is to forget about your diabetes self-care, you'd better find employment with a low level of stress.

The issues become more subtle when you consider job demands that go beyond concerns of physical condition or stress. People worry about whether their diabetes is compatible with long hours, shift work, irregular hours, and unpredictable exercise. They worry especially about jobs that require a high level of intellectual function on which much depends. Can you climb to the top of your organization, with all that this entails, even though you have diabetes? Absolutely! But again, you have to consider your own personality. If you love the challenge and can work variety into your self-care, go for it. There is certainly no ceiling on the amount of personal responsibility or intellectual demand a person who has diabetes can manage.

Real-Life Scenarios

Kurt has Type 1 diabetes that is quite unstable, with glucose levels that fluctuate widely if he is not very careful, and sometimes even when he is. He is assigned to the graveyard shift at an automobile plant, working nights five days a week, sleeping from 9 a.m. to 4 p.m. On Saturdays and Sundays he lives "normal" hours so he can see his family. Kurt's blood glucose goes haywire because he can't get his insulin doses timed properly with these shifting hours.

Shift work, with changing hours of sleep, often causes a problem for people who have diabetes. One solution, the most intensive, is either to be on an external insulin pump or to follow a regimen consisting of long-acting insulin and a dose of rapid-acting insulin before each meal. This way, you can maintain a day-and-night low level of insulin (with a basal rate on the pump or with long-acting insulin) while covering each meal, whenever it is eaten, with rapid-acting insulin. You can also request a reasonable accommodation to be moved to a different shift, but keep in mind that the courts don't always agree that this is a reasonable accommodation and you may need to negotiate with your employer to make this change.

Marcia is a law enforcement officer who carries a gun in her daily work. Admittedly, she has never used it in action over a long career in police work. But she is concerned that if an insulin reaction were to occur at the wrong time, someone could get hurt.

It is a realistic worry that almost everyone taking insulin has at one time or another: that they will have an insulin reaction when they are driving a bus, arguing a case in court, doing brain surgery, or driving their kids to school. An easy answer is to say that no one's risk is ever zero and that no one ever knows when any type of health emergency might occur—a heart attack, epileptic seizure, or whatever. But that's not a good answer, because taking insulin *does* increase the risk of hypoglycemia. There are many practical steps you can take to avoid catastrophic insulin reactions. We went into this in much more detail in Chapter 5, but here are a few reminders to carry with you into the workplace:

—*Know if you are at risk.* What treatment are you on? (Insulin is always more likely to cause hypoglycemia than pills, for instance.) Are you always aware when your blood glucose goes low, or does it sometimes sneak up on you without warning? Have you ever become confused and required the help of another person to treat your hypoglycemia? If you answer yes to either of these questions, you are at special risk; if your answer to both is no, the risk is much less.

—*Know when your most vulnerable times are.* Does your blood glucose tend to be on the low side before lunch or late in the afternoon? Even if it is not frankly low at these times (for example, not in the 50s but in the 70s), recognize that you are cutting it close and that one day you may run very low at that same time.

—*Keep a source of concentrated sugar with you at all times.* This is just common sense, but it is absolutely essential if you take insulin.

—*Consider telling some of your coworkers what an insulin reaction is and how to treat it.* By talking it over with them, you make it possible for them to offer help (by giving you some sugar) if you have a hypoglycemic reaction. If they have no idea what is going on, your reaction could be more traumatic for them than it is for you! Of course this can be tricky, because your coworkers could tell your boss and you might not want your boss to know. Letting others know you have diabetes and take insulin is not required legally, but it is a safer personal option.

—*Anticipate the times when you'll want to be sure your blood glucose is okay.* Check it just before you drive the kids to school, kick off a key sales meeting, or prepare to do brain surgery.

Theresa is skating on thin ice at her job. She developed Type 2 diabetes a few years ago, just a year after starting this job. Her attendance record, never that good, got worse. Between visits to doctors and a liberal assortment of days off for colds, allergies, and cramps, Theresa is nervous that her supervisor is just about fed up with her frequent absences.

In Theresa's case, we see the supervisor's point. You may need to do some schedule juggling, stacking up several doctors' appointments into one morning, or taking just an hour off at the end of the day. Having diabetes may mean coming to work when you are not feeling 100% perfect. In the worst case, if complications really preclude full-time work, you'll need to consider working part time or requesting an alternative work arrangement, such as telework. If you need extra time to attend doctors' appointments or to deal with hypoglycemia in the morning, you may be entitled to medical leave (which does not have to be paid) under the Family Medical Leave Act or even as a reasonable accommodation under the Americans with Disabilities Act or state antidiscrimination law. A person who has diabetes hopes for understanding, but employers are not required to keep a worker who can't get the job done.

Tom sees that his coworkers are sloppier than he is, that they don't do their work as neatly or completely, show up and leave work at will, and are generally undisciplined. But he is the one with diabetes, and his supervisor is always bugging him about whether he is able to do his work.

Chances are that Tom's supervisor is almost completely ignorant about diabetes and may well be prejudiced against it. Tom's challenge is to convince his employer that he is doing the job well—better than average, in fact. There may be a point at which the supervisor can actually learn something about diabetes. But if the supervisor isn't interested, Tom should just concentrate on showing her that diabetes is not a factor in his job performance.

. . .

Having diabetes is readily compatible with the vast majority of work settings and potentially compatible with anything. But we know this is the rosy view. We know that you have to think about many things that your colleagues at work can ignore: timing of your meals, work schedules, extra doctors' appointments, unexpected out-of-range blood glucose numbers, and so on. You can do it, but you will have to work that much harder to succeed.

If you are looking for a job or considering a change, be aware of which areas of employment are most compatible with you and with your diabetes. You can anticipate special problems in the military and commercial piloting, for example. While diabetes will inevitably play a role in your employment decisions, we hope it will not dominate them.

There are many things you can do to ensure that you do your work safely and competently. If, despite your best efforts, you encounter illegal job discrimination, you'll be faced with a personal choice between confronting it and sidestepping it. Either course of action is honorable. If you decide to fight it—or just want to learn more about your rights or how to negotiate a resolution—you'll find expert legal advocates at the American Diabetes Association who can help you. Call them at 1-800-DIABETES.

Whatever your employer or your coworkers think, you should know in your heart that diabetes is just one of your personal characteristics. It shouldn't define you in the workplace anymore than it should define you throughout life.

There is even a positive side to diabetes in the workplace, especially from the employer's point of view. The traits required to effectively manage diabetes are enormous strengths in the work environment. They are exactly what employment offices yearn for. And, in fact, they are very common traits among people who have diabetes. So it is really no surprise that people with diabetes are usually excellent employees. As you know, the world is studded with outstanding, successful people who have diabetes, including actress Mary Tyler Moore, baseball player Catfish Hunter, singer Nick Jonas, Supreme Court Justice Sonia Sotomayor, and thousands more. Self-discipline is a key to success, and people with diabetes usually have it. On the whole, they make excellent employees. The world should know that.

Take Home Messages

- At work, the goal is to be able to do your job while managing your diabetes for both long-term health and short-term safety.
- The Americans with Disabilities Act, the Rehabilitation Act of 1973, and state antidiscrimination laws form the basis of your legal rights as they relate to employment and diabetes.
- A potential employer *cannot* ask you specifically whether you have diabetes or otherwise seek to obtain information on your health status.
- Today, there are many fewer jobs that have a blanket ban excluding people who have diabetes.
- While you're on the job, you have to think about many things that your colleagues at work can ignore: the timing of your meals, work schedules, extra doctors' appointments, unexpected out-of-range blood glucose numbers, and so on.

Complications

The complications of diabetes, in both the short run and the long run, are what make it such a frightening disease. If there were no complications, the high blood glucose would just be an abnormal result on a lab test. But of course we all know that diabetes can cause serious complications. What many people with diabetes *don't* understand is that the complications are far from inevitable and can be very successfully managed. The horror stories you may have heard probably happened before the modern era of diabetes care, or they happened to people who did not take advantage of what is now available.

Part IV describes the various complications of diabetes. There are two broad categories: immediate (or acute) and long-term. Acute complications are directly and immediately due to high blood glucose. They come on in a matter of minutes or hours when the glucose goes up and disappear as the glucose comes back down. Most commonly they include thirst, frequent urination, blurred vision, fatigue, weight loss, and, in women, vaginal yeast infections. In the extreme they lead to ketoacidosis or hyperosmolar coma.

The long-term complications occur only over many years or decades of diabetes and are not so easily cured. They can affect the blood vessels, eyes, kidneys, nerves, legs, and feet. For good reason, the long-term complications of diabetes are feared. But a great deal of misinformation is spread about them. We want to clear this up and tell the facts as they are.

Throughout most of the twentieth century, the long-term complications were so common that doctors and patients alike began to consider them almost inevitable. Looking back, though, we can see that people who took extremely good care of themselves, even with the primitive tools then available, did best in avoiding the complications.

Today, we know for sure that you can stack the deck in your favor. Good control of blood glucose over the years matters. You *don't* have to share the grim prognosis of previous generations with diabetes.

Even when a particular complication (such as nerve damage or eye disease) is detected, good management can keep it from becoming a serious problem. If you do develop complications, there is much that can be done to limit the damage, reducing the chance that the complications will become disabling. Together with you, we are in the business of eliminating the complications of diabetes.

20

Systemic Symptoms

- "I'm tired all day, and then at night I don't get any rest because I'm up to go to the bathroom every three hours."
- "Blurry vision, feet tingling—I'm a wreck just worrying about what it all means."
- "I'm motivated to keep my sugars in control now, because I just don't like the way I feel when they're high."

Too high a blood glucose makes you feel bad. Some of the feelings, such as fatigue, may be so subtle you don't notice them. Others, such as a cottony dry mouth and painful feet, are unpleasant, making it difficult for you to go about your daily activities. In this chapter we discuss the *systemic symptoms* of uncontrolled diabetes (summarized in Figure 25), meaning those symptoms due to high blood glucose that affect the body as a whole and go away as soon as the glucose levels are improved. After reading this chapter you may realize that you're bothered by these symptoms more often than you thought. That's actually good news because, by learning how you feel when your glucose is high, you can set yourself on a course to feeling better fast.

We also discuss the dangers of becoming overly focused on high blood glucose as the cause of all your symptoms. You may forget that there are plenty of other reasons why you, or anyone else, might feel sick. Finally, we describe instances where you need to ramp down self-imposed stress and realize that the episode is transient and you're doing what you should to keep your numbers under control.

First, a definition: *symptoms* are what a person feels. It's always helpful to think clearly and specifically about your symptoms. Saying "I just feel terrible" isn't nearly as helpful as pinpointing *in what way* you feel terrible: "I feel terrible because I'm so thirsty" (or so feverish, or have such a headache,

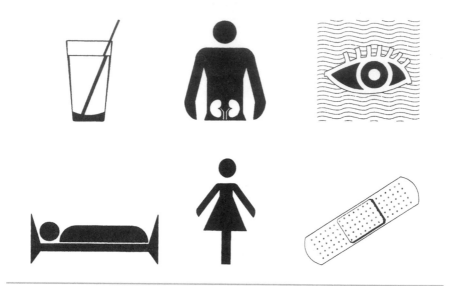

Figure 25. High blood glucose can make you feel miserable. The symptoms are thirst, frequent urination, blurry vision, fatigue, vaginal infections, and sores that don't heal.

or whatever). Thinking clearly about your symptoms will help you and your health care professional identify what's causing them.

Thirst and Frequent Urination

The blood thickens when the glucose is high. Think of a high concentration of glucose as making the blood more like syrup. The brain registers this thick blood as a sign of dehydration and sends you the message to drink fluids in order to dilute (thin) your blood back to normal. When you drink gallons of water, your kidneys get rid of the water by making large quantities of urine. After the blood glucose rises above 180 mg/dl, the kidneys can no longer prevent glucose from spilling into the urine. This draws even more water into the urine, leading to more dehydration.

Thirst and frequent urination—*polydipsia* and *polyuria*—can be severe. We have known people to urinate as often as every half-hour and drink one glass of water after another. (This situation is made much worse, of course, if the person is drinking a liquid that contains sugar, such as soda or orange juice.) Being thirsty can make you very uncomfortable. One woman was so thirsty she cupped water in her hand from the faucet and continuously brought it to her mouth. By the time she came to our clinic, her lips were chapped and raw.

Symptoms of thirst and frequent urination aren't always that obvious. Your diabetes may be well controlled much of the time. But even with well-controlled diabetes, mild symptoms can arise with a temporary increase in blood glucose after a particularly large meal or too little insulin. A slightly dry mouth or greater than normal thirst may be your only clue that your glucose is creeping up. Check and see. The glucose level usually has to be well over 200 mg/dl (and more often over 250 mg/dl) to cause thirst.

We should note here that not all frequent urination is due to high blood glucose. Try to determine whether you are actually urinating large volumes or just urinating frequently. Frequent trips to the bathroom to void small amounts of urine, especially if there is pain, blood in the urine, or (in men) difficulty starting the stream, are more likely due to a urinary tract infection or prostate problem than to diabetes.

Blurred Vision

Blurred vision can be scary. You know that diabetes can cause visual loss, and you may begin worrying that your time has come (even if you've had diabetes for only a few years, when serious diabetic eye disease rarely occurs). Actually, damage to the retina caused by diabetes (called diabetic retinopathy; see Chapter 23) results from *longstanding* high blood glucose; it is a long-term complication, not an acute complication. By contrast, blurred vision regularly occurs as a rapid—and quickly reversible—effect of high blood glucose.

Here's how it happens. The lens is a clear focusing device (like the lens of a camera) located toward the front part of your eye. It focuses your vision, automatically changing shape when you move your gaze from near to far. When you look out at a distance, the lens flattens out. When you look at something close up, it becomes rounder. If your blood glucose is high for several days or more, the lens swells up and can't change shape as easily. Then, whether you're looking near or far, it's as if you're wearing the wrong pair of glasses. Things are out of focus, blurred. Some people who wear glasses and have high glucose levels start seeing better without their glasses. In the extreme, vision can be severely limited when glucose levels stay quite high. Fortunately, the lens regains its elasticity fairly quickly with stabilized blood glucose control. Most people will see an improvement in vision within a few days, although it can take up to six weeks for the lens to return completely to normal. It's important to realize that if your vision is blurry because of uncontrolled diabetes, this is not the time to get your glasses changed. If you do, chances are you'll just have to have them changed again in a week or so. It's best to wait until your blood glucose levels have been in a good range for several weeks before having your prescription checked.

Blurred vision is often the symptom that leads a person with diabetes to seek medical care in the first place. It may also get your attention following a few days of high blood glucose as the result of an illness. But almost always, blurred vision in someone without definite, established retinopathy is a temporary problem that will respond to better blood glucose control.

Fatigue

One of the most bothersome symptoms of high blood glucose is fatigue. It is generally caused by a lack of insulin or insulin function. Remember that without insulin, glucose is not taken up normally by your cells to be converted to energy; this causes the glucose to stay in your bloodstream and build up to a high level—resulting in the sensation of your body running out of gas. You may be eating, but if glucose is not getting into your cells, eating isn't doing you any good.

Fatigue from high blood glucose can be mild or severe. When it is mild, it is often ignored or attributed to age, overwork, or stress. In the extreme, some people become so fatigued that they fall asleep during a conversation. Insulin users often notice some transient fatigue after a meal, particularly if it is large and not enough insulin is taken, until the insulin "catches up" with the food and moves the glucose into the cells.

It shouldn't be hard to tell the difference between the fatigue of high blood glucose (hyperglycemia) and the fatigue that results from low blood glucose (hypoglycemia). Low blood glucose occurs when you're taking pills that stimulate your body to make insulin and you haven't eaten in a while or when you haven't eaten enough food for the amount of insulin you've taken to cover the meal. In addition to fatigue, hypoglycemia usually causes other symptoms, like sweatiness, shakiness, palpitations, or trouble thinking clearly. High blood glucose, on the other hand, is more likely to worsen in the few hours *after* a meal or when you are sick. The fatigue due to high blood glucose creeps up on you; it doesn't come on in a matter of a few minutes.

The best way to determine whether your blood glucose is running high or low is to test it. But if you don't have a meter close by, you should eat or drink something sweet and see if the symptoms go away (in which case, they were due to hypoglycemia). As a person who is knowledgeable about his or her diabetes, you will learn to tell your highs from your lows.

Weight Loss and Hunger

Weight loss and hunger occur for the same reason as fatigue—a lack of insulin or insulin function. As the glucose level rises in the blood, it spills into the urine. It may come as a surprise to you, but glucose in the urine actually amounts to a significant drain of calories. If you need, say, 1,800 calories a day to maintain your body weight, and you eat 1,800 calories but lose 300 of them in your urine, that's like eating only 1,500 calories. You will lose weight. Eating doesn't do any good if the calories you take in just pass out of your body through the urine.

Weight loss out of proportion to dieting, then, is not a good sign. This may be a tricky point to recognize. Does the weight just seem to melt away now, even though in previous years you had difficulty losing weight? Are you not really following a calorie-restricted diet but getting terrific weight loss results? If so, check your glucose. It may be high (200s, 300s, 400s). If it is allowed to continue, this situation will surely get worse, not better. High blood glucose levels are definitely not the recommended way to lose weight.

Excessive hunger, called *polyphagia*, is the third symptom of the triad that also includes polydipsia (thirst) and polyuria (excess urination). Since glucose can't get into cells to be burned for energy, your body can feel starved. Hunger may be the hardest symptom to pin on high blood glucose. First of all, it is much less common than thirst and excess urination. Second, hunger is more psychological than physical: most people feel hungry if they see some food that looks or smells appetizing, no matter what their blood glucose is. Third, like fatigue, hunger is a common feeling when your blood glucose is low, not high. So, again, test your glucose when in doubt or until you have learned to recognize your symptoms accurately. Reacting to every "pang of hunger" may be exactly the *wrong* response.

Infections

High blood glucose increases the risk of infections, for two reasons. First, the fungi and bacteria that cause infections thrive in a high-glucose environment. Second, the immune system, which fights off infections, doesn't work as well in the presence of high blood glucose.

The most common infection seen in out-of-control diabetes is a fungus (yeast) called candida or monilia. It is the organism that causes an infection all too familiar to many women—a vaginal yeast infection. Many women are diagnosed with diabetes by their gynecologist when they keep coming back with yeast infections. Men can also get yeast infections in the groin or on other areas of skin. Yeast infections are effectively treated with creams, ointments, and suppositories, but they will keep coming back unless there is an improvement in blood glucose control.

Other common infections associated with high blood glucose include urinary tract infections (especially in women), gum infections, infections of wounds, and infections of the extremities, especially the feet. Foot infections have the potential to become serious. People with diabetes are also more likely to get a secondary bacterial infection complicating a viral respiratory infection, such as bronchitis following the flu. That's why we recommend flu shots for all our patients with diabetes.

We are often asked whether having high blood glucoses in the hospital after a surgical operation will keep a person from healing or even cause an infection. It is true that having very high glucoses (for instance, over 300 mg/dl) continuously for days at a time can slow down healing. But this has to be balanced with the more immediate danger of severe hypoglycemia during the hospitalization, when you may not be eating well. We don't expect perfect blood glucose control from people who are recovering from surgery; in fact, we tend to relax control a bit in the postoperative period and aim for glucose levels of 100–180 mg/dl.

Cloudy Thinking

Many people notice a change in their thinking with high blood glucose. Some people describe it as "being full of cobwebs" or "not being able to track a conversation as well." Others describe moodiness, especially lacking interest or feeling depressed. High blood glucose makes work and study difficult. One woman said she became aware of how much high blood glucose was affecting her thinking only after her control improved with an insulin pump. Her grades at college jumped from a low B average to mostly A's. Moodiness and irritability are definitely associated with high blood glucose. When control is improved, family members often notice the difference: "Sam's back to his old self again. He's happier and interested in doing things!"

Increase in Nerve Pain

Many people with diabetes feel the effect of high blood glucose on their nerve fibers. They may have had a tingling or burning sensation in their feet even before the diagnosis of diabetes was made. Pain from their established neuropathy (nerve damage) may worsen when the blood glucose is high. While the sensations are more common in the lower extremities, some people experience pain in their hands as well.

Neuropathic pain (nerve pain) usually improves with improvement in blood glucose control, but if neuropathy is established, it won't resolve completely. Think of painful nerves as being like static on a radio: you can improve the sound quite a bit just by tuning into the station properly (like tuning up your blood glucoses), but if the radio is old and dusty (like your nerves when years of damage have caused neuropathy), reception won't completely return to normal even with fine-tuning. Chapter 25 describes the medications used to relieve nerve pain if it is interfering with daily functioning.

The Differential Diagnosis

For people who have diabetes, one mistake that's sometimes made is seeing everything as related to blood glucose control. Although it's a good idea to pay attention to your glucose levels and to explore options for control, it's not so good if you ignore other illnesses, always assuming that "it's just my diabetes." Professionals may fall into this trap, too. Our treatment of Stanley is a case in point.

We were sure that Stanley, a retiree, had high blood glucose when he described his frequent urination, which interrupted his woodworking activities and awakened him four times at night. He said he was tired all the time (who wouldn't be, waking up every other hour all night?), and we focused entirely

*on his blood glucose control. Imagine our surprise when his hemoglobin A1c
test result was excellent and his blood glucose monitoring confirmed that his
glucose levels were mostly just fine.*

It turned out that Stanley's symptoms were caused by an enlarged prostate and some nerve damage to his bladder. He was urinating frequently because he couldn't empty his bladder completely. Only when he was treated
for the prostate problem were the symptoms relieved.

How can you tell whether it's your diabetes or something else that's causing a particular symptom? Think about the *differential diagnosis*: what are
the different possibilities? Just about every symptom can have more than
one cause, and the list of possible causes is called the differential diagnosis. You may not know all the possible causes of a particular symptom, but
there's one easy way to tell if a current symptom is due to high blood glucoses: check your glucose. And confirm your impressions with your health
care provider. Don't postpone testing when there's an easy way to confirm
(or not) your suspicions. Too many people put themselves through needless worry over something like blurred vision, which turns out to be easily
reversed and managed.

How Serious Is It?

If you have diabetes, you will have high blood glucoses at least once in a
while. Diabetes cannot be controlled perfectly. But how serious is a particular episode of high blood glucose? Generally, it is serious if it is longstanding or if it produces severe symptoms. Checking the hemoglobin A1c is an
easy way to determine whether the high blood glucose has been persistent.
The A1c is a measure of average blood glucose over the past two to three
months. If the A1c is above your target, usually over 7%, investigate further by doing more intense self-monitoring of blood glucose and by keeping
careful records. You may find a pattern for your high blood glucose levels.
Maybe you've gone overboard with afternoon snacking, or maybe your glucose goes high regularly after supper. But if there is no obvious pattern, or
if you are having trouble getting your blood glucose levels back on track,
get in touch with your health care professional to collaborate on some new
self-care strategies.

Even if your A1c is within your target range, an acute episode of high
blood glucose with severe symptoms should not be ignored. Infection, se-

vere stress, or a bottle of insulin that's gone bad all can cause a rapid deterioration in blood glucose control. Get the blood glucose down! If you are unable to get it down quickly, if you have ketones, or if symptoms progress, get in touch with your health care professional or go to the emergency room immediately.

In the end, there will be some glucose levels that you can't explain. Focusing excessively on the odd bounces will only lead to frustration. We always ask our patients to look for *patterns* and not to fret about every single value.

Listen to what your body tells you about your glucose. In the process you may discover why you have that thirst in the evening that leads you to drink several diet sodas when no one else seems thirsty. You may find out why on some days you just don't have any energy or any patience. You may learn why you are losing weight so easily. Listening to your body will let you hear an early alarm that something is wrong and needs your immediate attention.

Take Home Messages

- Too high a blood glucose makes you feel bad. Some feelings, such as fatigue, may be subtle; others, such as painful feet, can make it difficult to go about your daily activities.

- Other symptoms of high blood glucose include dry mouth and thirst, blurred vision, hunger and weight loss, an increased risk of infections, and cloudy thinking.

- Not all symptoms that are commonly related to high blood glucose are necessarily caused by high blood glucose. If you have these symptoms and your blood glucose levels are not high, be sure to talk to your health care provider about other possible causes.

- Everyone with diabetes has high blood glucose levels from time to time. High blood glucose is most serious when it lasts for weeks and months. Your hemoglobin A1c test results are a good way to tell what your average blood glucose control has been over the past two or three months.

21

Diabetic Ketoacidosis and Hyperosmolar Coma

- "I was in the hospital once for diabetes, but I don't have a clue whether it was diabetic ketoacidosis."
- "I used to check my ketones all the time, and sometimes they were a little bit positive. I really don't understand what that all means. What's more, I don't know if it matters."
- "How high can the blood glucose go, and what happens when it gets there?"

Diabetic ketoacidosis and hyperosmolar coma may seem like the sort of long scientific terms that you never really wanted to understand. But these conditions can definitely be dangerous and are completely preventable. So let's try to make sense of them.

Diabetic Ketoacidosis

Doctors generally refer to *diabetic ketoacidosis* as DKA. We think it is important for you to understand what DKA means, why it happens, what to do about it, and how to prevent it.

What Is DKA?

As the name implies, diabetic ketoacidosis involves high levels of *ketones* (also called *ketoacids*) building up in the bloodstream. Ketones are the chemical by-products of fat breakdown, just as ashes are the by-product of burned wood. Some amount of fat breakdown is always taking place in the human body, and there's always some normal amount of ketones in the blood. Ketones build up in the blood only when fat breakdown is increased—for example, when you don't eat for 12–18 hours. When blood ketone levels are high, ketones spill into the urine, just as glucose does when blood glucose levels are high. A small amount of ketones in the urine (called *ketonuria*) is not unusual. But it is important to understand the central role that insulin plays in the control of ketone production and disposal because too high a level of ketones in the blood will cause ketoacidosis.

As we've said in earlier chapters, insulin is needed to allow the body's cells to take up and burn glucose. With the right amount of insulin (in a person without diabetes), as soon as the blood glucose rises, as it does after a carbohydrate-containing meal, the body uses that glucose as fuel and keeps its fat stores for later use, when no carbohydrate fuel is available from the diet. So, glucose (carbohydrate) is the preferred fuel, and when it is available it is used; fat is the main backup, storage form of energy. In this normal situation, if no carbohydrate has recently been eaten, there's relatively little glucose in the blood, the insulin level goes down, and the body turns to fat for energy. Blood ketones increase a bit from the fat breakdown and may spill over into the urine.

The problem develops if your pancreas isn't making nearly enough insulin (as in untreated Type 1 diabetes) and you don't get enough insulin by injection. The glucose builds up in the bloodstream but is not used for fuel (since there's no insulin to help it enter the cells). The body must turn to its fat stores for energy, increasing ketones in the blood.

When ketones rise to a high level, not only do they spill into the urine but they also can cause your whole body to become too acidic: in other words, you have *acidosis*. That's because the ketones are actually acids (hence the term *ketoacids*). If your health care professional thinks you may have DKA, he or she will look for the presence of too high a level of ketones in your blood and urine and the presence of acidosis.

What Are the Common Causes of DKA?

For a person with Type 1 diabetes, DKA is caused by having far too little insulin in the blood. People newly diagnosed with Type 1 diabetes may experience DKA because the diagnosis wasn't recognized until insulin levels had already become severely low and glucose levels markedly high. Too little insulin can also result from missed insulin injections due to neglect or a particularly extreme case of denial or anger. If improperly stored or outdated, insulin can go bad. Rarely, people run out of insulin in places so remote that they cannot get a new supply. Whatever the cause of not getting nearly enough insulin when it's needed, anywhere from a day to a few days later, the person with Type 1 diabetes will develop DKA.

If you have not stopped taking your insulin, the other major cause of DKA is a need for insulin that's much greater than the amount being taken. There are many temporary stressful situations that increase your need for insulin. Stress hormones released during an illness will counteract the actions of insulin, increasing your insulin requirements. The most common illnesses are infections, such as stomach viruses that cause nausea or diarrhea, urinary tract infections, or the flu. Usually, if you are taking your normal doses of insulin while ill, your glucose levels will run high, but DKA doesn't develop. DKA is more likely to develop if you skip your insulin because you are too ill to eat. More stressful illnesses, such as pneumonia or a heart attack, can certainly push a person with diabetes into DKA because of overwhelming levels of stress hormones.

A common cause of DKA is the mistaken impression that when you are sick and not eating well, you should not take insulin. The opposite is often closer to the truth: illness *increases* your need for insulin, and omitting your insulin during the stress of an illness can very easily lead to DKA.

What Are the Symptoms of DKA?

Diabetic ketoacidosis can make you very sick and can even be fatal. What clues should you look for that suggest you may have DKA? First, your blood glucose will be high. In all likelihood you'll be feeling the symptoms of thirst, frequent urination, and fatigue. Second, ketones make you feel nauseous and usually cause vomiting. Finally, DKA can progress to the point that you are more or less bedridden with weakness, fatigue, dehydration, abdominal pain, and nausea.

A more specific sign of DKA is called air hunger (or Kussmaul respiration). Breathing hard (as you would after strenuous exercise) is the body's way of getting rid of excess acid by exhaling more carbon dioxide. The person with DKA, then, tends to breathe deeply and rapidly, just as if he or she has been exercising.

DKA can sneak up on you. It can be mistaken for the flu, or it can be a complication of the flu or some other illness. If you have Type 1 diabetes and you are feeling sick for whatever reason, check your blood glucose and test your urine ketones regularly—it could be DKA. If you have Type 2 diabetes, you are unlikely to get DKA unless you're under severe stress. But rather than thinking of DKA as occurring only in Type 1 diabetes, it is better to think of it as very badly undertreated diabetes of either type. If your blood glucose is up, you're not feeling well, and you're spilling ketones into your urine, be sure to take your insulin, consider adding some extra rapid-acting insulin, and contact your health care professional if things do not improve soon.

How Is DKA Treated?

The person with DKA is treated under medical supervision, usually in a hospital. The basic elements of treatment are simple enough: provide insulin, replace fluids, and check that the electrolytes (especially potassium) do not fall too low. The health care professional will probably want to start an intravenous line, to be sure fluids and insulin get into the body rapidly. For the first 24 hours, most persons with DKA are admitted to the intensive care unit because each of these treatments has to be carefully monitored.

With proper medical attention, DKA is almost always successfully treated (the death rate is well below 5%). But without treatment, or if treatment is delayed much too long, it can be fatal.

Can DKA Be Prevented?

Diabetic ketoacidosis can definitely be prevented. In fact, we consider DKA to be the result of a major breakdown in routine diabetes care. At least in theory, there is no reason for anyone to develop this condition. Consistent insulin dosing prevents DKA from developing.

Simply put, good self-care is the key to prevention. Check your blood glucose regularly, and check more often when you are sick. Take insulin regularly, even when you are sick. Have the urine test strips available to check for ketones, especially when you are sick. If there are ketones in your urine stream, the end of the strip will change color. Act on the results: when ketones are present and your glucose level is high, if you take insulin, you will need more than usual to bring the glucose down. Take extra rapid-acting insulin to treat the high glucose, and test again in one to two hours. How much insulin to take depends on your situation, but it is a reasonable estimate to take as much as 10% of your usual daily requirement every two hours when ketones are present and blood glucose levels are high, until your glucose starts to come back down.

If you do have an episode of DKA, it's worthwhile thinking about how it happened so you can avoid it the next time. Did something happen that caused you not to take your insulin for a period of time? Did you not realize until too late that you had a bad bottle of insulin? Did you not increase your insulin enough when you were experiencing some sort of stress, such as the flu? Asking yourself these questions will help you prevent DKA from happening again.

Hyperosmolar Coma

Hyperosmolar coma means "coma due to too thick blood." You can see for yourself what this means by pouring syrup into a glass of water until the water visibly thickens. This is what happens in hyperosmolar coma: the blood glucose goes up so much that the blood is actually thicker, or hyperosmolar.

How high do blood glucose levels go? In hyperosmolar coma, the glucose level almost always exceeds 1,000 mg/dl and can reach 1,500 or 2,000 mg/dl. As the blood glucose goes up, the person urinates frequently and becomes dehydrated. A vicious cycle is set up in which the blood glucose goes up, dehydration follows, and the blood glucose increases still more. Many conditions, such as fever, severe burns, or too many diuretic pills, can contribute to hyperosmolar coma.

Hyperosmolar coma most often occurs in people who have Type 2 diabetes. In Type 1 diabetes, DKA develops well before blood glucose rises to the astronomically severe level of over 1,000 mg/dl. People most likely to go into a hyperosmolar coma are those without access to water, usually older or ill persons who are physically unable to get water on their own or can't tell someone how thirsty they are.

Hyperosmolar coma is a medical emergency: it is fatal if not promptly treated in a hospital. Because dehydration is such a central part of the problem, large amounts of intravenous fluids have to be given, along with insulin.

Prevention of hyperosmolar coma depends on catching it before it becomes severe. Taking even basic measures such as increasing water intake and treating a rising blood glucose with insulin is usually enough.

Take Home Messages

- Diabetic ketoacidosis (DKA) is a serious condition, most common in people with Type 1 diabetes. It occurs when a person is taking far too little insulin.
- DKA can be caused by not taking insulin for a day or longer or not taking enough insulin when insulin needs are higher than usual, such as during periods of illness or very high stress.

- DKA can be avoided by checking ketone levels whenever blood glucose levels are high and taking extra rapid-acting insulin if ketone levels are elevated.
- Hyperosmolar coma is another serious condition, most common in people with Type 2 diabetes.
- Hyperosmolar coma can be avoided by checking blood glucose levels and taking extra rapid-acting insulin and drinking lots of water if the glucose levels are high.

Hardening of the Arteries

- "I had a heart attack at a pretty young age—I was just 55. My doctor said it was due to diabetes. But I thought that was something that happens to much older men."
- "My teenager has diabetes, and everyone keeps talking about foot care and cholesterol in the arteries. I don't understand whether this is really a problem for him or when it will happen."

Hardening of the arteries (*arteriosclerosis*, also called *atherosclerosis*) results when fat deposits, or plaques of cholesterol, develop within the walls of arteries. The best analogy for arteriosclerosis is rust building up inside a pipe. Like rust in a pipe, hardening of the arteries is commonly associated with aging and can cause a blockage, with many potential consequences. If the artery is partially blocked, the blood flow getting through may be marginal; if it is entirely blocked, no blood gets through. In this chapter we talk about what causes hardening of the arteries and how best to prevent it. We discuss which parts of the body are most often affected, the symptoms, and the effect. Finally, we describe what can be done about arteriosclerosis when it does occur.

Risk Factors for Arteriosclerosis

As is becoming increasingly clear, the causes of hardening of the arteries are more complicated than just the amount of cholesterol in the blood. Taken together, the things that increase your chance of having hardening of the arteries are called risk factors. Having a risk factor for a problem doesn't mean you'll get the problem, but it does mean that you have an increased *chance* of getting it.

There are five major risk factors for arteriosclerosis, most of which you probably know about already: high LDL cholesterol (or low HDL cholesterol) levels, untreated high blood pressure, smoking, poorly treated diabetes, and a family history of heart disease (coronary artery disease) at a young age. Aging and menopause also increase the risk. The risk factors are additive, meaning that the more of these risk factors you have, the more likely you are to develop arteriosclerosis at a young age, and the fewer you have, the less likely you are to have this problem.

High LDL Cholesterol (Hypercholesterolemia or Hyperlipidemia)

It's easy for your health care professional to check the levels of your blood cholesterol and other blood lipids (fats). Total cholesterol is the total amount of cholesterol in your blood. It can be subdivided (broken down or fractionated) in a "lipid profile" into LDL cholesterol, triglycerides, and HDL cholesterol. The LDL cholesterol is called "bad cholesterol" because it is the fraction of total cholesterol that, when elevated (for example, over 100 mg/dl), increases the risk of arteriosclerosis. HDL cholesterol, or "good cholesterol," on the other hand, protects you from hardening of the arteries. High levels of HDL cholesterol (over 60 mg/dl) decrease your chances of developing heart disease, foot problems, and stroke; low levels (under 55 mg/dl for women, under 45 mg/dl for men) increase your risk.

Finally, there's the triglyceride part of the lipid profile. There is still some debate about how important high triglyceride levels are, but most experts think that high levels do increase the risk of heart disease for people who have diabetes. Furthermore, very high levels can increase the risk of pancreatitis. People with high triglycerides also often have low HDL cholesterol.

A national panel has published recommendations for each of the blood lipid levels (see Table 15). As you can see, the recommended lipid levels and treatments depend on how many risk factors you have.

Your total cholesterol can be accurately measured whether or not you have eaten before the test, but lipid fractionation must be done after fasting for at least 12 hours. The first step in treating abnormal lipids (hypercholesterolemia or hyperlipidemia) is always a good cholesterol-lowering diet. This diet is lower in total calories for those who are overweight, low in saturated and trans fats, high in foods containing omega-3 fatty acids, high in fruits and vegetables, and rich in high-fiber carbohydrates. A dietitian can help draw up a diet plan that is best for you. If this doesn't work, effective pills are available.

Table 15   Coronary Artery Disease: Evaluating Your Risk and Choosing Your Treatment

---

Evaluating Your Risk

You are at *very high risk* if you have *already been diagnosed* with coronary artery disease (heart attack or angina), stroke, TIA (transient ischemic attack), or poor circulation to the feet (peripheral vascular disease).

You are at *high risk* if you have diabetes and *one* or more of the following risk factors:

- You are a man over 50 years old
- You are a woman over 60 years old
- You smoke cigarettes
- You have, or have been treated for, high blood pressure
- You have an LDL cholesterol over 100 mg/dl
- Your HDL cholesterol is lower than 40 mg/dl
- Your father or a brother had a heart attack before the age of 55
- Your mother or a sister had a heart attack before the age of 65

You are at *low risk* if you have *none* of the above risk factors in addition to having diabetes. If your HDL cholesterol is over 60 mg/dl, you are at *low risk* unless *two* of the above risk factors are present in addition to diabetes.

Choosing Your Treatment

Based on your LDL cholesterol values and whether you are at low, high, or very high risk, you and your doctor should consider treatment according to the following guidelines:

- Always follow a diet low in saturated fat.
- Use *pharmacological* (pill) treatment with a statin based on the following criteria for risk group and LDL cholesterol level, after dieting:

Low risk	LDL over 100
High risk	Any LDL; treatment goal is less than 100
Very high risk	Any LDL; treatment goal is less than 70

Source. Copyright 2013 American Diabetes Association. From *Diabetes Care®* 36 (2013): S11–66. Modified by permission of the American Diabetes Association.

Note. To complete this evaluation, you need to know your blood lipid levels of LDL cholesterol and HDL cholesterol.

Untreated High Blood Pressure (Hypertension)

Blood pressure, like blood glucose, is one of those measurements that change from minute to minute. Also like blood glucose, it is hard to measure blood pressure continuously. So when you go to your health care provider's office, a single high reading may be due only to your momentary stress from being in the examining room ("white coat hypertension"). But a high reading should be rechecked so that persistent high blood pressure is not missed or minimized. Hypertension is a very strong risk factor for hardening of the arteries, eye disease, and kidney damage.

As with high cholesterol, diet is the first step in treating hypertension. The mainstay of dietary treatment for high blood pressure is to cut down on salt intake. Weight control and exercise are also very effective. If these measures don't work, you may need oral medications. Several classes of pills are available. The thiazide pills (such as hydrochlorothiazide) are often used and are effective, but they can worsen your diabetes control if used in doses that are too high. Likewise, the beta-blockers may decrease your awareness of insulin reactions, though they have not been shown to increase the risk of severe low blood glucose reactions.

Numerous studies have found that the ACE (angiotensin-converting enzyme) inhibitors and ARBs (angiotensin receptor blockers) are effective not only in controlling blood pressure but also in slowing the progression of kidney disease. The ACE inhibitors are now generally recommended as the first-line drugs to control high blood pressure in diabetes, especially for people who have some evidence of kidney disease, such as protein in the urine. A persistent dry cough is the most common side effect of ACE inhibitors, but this usually goes away shortly after you stop taking the drug. The ARB class of drugs do not cause a cough and are usually the next choice of drugs to control hypertension in persons with diabetes. It is common for someone to need two or three different drugs for the blood pressure to fall below 140/80, the usual target.

Smoking

Long known to cause lung cancer, cigarette smoking is also well known to increase the risk of heart disease. Obviously, the best approach is to avoid smoking in the first place. Quitting is difficult, to say the least. Also, people have a strong tendency to gain weight when they first quit. But even for people with Type 2 diabetes, who often have a weight problem, the health benefits of stopping smoking far outweigh the effects of weight gain. The effect of smoking on risk for heart disease disappears within a few years of quitting. So put "quit smoking" high on your to do list if you have diabetes and you smoke.

Diabetes

Long-term high blood glucose levels definitely increase the risk of arteriosclerosis. Diabetes is considered a coronary heart disease "risk equivalent." This means that the risk of developing coronary heart disease (a heart attack) for persons with diabetes is the same as that for someone without diabetes who has had a prior heart attack. The risk of having a heart attack or stroke is increased twofold for men and fourfold for women who have diabetes. So the protection from heart attack or stroke afforded by being female is lost if you have diabetes. Research studies have now shown that improved diabetes control over many years reduces the risk of cardiovascular events (heart disease, strokes, and peripheral vascular disease) in both Type 1 and Type 2 diabetes. Poorly controlled diabetes also increases the chance that your lipid levels will be abnormal. If you practice diabetes self-care in the broadest sense—improving your diet, exercising regularly, and taking diabetes medications as prescribed to get your blood glucose levels into target ranges—you'll considerably reduce your risk of developing early or accelerated arteriosclerosis.

Family History

This is the one risk factor that is out of your control, since you can't pick your parents. But you should be especially mindful of the need to reduce your other risk factors if your father or a brother had significant heart disease or sudden death before the age of 55, or your mother or a sister did so before age 65.

Heart Disease, Peripheral Vascular Disease, and Cerebrovascular Disease

The three major areas most often affected by hardening of the arteries are the blood vessels supplying the heart, the legs, and the brain. Heart disease—angina pectoris and heart attacks—is the most common of these problems.

Heart Disease

To understand heart disease, you have to understand something about the heart. It is a large muscle that pumps the blood to the rest of your body. Like all muscles, it has its own arteries that provide its blood supply. These arteries, called coronary arteries, are essential to the function of the heart as an effective pump. When a coronary artery is fully blocked, unless there is an alternative supply of blood for the part of the heart normally supplied by that artery, some heart tissue dies. Coronary arteries are often partially or completely blocked by arteriosclerosis (Figure 26).

Think of a rural county where a town depends on supplies trucked in on a single road. If a storm comes along and destroys that road, unless alternative supply lincs can be opened up, the town goes without supplies. The

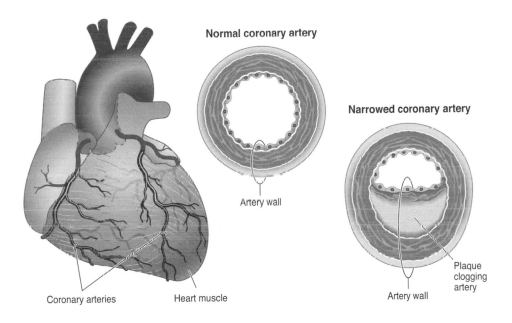

Normal coronary artery

Narrowed coronary artery

Artery wall

Plaque clogging artery

Coronary arteries   Heart muscle   Artery wall

Figure 26. The heart is a big muscular pump that needs its own supply of blood to remain healthy. The coronary arteries carry out this function. If they become clogged, they cannot perform this function as well. If an artery becomes completely occluded, the heart muscle will be injured—a heart attack.

amount of damage done to the town depends on how big the town is and how long it's left without supplies. But unless supplies are restored quickly, there will be pain and damage in the town.

When a coronary artery is partly blocked, enough blood may get through to keep the heart beating normally when the person is at rest. But when the heart has to pick up its speed—for example, during exercise—this partly blocked artery can't open up enough to let an adequate amount of blood through. The symptom produced by this marginal blood flow is chest pain with exercise, called *angina pectoris*. This pain is often quite characteristic: when you walk quickly, carry groceries, or even become very emotional, a deep, tight pain develops in your chest, jaw, or left arm. It goes away as soon as you stop the exercise and calm down—in other words, when your heart rate returns to normal. There are many less typical forms of angina, including a burning sensation, a heaviness in the chest, or even shortness of breath with only mild exercise. So, if chest pain develops when your heart rate increases or you easily become short of breath, you should definitely see a health care professional to find out whether it's due to a coronary artery blockage.

If a coronary artery, large or small, becomes completely blocked (usually by a small blood clot on top of a plaque), it will cause some of the heart tissue to die. This is called a heart attack or *myocardial infarction*. The chief symptom is usually an angina-like pain that does not go away even with rest. If the area affected is big, the heart attack is severe; if a small artery is affected, the heart attack is mild.

Whether the heart attack is mild or severe, the outcome depends mainly on how quickly it is treated. Doctors these days often give heart attack patients drugs that break up blood clots and reduce the blockage. They then monitor these patients for signs of continued inadequate blood supply to the heart, irregular heart rhythms, or signs of bleeding. These treatments are more successful if the person is seen by medical professionals within an hour of when symptoms begin. Since early treatment significantly affects outcome, if you have any persistent chest pain (pain lasting over about 15 minutes), especially if accompanied by sweating, faintness, or pain to your left arm, you should be evaluated *immediately in an emergency room setting*.

In addition to the immediate medical treatment of heart attacks, which is usually very successful, surgical procedures are often done. In one technique, called a *coronary angioplasty*, the inside of a blocked artery is opened by inflating a balloon. This is often followed by placing a stent into the narrowed artery to make sure it stays open. Some stents release medications that prevent clots from developing in the area of the stent, a so-called drug-eluting stent. More commonly, when more than one blood vessel is blocked, the blocked arteries are bypassed by putting in new vessels during *coronary bypass surgery*. Recent trials have found that bypass surgery may be more effective than angioplasty for people who have multiple blocked coronary arteries. Given modern medical care, people can live long, productive lives after suffering a heart attack.

The higher rates of heart disease among people who have diabetes could be explained in part by another factor, one we mentioned earlier in the book: the disproportionately high rate of depression among people with diabetes. We do not fully understand how diabetes, depression, and heart disease affect one another, but we do know that depression is linked to a variety of known heart disease risk factors such as high blood glucose and cholesterol levels, smoking, decreased physical activity, and unhealthy eating.

In the Look AHEAD trial, which we've discussed in earlier chapters, study participants with more depression symptoms were more likely to have elevated heart disease risk factors, including those just noted above. In another study, people with diabetes were much more likely to die after a heart attack if they were depressed than if they were not depressed.

The relationship between heart disease and depression almost certainly goes both ways. Being depressed can increase a person's risk for heart disease, and having heart disease increases the likelihood a person will be depressed.

Hardening of the Arteries in the Legs (Peripheral Vascular Disease)

Just as arteriosclerosis can affect coronary arteries, it can also affect the long arteries going to the legs and feet, a condition known as peripheral vascular disease, or PVD. The symptoms are somewhat similar. When the leg vessels are partially blocked, enough blood usually gets through except during increased exercise of the leg muscles. During such exercise as walking briskly, the muscles (usually of the calf or thigh) don't get enough blood, and they hurt. This is called *claudication*. As with angina, the pain (usually a cramping of the calf) stops soon after the person stops exercising.

Complete blockage of an artery in the leg can cause gangrene. This does not happen very often, partly because other, more open arteries in the leg can bypass the block and supply blood to the lower portion of the leg. A foot can also get into serious trouble when some degree of vessel blockage coexists with severe nerve damage and then some sort of trauma to the foot causes a break in the skin. An open area of skin that is poorly supplied by blood makes it much easier for an infection to set in (see Chapter 26).

As with the coronary arteries, there are several surgical approaches to correcting severe blockage in a leg artery. An angioplasty procedure can be done to open up the artery, or an artificial artery can be put in place to by-pass the blocked one.

Hardening of the Arteries to the Brain (Cerebrovascular Disease)

Essentially the same problem that takes place in the heart and the legs can happen to arteries supplying blood to the brain, causing cerebrovascular disease. Again, mild symptoms may appear with a partial blockage, before any complete blockage occurs. In medical terms, the symptoms of partial blockage are called *transient ischemic attacks* (TIAs).

The symptoms of partial blockage usually include temporary neurological problems, such as a numb arm or the loss of ability to speak clearly. They last only a matter of minutes, but they usually recur. Complete blockage of an artery to some part of the brain causes a stroke: a particular part of the brain is starved of blood and dies. (There are several other causes of strokes that are not specifically related to diabetes or to arteriosclerosis, such as a hemorrhage into the brain or the blocking of an artery by a blood clot that has traveled from the heart, called an *embolism*.)

A disturbing and essentially untreatable condition may develop when many arteries in the brain, large and small, are partially blocked by hardening of the arteries. This problem, called *diffuse cerebral arteriosclerosis*, can cause a gradual decline in mental function or even multiple small strokes without any one blockage being identified. It is one cause of senility or a gradual falling off in someone's ability to function.

A surgical endarterectomy (a stripping away of the clot in an artery) can clear a partially blocked artery in the neck (the carotid artery), if a block located there is causing the TIAs. It is not possible, however, to bypass arteries located in the brain.

. . .

Hardening of the arteries, or arteriosclerosis, is a common feature of aging and occurs to some extent in all of us as we grow older. Diabetes is one of the five major risk factors that increase the rate of progression of arteriosclerosis. To reduce your chances of developing accelerated or early hardening of the arteries, you not only should work to control your diabetes but should also be aware of your cholesterol level and your blood pressure. And you should definitely stop smoking.

If blockage of an artery becomes severe, it can cause angina or a heart attack, claudication or gangrene in the feet, and TIAs or a stroke. But there are preventive approaches that will significantly reduce the likelihood of developing any of these problems. If the problem already exists, there are medical and surgical approaches that can help correct it.

Take Home Messages

- Hardening of the arteries (arteriosclerosis) results when fat deposits develop within the walls of arteries.
- There are five major risk factors for arteriosclerosis: high LDL or low HDL cholesterol levels, high blood pressure, smoking, high blood glucose levels, and a family history of heart disease.
- Heart disease is the most common form of arteriosclerosis; it is more common among people who have diabetes than in the general population.
- Hardening of the arteries in the legs (peripheral vascular disease, or PVD) is another common problem. A sign of PVD is cramping in the calf or thigh muscles during exercise such as brisk walking.
- Hardening of the arteries in the brain (cerebral vascular disease), like hardening of the arteries in the heart or legs, can be partial or complete.
- The best approach is always to try to prevent the development of arteriosclerosis, but if it does develop, there are effective treatments for treating hardening of the arteries in the heart, legs, and brain.

Diabetic Eye Disease

with Sharon Solomon, M.D.

- " I didn't realize the damage I was causing to my eyes when I let my blood sugars run high all those years. Will I go blind?"
- "Ophthalmologists, lasers, yellow dyes. I don't get it. I don't have problems with my vision, and I don't understand why I should keep seeing eye doctors unless I have problems."

Diabetic eye disease is among the most feared long-term complications of diabetes, and for good reason. Over the years it has been the most common cause of blindness in adults (with or without diabetes) aged 20–64 years, and even today many people who have diabetes require treatment for the effects of diabetes in their eyes.

But the subject also suffers from far too much misinformation. To begin with, visual impairment is *not* inevitable. Good blood glucose control dramatically increases your chances of maintaining excellent vision throughout your life. Even if you do develop eye disease, it *is* treatable. Found early (see Figure 27) and treated properly, most diabetic retinopathy never causes impairment of vision.

Understanding how diabetes affects the eyes and what to do about it is not that complicated. A little knowledge can put you on the right track to avoid visual impairment in your lifetime with diabetes.

How the Eye Works

The basic function of the eye is to focus an image of something you're looking at (say, an eye chart) on one spot on the back of your eye. The "photographic plate" that picks up the image and transmits it to the brain is called the *retina*. (See Figure 28 for an illustration of the structures of the eye.)

To get an image focused properly on the retina, the light rays reflected from the object being observed first pass through the outermost clear covering of the eye (called the *cornea*) then enter through the *pupil* (the black spot in the middle of the eye that is really a hole in the *iris*, the colored part of the eye). Inside the eye, the light rays are focused by the *lens*. The lens is a common spot for eye problems, though not usually due to diabetes. If the lens is not strong enough to focus the light rays from the object all the way to the back of the eye, it may need help in the form of a contact lens or glasses. If the lens gets cloudy, like fog on your glasses, the light can't get through it clearly. This is called a *cataract*, and you may require surgery to

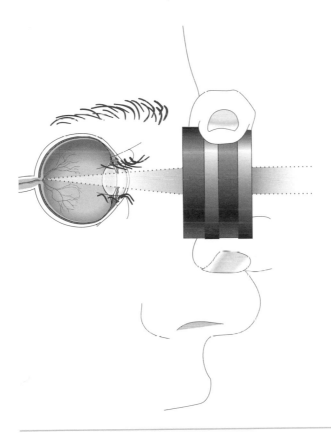

Figure 27. You can't see retinopathy by looking at the outside of the eye. The ophthalmologist must look through the dilated pupil to see the back of the eye and carefully examine the tiny veins and arteries for hemorrhages, outpouchings, or other abnormalities.

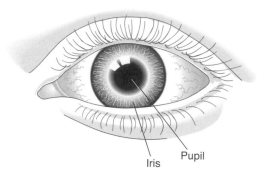

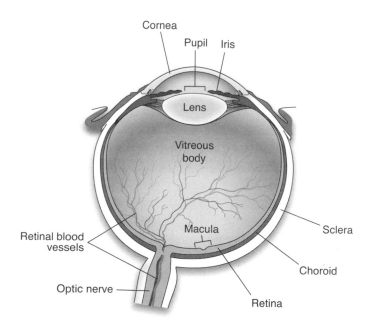

Figure 28. Anatomy of the eye.

replace your natural lens with a lens implant. With uncontrolled diabetes, cataracts can develop at an earlier age. If there is too much pressure in this front part of the eyeball, much like the overfilling of a tire, the condition is called *glaucoma* and definitely requires medical treatment.

After passing through the lens for focusing, the light rays cross through the gel (the *vitreous*) of the eye, whose purpose is to keep the eyeball spherical, like the air in a soccer ball, and to allow light to pass easily through the eye.

Finally, if all systems are working and all these layers of the eye are clear, the light rays are focused to form an image of the object on the retina, the thin tissue that lines the inner wall of the eye—but not just anywhere on the retina. The image needs to form exactly on one small area called the *macula*, which is especially rich in nerves and is the spot that gives you focused vision. Cells in the macula collect light from the outside world and send an image via the optic nerve to the brain, where vision—perception of the image—actually occurs. The macula is essential for reading and for discriminating fine details, such as the letters in a word or the details of a human face. The rest of the retina, lining the whole back of the eye, is used only for peripheral vision—to allow you to see things "out of the corner of your eye." By far the most important spot, then, is the macula. If the light rays forming the image reach the macula unimpaired, you have good, focused vision; if not, you won't focus well.

What Happens in Diabetes?

If a person's glucose levels have been high for a long time, usually more than several days, the lens of the eyes will swell. This is a common finding when individuals are first diagnosed with diabetes and their glucose levels have been high for some time. A swollen lens leads to blurred vision—or sometimes improved vision in persons who normally wear glasses. Vision changes such as these will go away after blood glucose levels fall back into a more normal range.

When caring for your diabetes, you and your eye doctor especially want to avoid severe bleeding into the vitreous gel. As you can imagine, if blood pours into this part of the eye, no light will get through to the retina. But bleeding into the vitreous (vitreous hemorrhage) doesn't just happen: it is the end result of a buildup of diabetic retinopathy that occurs over many years.

The first sign of diabetes in the eyes is almost always what is called *background retinopathy*. It usually starts after 5–10 years of uncontrolled diabetes, is very common, and is usually not dangerous in itself. To determine whether you have background retinopathy, the ophthalmologist will dilate (enlarge) your pupils with drops. To use a common analogy, if the doctor doesn't dilate the pupils, she is trying to see a whole room through a keyhole, and this cannot be considered a complete diabetes eye exam. Background retinopathy is seen as little red spots on the retina called *microaneu-rysms*, larger smudges called *microhemorrhages*, or yellowish deposits called *exudates* (see Figure 29). Don't be alarmed if the doctor comments on some "spots," or "small hemorrhages," or "diabetes in the eye," as these findings are quite common. In the United Kingdom Prospective Diabetes Study (UK-PDS), 37% of people newly diagnosed with Type 2 diabetes had retinopathy at the time of diagnosis, suggesting that their diabetes had gone undiagnosed for many years. Background retinopathy occurs in about 50% of people after 7 years of diabetes and in 90% after 15 years. The longer an individual has diabetes, the more likely he is to develop diabetic retinopathy. While diabetes and its complications can occur in all races/ethnicities, the National Health and Nutrition Examination Survey III of Type 2 diabetes showed that for people over 40 years of age, diabetic retinopathy was more common among non-Hispanic/Latino blacks (27%) and Mexican Americans (33%) than among non-Hispanic/Latino whites (18%). The reason for this is unclear.

The presence of background retinopathy alone is not a big concern. It does not cause any symptoms unless some fluid accumulates in the macula (a condition called *macular edema*), in which case treatment is considered. However, the main concern and the primary reason that background retinopathy should be monitored closely is that it can progress to the next stage, called *proliferative retinopathy*.

In proliferative retinopathy, tiny new blood vessels form, which are fragile and liable to break and bleed. These new blood vessels are the culprits that can impair vision by bleeding into the vitreous (see Figure 30).

When a major vitreous hemorrhage occurs, it causes a sudden loss of vision in that eye as blood fills up the vitreous. Often the blood will drain out of the eye over a few weeks or months, and vision will return. The bleeding can recur, though, and scars and clots can form that will pull the retina out of place, off the back of the eyeball (*retinal detachment*).

Figure 29. (*facing page*) A normal, healthy retina (*top*), showing the blood vessels that supply the center of the retina (the macula) and the optic nerve. A retina with diabetic retinopathy (*bottom*), showing exudates, bleeding, microaneurysms, and edema, all caused by leakage from damaged blood vessels into the macula, making the tissue swollen and unable to transmit a clear image to the brain.

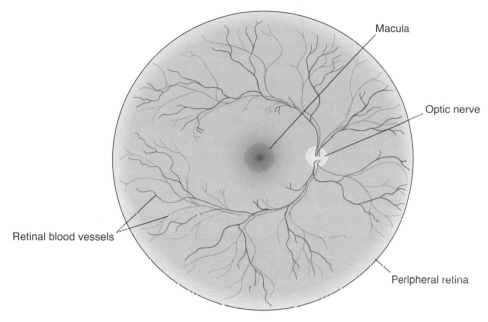

Macula

Optic nerve

Retinal blood vessels

Peripheral retina

Normal retina

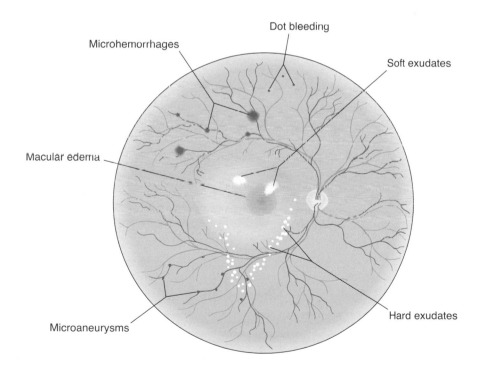

Dot bleeding

Microhemorrhages

Soft exudates

Macular edema

Microaneurysms

Hard exudates

Diabetic retinopathy

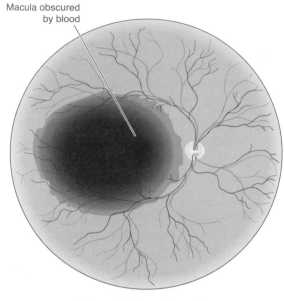

Macula obscured
by blood

Retina with vitreous hemorrhage

Figure 30. Vitreous hemorrhage in an eye with proliferative diabetic retinopathy. The large hemorrhage is sitting on top of the macula and blocking light from reaching the macula. Thus, no image is sent to the brain. The person cannot see clearly.

How Do I Know If I Have Diabetic Retinopathy?

People often assume, incorrectly, that because they do not notice any change in vision, they must not have any damage to their eyes from diabetes. By the time someone begins to notice vision loss from diabetic retinopathy, she has usually already developed a lot of damage to the retina. Given the highly effective treatments for diabetic retinopathy that can help preserve vision and, in some cases, restore vision, a regular eye examination is essential for persons having diabetes.

Detecting Diabetic Eye Disease: The Eye Examination

As we've mentioned, the early stages of diabetic eye disease usually don't produce symptoms, but it is extremely important to regularly examine for eye disease so that treatment can be started at the right time. There is no way for you to know the status of your eyes unless a qualified eye doctor examines them. Two questions arise at this point: who is a qualified doctor and how often should you be examined?

A qualified doctor is one who does this exam often and is used to looking for the subtle changes of proliferative retinopathy that signal trouble. We mentioned earlier that a good exam must be done with a dilated pupil (which is accomplished by putting in the drops that sting for a moment and make your vision blurred for several hours). Ophthalmologists (medical doctors who specialize in eye disease) are generally well trained to detect retinopathy and decide whether your eye has reached the stage when it requires laser photocoagulation (see below). Few other doctors, with the possible exception of diabetologists, are well qualified to detect diabetes in the eye.

Some optometrists (non-M.D.s) are competent to examine a dilated eye for diabetic retinopathy, although their main work is assessing eyes for glasses or contact lenses. General internists and family practitioners are usually much less experienced at detecting retinopathy, and other medical specialists usually are not trained to do such exams.

How often should you be examined? The standard recommendation is annually for people who have had Type 1 diabetes for five or more years and for everyone with Type 2 diabetes, since the onset of Type 2 is less accurately dated. Persons who are found to have mild nonproliferative diabetic retinopathy on a dilated examination can be seen anywhere from every nine months to once a year. Those with more advanced or moderate nonproliferative diabetic retinopathy should have dilated eye exams every six months, and those with severe nonproliferative diabetic retinopathy should be evaluated approximately every four months. Extremely close follow-up is recommended for people with proliferative diabetic retinopathy who are at risk for vitreous hemorrhage or retinal detachment, with exams as frequently as every two to three months. Pregnant women with diabetes are at especially high risk for progression of any preexisting retinopathy during pregnancy and should have a dilated eye exam during their first, second, and third trimesters.

Fluorescein angiography is used to detect any leaking vessels. The ophthalmologist (or assistant) injects a yellow dye into a vein in your arm and takes pictures of your retina in rapid sequence. The dye makes some people nauseated for a few minutes and turns the urine a bright orange-yellow.

The key point to remember is that diabetic eye disease is treatable if caught at the right time. The whole point of having regular eye exams performed by an expert is to pick up the changes at a stage when diabetic retinopathy can be successfully treated, before major bleeding occurs.

Treating Diabetic Eye Disease

Prevention of diabetic retinopathy through blood glucose control is the ideal, but if the eye disease does develop, it is rarely ever too late to intervene to stop the worsening of the retinopathy and to try to prevent further vision loss.

Photocoagulation

In laser photocoagulation, a laser beam is used to coagulate (clot) the fragile new vessels in the eye that cause a vitreous hemorrhage. Laser beams are used because they can be very finely focused and accurately aimed. Since the early 1970s, laser beams have been used to treat many types of eye problems, including those due to diabetes.

When laser therapy is done, the eye doctor dilates the pupil and numbs the surface of the eye with drops. A beam of light is then focused on a particular spot of the retina, and a laser burn is rapidly placed. The laser beam is then moved to another spot on the retina and another burn is placed. Up to hundreds of little spots, or burns, are placed on the retina in one sitting. Even so, you may need to come back for more.

There are generally two patterns of laser treatment for diabetic eye disease. In *panretinal photocoagulation*, the doctor places laser burns in a pattern throughout most of the retina, *except for the macular area* (see Figure 31). If you think about it, the macula (which is where the focused image forms) is the very spot that the ophthalmologist wants to *protect*, not touch with a laser burn. The second pattern of laser treatment is called *focal photocoagulation* and is used to touch up just a few leaking spots that have caused or are at risk of causing macular edema. Laser photocoagulation is done to decrease the risk of vision loss from vitreous hemorrhage or retinal detachment.

Does laser therapy hurt? Most people report no pain or only minor discomfort with laser photocoagulation, although sometimes it does seem to "hit a nerve." If the procedure is painful, the doctor can put a local anesthetic in the back of the eye, much as a dentist uses Novocain. Fairly often, there is some mild aching after the treatment.

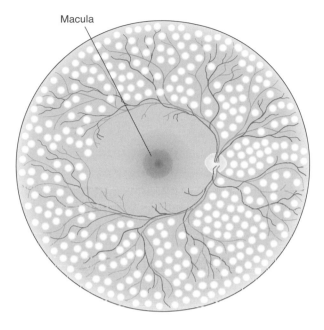

Macula

Figure 31. Panretinal laser photocoagulation. A laser burn is placed in all quadrants of the peripheral retina outside the macula, causing the new retinal blood vessels to disappear and decreasing the risk of vitreous hemorrhage and retinal detachment.

How does laser therapy work? The answer to this question is not completely clear. One thought is that the laser is burning out the fragile little blood vessels that cause the bleeding, essentially clotting them off to prevent bleeding. It is also thought that burns placed in the peripheral retina decrease the amount of a chemical called VEGF (vascular endothelial growth factor) that is produced by the retina in persons with diabetes. The burns lead to the growth of fewer new blood vessels and thus decrease the risk of vitreous hemorrhage and retinal detachment.

Does laser therapy work? There is no doubt about the effectiveness of laser photocoagulation. Several large, well-conducted studies have shown that laser photocoagulation works and that its benefit is lasting. If done at the right time, the treatment reduces the rate of severe visual loss by as much as 90% and possibly more. This treatment is worth taking advantage of, and it is the main reason that every person with diabetes should have eye exams as recommended.

Vitrectomy

Vitrectomy is a surgical procedure in which the gel of the eye (the vitreous) is removed and replaced with a clear solution. It is done only when there has been repeated bleeding into the vitreous and vision is cut off by scars or other debris that block the transmission of light through what should be a clear gel.

Since it is done only after a vitreous hemorrhage has occurred and has not cleared on its own, vitrectomy should be thought of as a last effort to save vision in an eye that is not otherwise likely to be useful. Its success rate varies considerably, depending on the amount of damage that has already occurred and whether vitreous bleeding recurs after the vitrectomy.

Intravitreal Delivery of Drugs

For many decades laser photocoagulation of leaking blood vessels in the macula was the main treatment for macular edema. In recent years some studies have shown that intravitreal delivery of drugs that block chemical signals that cause blood vessels to become leaky in the first place works even better. These drugs, known as anti-VEGF agents, are injected into the vitreous cavity of the eye, using topical anesthetics, during a routine office visit (see Figure 32). Persons often need monthly injections until the macular edema resolves. This treatment has proved very successful in returning the swollen retina to normal and has been shown to produce a lasting improvement in vision (see Figure 33).

Prevention of Diabetic Eye Disease or Its Progression

The Diabetes Control and Complications Trial (DCCT) and the UKPDS showed that tight blood glucose control could both dramatically reduce the risk of developing retinopathy when none existed to begin with and reduce the risk of worsening eye disease when some eye involvement was present

---

facing page

Figure 32. (*top*) Intravitreal injection of an anti-VEGF (vascular endothelial growth factor) agent.

Figure 33. (*bottom*) A, normal macula. B, macula with large spaces that represent edema.

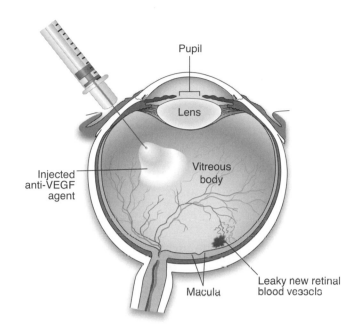

Pupil

Lens

Injected
anti-VEGF
agent

Vitreous
body

Macula

Leaky new retinal
blood vessels

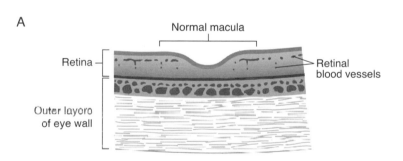

A

Normal macula

Retina

Retinal
blood vessels

Outer layers
of eye wall

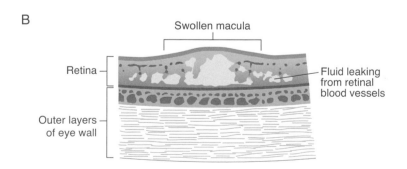

B

Swollen macula

Retina

Fluid leaking
from retinal
blood vessels

Outer layers
of eye wall

at the start. These findings have practical implications: good diabetes care, keeping your blood glucose in a good range, is effective not only early in the course of diabetes but also later on. Even when you are diagnosed as having diabetic retinopathy, it is not too late to begin efforts to improve your glucose control. Your chances of maintaining good vision are considerably better if you control your diabetes well.

There is evidence that stopping smoking and controlling blood pressure also improve your chances for avoiding visual loss. Finding out about and treating other eye conditions, particularly glaucoma, is also very important to maintaining good vision.

You can take two important steps to prevent diabetic eye disease: control your blood glucose well throughout your life with diabetes and have regular eye exams by an expert in the field. With these two measures, there is every reason to think that cases of visual impairment from diabetes will become fewer and fewer.

Recent research also shows that depression plays a role in diabetic eye disease. We've known for some time that depression is associated with higher blood glucose levels, a major risk factor for diabetic eye disease. Now, new studies have established a direct causal link between depression and eye disease in people with diabetes: patients who were depressed had a significantly higher risk of developing eye disease (retinopathy). This suggests that improving depression treatment for people with diabetes could contribute to preventing diabetic eye disease.

Take Home Messages

- Diabetes-related changes in the eye known as diabetic retinopathy are common.
- Retinopathy is more likely to develop the longer someone has diabetes and the less well the diabetes is controlled.
- People diagnosed with diabetes who maintain excellent control of their blood glucose and their blood pressure can maintain excellent vision throughout their lifetime.
- Regular dilated eye examinations enable the ophthalmologist to detect retinopathy and to more closely follow up on and treat it, thus greatly reducing the likelihood of vision loss.

24

Diabetic Kidney Disease

- "What's the relationship between the kidneys, high blood pressure, and swelling in the ankles?"
- "I was told that I have protein in my urine. What is the significance of that, and can I do something about it?"
- "What is involved with dialysis? Different people I've heard of seem to do it completely differently."

The Diabetes Control and Complications Trial (DCCT) was the first study to prove that intensive control of blood glucose levels greatly reduces the incidence of diabetic kidney disease in persons with Type 1 diabetes, as well as reducing progression of this kidney disease in those who already have it. Many other studies have shown that this is also the case for persons with Type 2 diabetes. But most people who have diabetes never develop diabetic kidney disease. No more than about one-third of people with Type 1 diabetes ever show a sign of kidney involvement, no matter how long they live, and a recent study even found that as few as 9% of Scandinavians with Type 1 diabetes developed kidney disease.

So, you may never face the problem of diabetic kidney disease, called *diabetic nephropathy*, but it is a possible long-term, serious complication of diabetes. Research shows that diabetic nephropathy can have an extremely adverse effect on a person's mental and physical quality of life. This being so, there are steps you can take to improve your chances of avoiding this complication or of controlling it if you already have it.

The Kidneys

A major role of the kidneys is to clean the blood of waste products. As the blood circulates through the body, it flows through the kidneys, which consist of millions of little filters, like the paper filters in a coffee machine. The filters clear the waste products from the "dirty" blood into the urine, with the "cleaned" blood returning to the bloodstream.

Another crucial role of the kidneys is to regulate the body's salt and water balance. Our normal body fluids are just about as salty as seawater. We drink fresh water and we eat salt, and the kidneys have the job of making sure that our body fluids maintain just the right amount of water and concentration of salt. They either spill out excess salt and water or conserve them, getting the balance just right. Kidneys are especially sensitive to fluid volume. You can check this out for yourself: drink a big bottle of water very quickly, and presto!—the kidneys will get rid of it by producing a large volume of diluted urine.

By controlling the water and salt content of the body, the kidneys also play a key role in regulating blood pressure. If your body retains salt and fluid, the blood vessels become overfilled, like the pressure in an overfilled balloon. This is called high blood pressure, or *hypertension*. On the other hand, when the vessels are seriously underfilled—for instance, when you lose a lot of blood or become overly dehydrated—blood pressure may fall dangerously low and you may go into shock. Well-functioning kidneys keep your fluid level and blood pressure normal.

What Goes Wrong with the Kidneys in Diabetes?

Kidney damage due to diabetes is classified along with diabetic eye disease as a *microvascular*, or small blood vessel, complication. In diabetic nephropathy, the little filters of the kidneys (called *nephrons*) develop thickened borders and eventually clog up entirely. If this is going to happen, it probably starts within the first 10 years of getting diabetes. But we don't know about it until later because we can't see the kidneys as easily as we can see the retina of the eye. (To look at the nephrons under a microscope, we'd need to perform a kidney biopsy, which is not a common procedure.)

The first clue that diabetic nephropathy is developing is usually the appearance of protein in the urine, called *proteinuria*. Proteinuria means that the kidneys' filtering system has become leaky. It's as if the same paper coffee filter has been used over and over again, eventually developing holes and letting the coffee grounds fall through. Instead of coffee grounds, the kidneys leak protein.

There are several different ways to test for protein in the urine (see Table 16), all of them using a urine sample. The *least sensitive* but *easiest* test is to dip a reagent stick into a urine sample. Significant protein in the urine will change the color of the stick. The *most sensitive* is a test for *microalbuminuria*, which can measure even tiny amounts of the protein albumin in the urine. Large amounts of albumin in the urine (macroalbuminuria) indicate a greater degree of kidney disease from diabetes. Urine protein measurements can be done on a "random sample" (which means you urinate into a cup without worrying about the time the urine is collected). The *most accurate* assessment is a timed sample. You collect in a bottle all the urine you make for some fixed period, usually 24 hours. The timed sample measures the total amount of albumin or the total amount of protein put out by the kidneys in the 24-hour period. This test also provides a very good idea of how the kidneys are working by measuring what is known as *creatinine clearance* (see below). Exercising during the period when you're collecting a timed sample of urine may cause some protein to be jarred through the kidneys into the urine without any abnormality at all, so it's a good idea to avoid exercise during a timed sample.

Significant amounts of protein in the urine, on repeated measurements, are an abnormal finding. To understand the meaning of a urine protein result, a few rules of thumb are helpful. If proteinuria is present in one sample but not on a repeat test, the finding may not be significant. The hallmark of diabetic nephropathy is *persistent proteinuria* (documented more than

Table 16   Tests for Protein in the Urine

Test Name	Sample Collection	Normal Values*
"Dipstick"	Random urine sample	Negative
Microalbumin	Random urine sample	Less than 30 mg/gram creatinine
24-hour microalbumin	24-hour urine collection	Less than 30 mg/24 hours
24-hour protein	24-hour urine collection	Less than 150 mg/24 hours
Creatinine clearance	14-hour urine collection	More than 100 cc/minute

*Normal values differ for different laboratories. The figures used here are estimates.

once), not just a single occurrence. A current bladder infection or a history of kidney disease independent of diabetes (some people have a condition called *nephritis* in childhood) may also cause elevated urinary protein. But when protein is found in the urine in two consecutive samples and there is no other known cause, it usually does mean that diabetic nephropathy is occurring, and measures should be taken to slow or halt its progression.

Treating Diabetic Nephropathy

There are four general approaches to slowing the progression of nephropathy: blood pressure control, blood glucose control, diet, and cholesterol control.

Blood Pressure Control

We've mentioned that kidney problems can cause high blood pressure (hypertension). But the opposite can also happen: high blood pressure may worsen kidney problems. So the single most important thing you can do to slow the progression of kidney disease is to interrupt this vicious cycle of high blood pressure and kidney damage by controlling your blood pressure.

What is normal blood pressure? For persons without diabetes, blood pressure is considered normal when it falls below 140/90. (The first, higher number in a blood pressure measurement is the *systolic pressure*, and the second, lower number is the *diastolic pressure*. When taking a blood pressure reading, the systolic number is the reading when you begin to hear the pulse sounds; the diastolic reading is when you stop hearing them.) For persons who have diabetes, most guidelines support aiming for a blood pressure of less than 140/80. There is even evidence that lower blood pressure levels may protect you from strokes and death. Studies find fewer strokes and a lower death rate in people with diabetes when the systolic pressure is less than 130, but no change in heart attack rates and many more serious medication side effects. For this reason, your physician may recommend keeping your systolic blood pressure below 130 especially if you are younger and tolerating blood pressure medications well. When your blood pressure is less than 140/80, you are less likely to develop microalbuminuria, less likely to have microalbuminuria worsen a lot in the future, and less likely to develop kidney failure. Please keep in mind that most individuals with high blood pressure need more than one blood pressure medication to get their pressure under control.

Many people think that when it comes to blood pressure, the lower the better. The only concern about blood pressure being too low is if you become dizzy as you stand up or go about your regular daily activities. In this condition, called *orthostasis*, which is sometimes caused by neuropathy, blood pressure is too low and not enough blood is getting to your head. Otherwise, if your systolic blood pressure is, say, 100–140 and your diastolic is 60–80, that should be fine.

There are lots of things you can do to help lower your blood pressure. If you're overweight, losing weight is helpful. Decreasing your intake of sodium, a component of common table salt, and increasing potassium intake have been shown to lower blood pressure. Moderating alcohol intake and increasing physical activity are also effective in lowering your blood pressure.

We noted in earlier chapters the use of *ACE (angiotensin-converting enzyme) inhibitors* to treat high blood pressure, and they are also used to treat kidney disease in diabetes. There are many ACE inhibitors, each with different side effects and different durations of action. An older one, captopril, is taken three times daily. Most others, including lisinopril and enalapril, are longer acting and can be taken once a day. An occasional side effect of these medications is a dry cough, less commonly a rash, and rarely angioedema (swelling under the skin) with tongue swelling and hives. These effects all go away after the medication is stopped. Another, newer class of blood pressure medications (though available for a long time now) that work like ACE inhibitors—and do not cause a dry cough—are the ARBs *(angiotensin receptor blockers)*.

The ACE inhibitors and ARBs block a key chemical reaction in the kidneys' control of blood pressure—a reaction that is often overactivated in diabetes, causing high blood pressure. Large research trials have shown that if people with diabetes have proteinuria, they do better with ACE inhibitors and ARBs than with other medications used to treat hypertension. In our practice, we recommend ACE inhibitors as the first choice to treat high blood pressure, and we prescribe them when a person with diabetes has proteinuria even without hypertension. So far there's not enough evidence to suggest using them when a person has neither hypertension nor proteinuria.

It is important to keep in mind that blood pressure, like blood glucose or heart rate, is not static: it doesn't just stay at one level minute to minute, hour to hour, day to day. As a person who has diabetes, you are used to this concept because you've seen your blood glucose levels bounce around. If you have hypertension, it makes sense to test your blood pressure regularly, not to rely on one test at home or in the doctor's office.

You've probably heard the term *white coat hypertension* (which we mentioned in Chapter 22), referring to the fact that a visit to your health care professional can temporarily raise your blood pressure. White coat hypertension really does happen to some people, but sometimes it's just an excuse for ignoring high blood pressure. To find out, you have to check your blood pressure repeatedly at other times. Ask a nurse at your workplace or a well-trained family member to check your pressure, or use a blood pressure cuff at a reliable supermarket or drug store. You may also want to learn to do it yourself, possibly with an automatic device you can use at home. Make sure you've been seated and resting comfortably for at least two minutes before having your pressure taken. Otherwise, if your adrenaline level is up, your blood pressure can be higher than usual and you can get a falsely high reading. That being said, *be sure not to ignore high blood pressure*, especially if you have diabetic nephropathy.

Blood Glucose Control

Throughout this book we have provided lots of reasons for controlling your blood glucose. Avoiding or slowing diabetic kidney disease is another good reason. The way that uncontrolled diabetes causes kidney damage is complicated, but, simply put, high glucose levels stick to and damage the cells that line small blood vessels in the kidneys and elsewhere in the body. This makes the blood vessels leak protein, which shows up in the urine, and later damages and scars the kidneys, making them lose function. The DCCT found that the lower the average glucose level, the better. There was almost no risk of kidney damage when the hemoglobin A1c stayed below 6%, very little chance of damage if it stayed below 7%, and then a greater and greater risk of kidney damage if the A1c stayed over 8% for many years. The greatest risk was for those with the highest average A1c. The DCCT also showed there was no special "danger" point. Therefore, we believe that your blood glucose control should be as good as you can make it, as long as you're not having too many or severe low blood glucose reactions (hypoglycemia).

High blood glucose affects the kidneys, like other parts of the body, over a long period of time. There is no reason to think that occasional episodes of hyperglycemia will have a serious effect. Rather, you should work on the averages, keeping your glucose control, on average, in as good a range as possible.

Diet

If you start showing signs of early kidney trouble, your health care professional may recommend—in addition to avoiding foods high in salt content to help control your blood pressure—cutting back on your protein intake. And he or she may recommend even greater protein reduction if you show even more loss in kidney function.

Cholesterol Control

High cholesterol levels seem to place people with diabetes at higher risk for kidney disease, probably because high cholesterol leads to blockage of blood vessels that supply the kidneys. Individual studies have shown that treatment with cholesterol-lowering drugs such as statins or fenofibrate can slow the rate of worsening kidney disease in those with diabetes. It also makes sense to screen for and treat high cholesterol levels in persons who have diabetes and kidney disease because they are also at a much higher risk for heart disease.

Kidney Failure

The progression of kidney damage (or nephropathy) can be hard to follow and hard to predict, at least until it is already quite severe. Proteinuria may precede kidney failure by as long as 10–15 years or more, especially if a person follows the treatment approaches described above and especially if the proteinuria is picked up early, as microalbuminuria.

Until kidney damage is severe, it's impossible to predict how soon complete kidney failure ("end-stage renal disease") will occur. Although advanced kidney damage most often proceeds to complete kidney failure, we do not agree with the approach that attempts to predict exactly when someone will need dialysis. We really don't know.

A test called the *creatinine clearance*, which involves collecting urine over a 24-hour period, provides a good indication of kidney function. Your care provider can also determine your glomerular filtration rate (GFR)—the rate at which your kidneys are filtering your blood—based on your blood creatinine level and your race/ethnicity, gender, and age. The GFR gives a close estimate of your creatinine clearance. A creatinine clearance result of 100 ml/minute or more is about normal. A creatinine clearance of 50 ml/minute suggests that the kidneys are functioning at about 50% of normal. Symptoms are not likely to occur until the rate is below about 20–30 ml/minute, and dialysis or transplantation is usually necessary when kidney function falls below about 10 ml/minute.

Nephropathy is largely a "silent" problem—one that does not make you feel ill. Its symptoms, when they do occur, occur very late. The first symptom may be ankle swelling, but don't panic if you have some ankle swelling: there are many causes, and some, such as premenstrual fluid retention, have nothing to do with diabetes. When kidney function becomes seriously impaired, the person develops anemia and usually feels much more tired. This will progress to more severe fatigue, itching, nausea, vomiting, and eventually less urine production. In that case the kidneys are no longer filtering out the toxins, which are building up to dangerous levels in the blood. The lab tests used to measure the waste products in the blood are *blood urea nitrogen* and *serum creatinine*.

People with failing kidneys should be told what is happening and what their options are well before their kidneys fail completely. They should have a chance to think over what is involved with each of the options. There are two options. When end-stage renal disease is reached—in other words, when the kidneys are essentially nonfunctional—only dialysis or kidney transplantation is possible. Otherwise, kidney failure is fatal. One comfort if you are facing end-stage kidney disease is that under current law in the United States, you automatically qualify for Medicare, which will pay for dialysis and transplantation. Without such coverage these extraordinarily expensive therapies would be out of financial reach for almost everyone.

Kidney Dialysis

Dialysis is a lifesaving approach that takes over the functions of the failed kidneys. It was introduced in the 1960s as a treatment that makes it possible for a person to live with end-stage renal disease. There are two ways to do dialysis: *hemodialysis* and *peritoneal dialysis*.

People receiving hemodialysis either go to a dialysis center several times a week or learn to do it with proper equipment at home. Either way, you are hooked up to a machine that takes your blood as it flows through an arm, runs it through a filtering apparatus, and returns it to the arm through another line. To make it easier for the blood to be drawn out of the arm and returned to the arm, a "shunt" is surgically placed in your forearm before the first dialysis treatment. The shunt is a large tube running from an artery in the arm to a vein. Beneath the surgical scar, a U-shaped lump is visible, which has a vibration that you can feel as blood rushes through the shunt.

People undergoing hemodialysis are usually not uncomfortable during the procedure. You sit in a special chair, reading or watching television, for a few hours. But you may feel below par for a while before dialysis, when the waste products have built up in your blood, and afterward, because the fluid shifts have been so abrupt. Anyone using hemodialysis must get it without fail. This treatment (in fact, any dialysis) requires a major and faithfully given commitment of time.

Peritoneal dialysis is done very differently. To start it, a tube is surgically placed through the skin into the abdominal cavity. This access line into the abdomen has to be kept very clean to prevent infection. With *chronic ambulatory peritoneal dialysis*, a large amount of liquid is made to flow through the tubing into the abdomen, swelling it up. A few hours later, the fluid is drained out, drawing with it the blood's waste products. A different approach, called *continuous cyclic peritoneal dialysis*, is somewhat more automated. Either way, with peritoneal dialysis there is no need to go to a dialysis center because you can do it yourself. It is not painful, but it does take time and a great deal of equipment (tubes, fluids, and so forth) stored in your home.

Most people do well on dialysis, often for many years. Because of the inconvenience, the chance of crises such as infections, and side effects such as disequilibrium after dialysis, many people look on it as an interim stage, hoping for a kidney transplant to provide a better solution.

Kidney Transplantation

Kidney transplantation is now done routinely at large medical centers, but it is major surgery that requires careful postoperative care. Unfortunately, not enough healthy kidneys are donated to transplant into all the people who need them.

A kidney that is to be transplanted is called a *donor* kidney; the person getting the donor kidney is the *recipient*. Donor kidneys have to be "matched" to the recipient to reduce the chance that the recipient's body will reject the new kidney. Matching is done by a series of tests, starting with the blood group (A, B, AB, or O) of the donor and the recipient.

On the whole, the chance that the transplanted kidney will survive is better if the donor is a close relative. Another reason that a related donor may be the best option is that the transplantation surgery can be planned electively rather than being dependent on finding a suitable donor and rushing the kidney to the recipient. Donating one kidney will not affect the long-term health of a healthy donor. Not every family member is suitable as a donor, however; the match may not be close enough or the donor candidate may have some kidney problem that makes it dangerous to give up a kidney and dangerous for the recipient to receive a potentially damaged kidney.

There are several other medical reasons, as well as social reasons, why a relative may not be available as a donor. In fact, most kidney transplant recipients do not have a suitable living related donor. Instead, the donor kidney is removed when someone, somewhere, has been pronounced brain-dead as a result of a sudden, catastrophic accident such as a motor vehicle accident or a medical event such as a severe brain hemorrhage. Organs are taken for donation only when the person has no chance of surviving and is essentially dead.

We want to clear up some common misconceptions by stating that you absolutely are not risking your life when you sign your approval as a potential organ donor (for instance, on your driver's license). There is no way your organs could ever be used if there were any chance at all that you would survive the current catastrophic event. Agreeing to be an organ donor simply means that if an exceedingly unlikely tragedy ever should strike you, parts of your body could at least provide life for someone else. Until more people sign on to be potential organ donors, there won't be enough donated organs to fill the need.

The system for identifying, analyzing, and transporting donor organs is well organized. Donor organs are computer-matched with people waiting for transplants. The person most in need—and with the best chance to make good use of the organ—gets the call. A dramatic set of events then unfolds rapidly. The donor kidney is removed from the donor, rushed to the recipient's hospital as the recipient is made ready, and transplanted into the recipient.

After the transplantation comes the process of circumventing the body's normal rejection mechanism. That is, a normal body recognizes when a foreign organ is put in and tries to reject it, so the recipient must take *immunosuppressive* drugs to suppress the body's normal immune defenses against the donor organ. Complications often arise in the posttransplant period, such as episodes of rejection or infections. But when the urine begins to flow again and the person can say goodbye to dialysis, this is a thrilling moment and a move back to a more normal life.

Combined Kidney-Pancreas Transplantation

At the same time that a kidney is transplanted into a recipient who has diabetes, or in a later operation, it may be possible to also transplant a pancreas. In this surgery the donor pancreas is placed in the lower abdomen. Since a working pancreas delivers insulin automatically, a successful pancreas transplantation, in essence, cures Type 1 diabetes.

Why, you will ask, don't we recommend pancreas transplantation to everyone, as soon as their diabetes is diagnosed, regardless of whether a kidney transplant is needed? The reason is quite simple: the surgery required, the postoperative risks, the need to suppress the recipient's immune system, and the chance that the pancreas will ultimately fail—all make pancreas transplantation, as currently done, a worse risk than controlling diabetes by other means. Organ availability is another factor: not nearly enough pancreases are available each year to provide for everyone with diabetes.

We understand that this is very disappointing for anyone who gets diabetes and wants what seems to be the quicker, easier fix of a pancreas transplant. But pancreas transplantation, for all the good it does in selected cases, does *not* provide an easy, safe alternative to treating diabetes conventionally. With the current state of the art, this procedure should be reserved for people who also need a kidney and therefore need immunosuppressive therapy anyway. Another relevant point here is that rejection of a trans planted pancreas can be detected earlier when a kidney from the same donor is transplanted at the same time. Blood tests pick up kidney rejection much earlier than pancreas rejection. Since the two organs will usually be rejected at the same time, rejection of the pancreas is picked up earlier (by signs the kidney is getting rejected) than when a pancreas is transplanted by itself.

The future of islet cell transplantation, in which only the islet cells are transplanted rather than the whole pancreas, is discussed in Chapter 31.

· · ·

Diabetic kidney disease, like so many of the long-term complications of diabetes, presents real challenges. The best news is that for most people who have diabetes, this complication will never develop, and when it does, its progression can be slowed significantly. Protein in the urine is the first sign.

Control of blood pressure (preferably with ACE inhibitors or ARBs), control of blood glucose, and restriction of dietary protein are the best ways to slow the progression of kidney insufficiency. But if your kidneys do fail, dialysis can keep you going and a successful kidney transplant can give you a new start.

Take Home Messages

- Most people with diabetes never develop diabetic kidney disease (diabetic nephropathy).
- There are four things you can do to protect your kidneys: maintain good blood pressure control, maintain good blood glucose control, eat a healthy diet (especially one low in salt), and maintain good control of your cholesterol levels.
- Protein in the urine (proteinuria) is the first sign of kidney damage. Doing the things noted above to protect your kidneys can help halt or slow the progression of kidney disease.
- For people whose kidneys are failing completely, there are several life-saving treatment options: kidney dialysis, kidney transplantation, and kidney-pancreas transplantation.

25

Diabetic Neuropathy

with Reshmi Srinath, M.D.

- "My feet feel funny—that's the only way I can describe it—my doctor says it's my nerves."
- "I rarely get an erection any more, and if I do, it doesn't last. I'm afraid my wife thinks I'm not interested in her."
- "Sometimes everything I eat just seems to stay in my stomach. I get bloated really quickly, feel nauseated all the time, and vomit. Forget blood glucose control at times like this—it's impossible."

Nerve damage due to diabetes is called *diabetic neuropathy*. The nervous system is extremely complex, and the symptoms of diabetic neuropathy can be distressing. In this chapter we want to help you understand how the nervous system works, what can go wrong with it in diabetes, and what can be done to prevent or treat the nerve damage.

Diabetic neuropathy is another long-term complication of poorly controlled diabetes. A person with newly discovered Type 2 diabetes may already have neuropathy, and if so, the diabetes has most likely existed undetected for some years before the diagnosis. Neuropathy rarely develops before 10 or so years after the onset of diabetes and sometimes later than that. One exception is when the high blood glucose itself causes the nerves to act up immediately, and the person feels better as soon as the blood glucose improves, whether or not there is any permanent damage to the nerves. It's important to distinguish this *acute* complication of high blood glucose from the *long-term* complication of diabetic neuropathy because the acute complication goes away quickly with proper diabetes control.

As with most long-term complications of diabetes, a lot has yet to be discovered about exactly what causes diabetic neuropathy and how to prevent or reverse it. People with high triglyceride levels, hypertension, and a history of smoking, as well as those with severely high blood glucose levels, are at greatest risk. There are thought to be two basic causes, each producing a very different kind of neuropathy. The most common kind of neuropathy is a gradual deterioration of the longest nerves due to years of high blood glucose. The less common kind is due to a sudden loss of blood supply to a segment of a nerve, like a mini-stroke outside the brain.

The Nervous System

Think of the body's nervous system as a massive telephone system, with each nerve being an individual line, all eventually joining one single large cable (the spinal cord) leading to a switchboard (the brain) that is immeasurably more complex than any telephone switchboard. Each individual nerve has a cell body with a nucleus, usually located in the spinal cord or brain, and then grows a long *axon*, like a single thread, that can extend all the way from the spine to a toe.

Every one of the billions of nerves outside the brain is specifically assigned either to incoming messages (the sensory nerves) or to outgoing messages (the motor nerves). The sensory nerves convey to the brain messages about body temperature, pain, position of a limb, and so on. The motor nerves deliver messages from the brain to the muscles. These messages may instruct muscles to make large, conscious movements, like "throw the ball" or "press the piano keys in sequence." Other motor nerves control completely unconscious, automatic actions, commanding the body to do such things as "speed up the heart rate," "widen the pupils," "move material through the intestines," or "breathe." These are called *autonomic motor nerves*.

The messages normally run quickly and smoothly along nerves, and to function properly everything has to work just right. Let's say the incoming lines carry the following message: "I'm resting my right hand down, and I feel warmth; my second finger is especially warm and—ouch! It suddenly hurts terribly!" The brain doesn't need to get involved when this alarm goes off. The message turns right around in the spinal cord, and your body receives a command to move fast and pull that finger off the top of the stove with lightning speed.

Think what happens if the part of the message signaling pain never arrives—if the nerve bringing the incoming signal, the sensory nerve, is damaged. The finger on the hot stove could suffer damage without the person even knowing it. Think also what could happen if the autonomic motor nerves didn't work right: the bowels might be underactive (constipation), sexual function might be affected, or the stomach might not move the food along properly into the intestine. These sorts of nerve defects can be a big problem in diabetic neuropathy.

The nervous system, then, consists of a complicated, delicate set of incoming and outgoing signals. Most often it is the incoming sensory nerves that are affected by diabetes. If they are irritated, it is like static on the telephone line, drawing attention away from normal conversation. If the nerve is nonfunctional, like telephone lines that have been cut down by a storm, the signal never gets through at all. Furthermore, once cut, nerves grow back only very slowly. So it makes far better sense to prevent nerve damage in the first place than to count on regrowing dead nerves.

Recognizing and Living with Diabetic Neuropathies

Peripheral Symmetrical Polyneuropathy

Peripheral symmetrical polyneuropathy, generally called *peripheral neuropathy*, is the most common diabetic nerve damage—occurring to some extent in many, perhaps most, people who have had diabetes for many years—and is more common if the diabetes has been poorly controlled. It can range from very mild to quite severe.

There are various theories about what causes the nerve damage. It may be due to swelling of the nerve cell or axon caused by an accumulation of the sugar sorbitol, or it may be due to the accumulation of "glycation end products," which are proteins essentially gummed up by glucose. Research is under way to find out whether blocking sorbitol accumulation will prevent or delay the onset of neuropathy, and other studies are looking at whether blocking the glycation end products will affect nerve damage.

Since gradual nerve damage first affects the nerves with the longest axons, its most common targets are the parts of the body farthest from the spine: the toes. This is why it is called *peripheral* neuropathy. But the same process can also affect the nerves that carry messages to the automatic functions of the body (the autonomic nerves), in which case it is called *autonomic neuropathy* (see below). All these forms of neuropathy develop slowly and are especially hard to reverse because, as we've noted, damaged nerves grow back only very slowly.

Symptoms and treatment. Peripheral neuropathy usually starts as numbness or tingling in the toes, progressing very gradually, over the years, up the ankle and leg. Sometimes the symptoms are barely noticeable and sometimes they are bothersome. Everyone describes the feelings differently: some people say it's like wearing thick-soled shoes, some report that they don't feel the movement of their toes as well as they should, while others say that their feet feel too sensitive. Tingling, burning, or sharp, shooting pains in the feet are common symptoms and are usually worse at night. Less commonly, people describe a sensation of feeling as though they are walking on pebbles. Some people aren't aware of any symptoms and are surprised when their health care professional finds their reflexes are not normal. Others report that even the feel of the bed sheets bothers them at night. The constant features of peripheral neuropathy are the location (almost always the toes and feet), the gradual onset, and the symmetry, since it usually occurs at least to some extent in both legs.

When peripheral neuropathy is severe, people experience either a great deal of discomfort or numbness. The painful stage usually doesn't last, as the feet become more and more numb. It is a blessing that the pain goes away, but if the numb foot is not well taken care of, it can be in great danger. Let's consider some examples.

> *Cheryl is 68 years old and for 10 years has known that she has diabetes. She suspects that she has had it for much longer, since she was diabetic during her last pregnancy, gained a lot of weight in her 50s, and was unusually thirsty for many years. She began having discomfort in her feet. At night she could hardly sleep, the pain was so bad. The pain never really went away, although a combination of pain medications helped somewhat. After suffering for a long time, Cheryl went to her doctor and received proper therapy.*

There are several approaches to treating painful peripheral neuropathy like Cheryl's. Mild pain may respond to the antioxidant alpha lipoic acid. Other effective medications include the antidepressants amitriptyline, desipramine, duloxetine, or venlafaxine. When prescribed for peripheral neuropathy, these antidepressant medications actually affect the nerves. Neuropathy is the result of structural damage to the nerves; psychological problems, which are every bit as real and serious as neuropathy, are not caused by nerve damage.

To treat painful peripheral neuropathy, a relatively low dose of amitriptyline or desipramine (25–50 mg/day) is initially prescribed, and then increased up to 150 mg/day if needed. The most common side effects include dry mouth and some drowsiness. Alternative medications for pain, such as the anticonvulsants pregabalin, gabapentin, carbamazepine, or valproic acid, are sometimes also prescribed along with the antidepressant drugs. A cream or ointment called capsaicin, composed of the ingredient that makes chili peppers hot, has been recommended, especially for those not able to tolerate the medications listed above. But it is hard to demonstrate whether the stinging effect of capsaicin that gradually deadens the nerve endings is actually effective. Finally, non-medication treatment such as local electric nerve stimulation may also be helpful.

> *James has had Type 2 diabetes for more than 20 years and never thought much about it. He went to his doctor every now and then but did not follow a diet or exercise regimen. He never pricked himself to do blood glucose monitoring (although he did have his own meter, which he never took out of the box). He was always a water drinker. At one point James began to notice a lack of sensation in his feet, but again he didn't think much about it. Later, he was alarmed to find that after wearing a new pair of shoes, he had developed a large ulcer on his big toe. It didn't hurt, but the doctor told him that the ulcer was due to peripheral neuropathy and that he needed to treat it with great care.*

When peripheral neuropathy causes the toes or feet to be numb, the danger is that they will be injured without the person even knowing it. A new pair of shoes, a longer-than-usual hike, stepping on something while going barefoot—all these are common causes of skin damage that can cause injury or an ulcer, which can become infected and ultimately could even require an amputation. (Diabetic foot problems are considered in more detail in Chapter 26.)

Lack of sensation is a danger. The nerves to the foot are there for good reason: they warn you about the pinching shoe, the pebble in the sock, or the tack you stepped on. When the nerves are damaged and you do not get that warning signal, you have to be very careful to take good care of your feet. We recall a patient who arrived home after work, took off his shoes, and found that his sock was bloody. It turned out his son's tiny metal toy had fallen into his shoe. Another of our patients, as he put his shoes back on after an exam in the office, found a comb inside the shoe and said matter-of-factly, "Oh, here it is—lost that two days ago." Numb feet can be dangerous!

People with diabetes should inspect their feet daily and discuss appropriate foot care with their health care professional. Comfortable, proper fitting shoes are important. A complete foot examination with testing for sensation, vibration sensation, and ankle reflex and assessment of blood flow are critical screening measures done in the doctor's office. The focus of care should be on blood glucose control, appropriate foot care, and treatment of pain.

Autonomic Neuropathies

The autonomic nerves control all those nerve functions that you don't have to think about: your heart rate, your stomach and bowel function, breathing, sweating when overheated, the opening of your pupils in response to low light levels, and, in men, erections. Just like the peripheral nerves, the long nerves that regulate these unconscious activities can be affected by diabetes. In fact, it is unusual for a person to have significant autonomic nerve problems without also having at least some evidence of peripheral neuropathy. When you consider the number of different functions the autonomic nerves control, it is not surprising that many different problems can arise if these nerves are affected by diabetes.

Erectile dysfunction. Erectile dysfunction (also called male impotence) is the most common of the autonomic neuropathies resulting from long-term diabetes. In males, achieving and holding an erection requires a complex series of interactions of the nerves and the circulatory system, and these interactions are easily disrupted. There are many causes of erectile dysfunction, but if none of the others exist, it may well be due to diabetes. After many years of having inadequately controlled diabetes, a man's sexual function can deteriorate. In women, the ability to have orgasms may be diminished by decreased sensation in the genital area, often called female impotence. (Male and female sexuality, including treatment options for problems with function, are discussed in Chapter 28.)

Intestinal involvement (enteropathy). Nerve impulses normally cause contraction of the muscles that surround the intestines to smoothly move the by-products of food digestion along the digestive tract. The loss of this smooth intestinal propulsion in persons with enteropathy generally leads to alternating bouts of diarrhea and constipation. The diarrhea may occur especially after eating and may become watery. It is not bloody, does not cause severe abdominal pain, and usually responds to simple over-the-counter antidiarrheal medications. Likewise, the constipation is usually not disabling and responds to cathartics such as prunes or over-the-counter laxatives.

Urinary retention. Sometimes the nerves to the urinary bladder stop functioning as well as they used to, and people retain some urine in their bladder even after voiding. If this problem is severe, the urine can back up to the kidneys, damaging kidney function, and can result in more frequent urinary tract infections. Often the condition causes no symptoms until it reaches the point where the person is not able to urinate at all. If you seem to be voiding only small amounts very frequently or often have to urinate urgently, you should be examined by a urologist. The urologist will use an ultrasound image to determine whether urine is left in the bladder after you have voided or to see how well the bladder muscles can empty water from the bladder.

Stomach involvement (gastroparesis). Although it is an uncommon neuropathy, gastroparesis can create real problems in longstanding diabetes. In gastroparesis, autonomic nerves that are responsible for emptying the stomach by squeezing food along from the stomach into the intestine are not functioning normally. The stomach becomes more like a slack bag that becomes filled with food and liquids but empties them poorly. Eating even a small meal can lead to a bloated, full feeling that may last for hours or be relieved only by vomiting. Nausea is common. Because the stomach empties slowly and erratically, it is especially hard to predict what the blood glucose will do following a meal, so diabetic control is often poor. And with this slower emptying of food from the stomach, people taking insulin may need to use the slower-acting Regular insulin rather than the rapid-acting insulins before meals. Studies show that gastroparesis can have a significantly adverse effect on a person's mental and physical quality of life. Fortunately, there are some effective treatments, including medications such as metoclopramide and a class of antibiotics that includes erythromycin and azithromycin, which help restore the stomach's normal movements. Occasionally, for people who do not respond to medications, it becomes necessary to insert a gastric pacer to cause the stomach to contract regularly or to insert a tube into the upper intestine, bypassing the stomach, to ensure appropriate nutrition and fluid intake.

Dizziness on arising (orthostasis). Autonomic nerves normally cause blood vessels in the lower body to constrict when you stand up, so that gravity doesn't pool all your blood into your legs. With autonomic neuropathy, though, this reflex may not happen. The result is that blood can pool in your lower body as you arise, causing you to feel dizzy because of a lack of blood in your head. There are medications that will cause your kidneys to hang on to more fluid, filling up the blood vessel tank more—but this approach may not be advisable, especially if you have any tendency toward high blood pressure, leg swelling, or heart failure. Usually we just advise people to get up slowly if they have been sitting or lying for some time, or to tense their leg muscles frequently while standing in place for a long time to help move fluid up the legs. Also, we advise patients to use specially designed compression stockings to keep the blood from pooling in the legs.

Sweating abnormalities. An unusual kind of autonomic neuropathy causes abnormal patterns of perspiration. Sometimes parts of the body do not perspire normally, and other parts perspire excessively. Occasionally this occurs on only one side of the body.

Single Nerve Involvements (Mononeuropathies)

Mononeuropathy is caused by sudden blood loss to a segment of a nerve, like pinching off one wire in a telephone line. The lack of blood supply is apparently like a mini-stroke to a peripheral nerve.

Symptoms. The symptoms are very different from those caused by the more common peripheral neuropathies. Mononeuropathies come on suddenly and do not affect the toes or feet symmetrically; instead they affect only one part of the body, supplied by a single nerve. The person may experience pain down the side of one leg, or from one side of the back right around the flank to the front of the abdomen, or in any other spot on the body. Sensory nerves are affected more often than motor nerves, but sometimes a cranial nerve can be affected, for example, causing an eyelid to droop.

Any number of conditions, from arthritis to sciatica, can cause sudden pain in one area, so diabetic mononeuropathy is usually diagnosed only after other problems have been excluded. It is very encouraging to know that mononeuropathies usually go away on their own within several weeks to six months or so.

Bell's palsy. This is a cranial mononeuropathy involving the cranial nerves that control the muscles on one side of the face. People with or without diabetes can develop Bell's palsy, but it is more common in people who have diabetes. Like the other mononeuropathies, this one usually resolves within weeks to months, although some people continue to have a droop on one side of their face for years.

Multiple single-nerve involvement (mononeuropathy multiplex). Mononeuropathy multiplex is an uncommon condition. As the name implies, it occurs when several or more single nerves are affected simultaneously. One classic if unusual example is when a whole series of nerves at the base of the spine are affected, causing the person to develop progressive weakness, especially of the hips and upper thighs, to the point where she or he cannot stand, climb stairs, or do physical work. Neurologists must be sure that some other disease or disk problem is not being missed, but if the condition is really mononeuropathy multiplex, it will resolve just like other mononeuropathies in a matter of six months to a year. The improvement can be dramatic in someone whose muscles were becoming alarmingly weak.

Take Home Messages

- The nervous system is so complex and sensitive that, not surprisingly, it can be severely affected by years of high blood glucose.
- The most common form of nerve damage (neuropathy) affects the longest nerves, those running to the feet. This peripheral neuropathy causes various degrees of discomfort, progressing to numbness. It does not reverse with treatment, so people must learn to accommodate to the lack of feeling in their feet by taking especially good care of them.
- Autonomic neuropathy affects automatic, unconscious nerve functions, causing such problems as erectile dysfunction and gastrointestinal symptoms. Like peripheral neuropathy, it develops over many years and does not reverse easily. Treatment of the symptoms is usually effective.
- The third main kind of neuropathy affects single nerves (mononeuropathy). It comes on relatively suddenly, affects only a limited area of the body, causes symptoms such as a droop on one side of the face or a sudden strip of pain, and reverses in weeks to months.

26

Diabetes and the Foot

- "My doctor keeps telling me to stop smoking to protect my feet. I know that smoking is bad, but what does that have to do with my feet?"
- "I'm young and I'm athletic. Is this foot care thing really that important?"
- "My feet feel like they're made of stone, and I feel like I'm walking on stones."
- "Now that I'm exercising regularly, the pain in my legs has gone away."

Most people associate diabetes with foot problems. Indeed, lower extremity complications are among the most frequent causes of hospitalization for persons who have diabetes, and half of all nontraumatic amputations occur in people with diabetes. These are sobering statistics, and yet amputations are largely avoidable with proper foot care and quick attention to problem areas.

In this chapter we focus on why diabetes increases the risk of foot problems, emphasizing how to evaluate your personal risk, then look in some detail at preventive foot care measures and treatment of specific problems. There's a big difference between *being at risk* for an amputation and actually *having* an amputation. A great many people develop some degree of neuropathy (see Chapter 25), but only a small fraction of them ever have their condition progress to where they need an amputation. Our purpose here is to help you limit foot problems so they do not progress to the point where they no longer respond to nonsurgical care.

Why are foot problems associated with diabetes? There are two reasons: peripheral neuropathy and poor circulation.

Peripheral Neuropathy and Poor Circulation

Diabetic *peripheral neuropathy* is damage to the peripheral nerves as a result of diabetes. As we discussed in Chapter 25, the symptoms are extremely variable and can range from tingling to mild or severe pain, from numbness to strange sensations such as feeling as if water is running over your feet when they aren't wet or a hypersensitivity to bed linens.

Although the pain and other odd sensations can be particularly bothersome or disruptive to daily life, the real danger is not to feel anything at all. It's numbness that gets people into trouble: if your foot is numb, you can't tell whether you've hurt it or not. We know a man who stepped on a golf tee and continued to play the entire game of golf, unaware that the tee had pierced his shoe and become embedded in his foot. If your feet are numb, not only do you have trouble feeling a serious injury like that but you may not feel when your shoes are too tight, the bath water is too hot, or there's a warm, inflamed area on your foot.

The other cause of foot problems is decreased circulation, or *peripheral vascular disease* (PVD). Circulation is the flow of blood to and from the tissues of your body through the pipelines, the arteries and veins. The blood brings nutrients, oxygen, and infection-fighting cells to keep tissues healthy. If the rate of circulation is decreased by the narrowing of arteriosclerosis (see Chapter 22) and the effects of smoking, the tissue gets less blood—and it complains. When blood flow is diminished because of PVD, there is a risk that small infections will not heal well.

Together, neuropathy (numbness) and PVD (decreased circulation) place the foot at increased risk for problems. Trauma can occur without your recognizing it, and infection can set in quickly. But you can compensate for these deficits with attentive foot care, greatly reducing the chance that neuropathy and decreased circulation will progress to a worse complication. On a positive note, young, athletic people like the one quoted above probably don't have neuropathy or a compromised circulatory system and therefore are at little risk for foot problems. Let's take a look at risk factors for foot complications.

What Is Your Risk?

Testing for Significant Neuropathy

The ability to feel trauma is probably the most important protection against serious foot problems. After all, that is a primary purpose of nerves: to alert the brain to a problem. But you generally don't lose sensation suddenly. The development of neuropathy is a gradual process. How quickly it develops and worsens is closely related to how poorly the diabetes has been controlled and how long you have had diabetes. Some people who have had well-controlled diabetes for over 50 years have little or no evidence of neuropathy, either by symptoms or on exam. People with mild nerve damage may notice they have to touch their feet a little harder in some spots to feel the touch. It may just be that you no longer have the increased sensitivity that used to bother you. More complete loss of sensation leads some patients to say that their feet feel as if they are made of stone. Poor sensation from the feet can also cause difficulty walking, leading to staggering when walking and further increasing the risk of foot injury.

Your health care professional can determine whether your level of sensation is still "protective," that is, still sensitive enough to detect trauma. This is sometimes tested by touching the toes very lightly. A more exact measure is the monofilament test, which is nothing more than pressing a three-inch piece of stiff nylon filament (like fishing line) against your toe, and your saying whether you feel it. If you cannot feel it, your risk of foot injury is definitely higher. Your doctor may also test for less specific evidence of neuropathy by checking your ankle reflexes with a reflex hammer, checking for position sense in your toes, or testing your ability to feel the vibrations of a tuning fork. Neuropathy due to diabetes is usually symmetrical, involving both sides equally. If symptoms or nerve function loss are on just one side, there may be a mechanical problem such as a disk in the spine pressing on a nerve. Nerve conduction studies may then be done to see where the nerve function drops off, which often helps show where the problem originates.

Testing for Significant Circulatory Compromise

Circulation can be assessed in several ways. One crude measure is simply to feel the temperature of the feet. With a decrease in the flow of warm blood to the foot, one foot may feel colder than the other. Note that we said *one* foot, which would indicate that a specific artery may be partially blocked. Don't be upset if your toes stay cold at night or your feet feel damp and cool. These signs are common in people without circulation problems. Loss of hair on the toes may be a sign of decreased circulation. However, more reliably, hair present on toes is an indication of good circulation in the feet.

A classic symptom of decreased blood flow to the legs is called *intermittent claudication*. In people with this condition, the calf gets sore or cramps when they walk briskly or uphill. The health care professional will want to feel your foot pulses to assess blood flow through your arteries at specific pulse points—a spot on top of your foot and a spot behind your ankle. If you test your own pulses, be aware that they may be hard to find even when blood flow is good, and they may not be present even in perfectly healthy people.

If there is reason to think your circulation is poor, blood pressure measurements can be done on the legs and compared with arm pressures to see whether there's a decrease. More sophisticated tests can also be done. One, called a Doppler test, looks at blood flow using an ultrasound probe. If surgery is being considered to address a circulatory problem, specialists may want to do an angiogram, running dye from your groin down through the leg arteries and taking X-rays to see exactly where the blockage is and how much there is.

Orthopedic Deformities

In assessing your risk, consider the shape of your foot. A normally shaped foot distributes weight evenly. Irregularity in bone structure can create increased pressure areas and possible tissue breakdown. Prior injury or advanced neuropathy can lead to muscle loss in the foot and create irregularities in the bone structure. Your doctor or a podiatrist can help you determine whether the shape of your foot is causing significant risk. The professional can also look for calluses or bunions that may cause problems.

High-Risk Habits

Harmful habits can contribute to your risk of foot problems. Smoking is the most important. In addition to increasing your risk for cancer and lung diseases, smoking contributes greatly to the risk of arteriosclerosis. Smoking a single cigarette causes decreased blood flow with a corresponding change in temperature in the extremities for up to an hour afterward. If you smoke, maybe you can even feel, or at least imagine, the blood flow to your feet being squeezed off with each cigarette. Smoking and diabetes are a very dangerous combination. Another harmful habit is wearing too-tight shoes that cause pressure points on your foot.

High Cholesterol and High Blood Pressure

Elevated blood cholesterol increases your risk of circulatory problems and thus foot trouble. Increases in the LDL cholesterol or decreases in HDL cholesterol are the main risks. High blood pressure over time also increases the risk for peripheral circulatory disease in the same way it increases the risk for strokes and heart attacks.

What Are the Common Causes of Foot Injury to the Person at Risk?

Evidence has accumulated in recent years that the worst outcomes—amputations—are almost always preceded by some recognized or unrecognized break in the skin of the foot. For the high-risk foot, dangers are always lurking: injury, pressure, repetitive stress, infection.

A dangerous break in the skin can come when walking barefoot or with thin-soled shoes. We mentioned a penetrating wound such as a golf tee poking through a shoe. Injuries from heat occur by stepping into a too-hot bath or onto a hot surface without first testing it with a sensitive area of your body or a thermometer. We know of a woman who burned the soles of her feet by walking on a beach on a sunny day, unaware of the intense heat of the sand. There have also been reports of heat injuries from the floors of motor vehicles on particularly long trips.

Sustained pressure concentrated on one spot on the foot can prevent blood flow to the area. Eventually, this lack of blood flow results in tissue breakdown or ulceration—a pressure sore. The most common cause of pressure sores is tight shoes, and the first tell-tale sign of a problem is a reddened area. If you can't feel that your shoes are too tight, the fitting at the shoe store may have been wrong in the first place. It's best to avoid fashionable but constraining shoes that put your feet in danger. High-heeled shoes with pointed toes compress the foot into an unnatural shape, and the high heels concentrate body weight toward the front of the foot.

Repetitive stress can create unnoticed inflammation in a vulnerable foot. Imagine you're on vacation and sightseeing on foot. If your sensation is normal, you will notice if your feet get sore from too much walking, and you will rest or maybe choose a bus tour for the next day. If your feet are numb, however, you may continue to walk day after day, unaware of the inflammation and tissue breakdown that might be taking place. An early sign of too much stress is heat radiating—heat that you can feel with your hand—from an area that appears red (see Figure 34).

A final danger to feet is infection. It may not be dramatic—just some cracks caused by athlete's foot, for instance. But further invasion of bacteria can occur through an opening in the skin created by any cause, and infections increase the demand for blood. In people with intact circulation, the body will probably be able to fight off small infections with or without prescribed antibiotics. If the circulation is decreased, however, it's harder

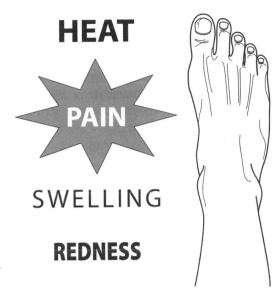

HEAT

PAIN

SWELLING

REDNESS

Figure 34. Warning signs of an infection of the foot.

for the body to fight the bacteria, and more aggressive measures may be needed to keep the infection from spreading.

Osteomyelitis is an infection in the bone. It's sometimes hard to diagnose because it doesn't always show up on plain X-rays. A bone scan or MRI may be needed to diagnose bone infection. Once established, osteomyelitis is hard to treat successfully because antibiotics don't get into the bone well. Scraping the infected area of bone (debridement) may be necessary. If the infection affects a relatively limited area, such as one small bone in the foot, it may be best to remove that bone or that toe to keep the infection from spreading.

Preventive Foot Care

Following preventive foot care measures is important for everyone who has diabetes. For persons with neuropathy or PVD, the foot becomes vulnerable to injury, pressure, stress, and infection. Prevention is the key to avoiding serious problems. We ask our high-risk patients to treat their feet like fine china: wash them and dry them carefully, inspect them, and give them the utmost protection. It's really not optional: if you have serious neuropathy or serious circulatory problems, you *must* practice prevention.

We'll look at each component of foot care separately. While the list may seem long, good foot care will become a simple habit once you've been doing it conscientiously for a few days or weeks.

Shoes

Shoes that protect the feet have hard soles and fit well enough to give all parts of your foot, including bony outgrowths, enough room without squeezing. Shoes should not be too loose, either, because loose shoes can cause a blister or ulcer if they slide back and forth on your foot as you walk. We recommend shoes made of leather, which breathes better and takes on the shape of the foot more readily than synthetic materials.

If you can't tell whether your shoes fit right, ask for assistance from a knowledgeable salesperson. Break in new shoes slowly, wearing them for only two to three hours at first, and inspect your feet afterward for areas of redness. It is best to alternate between two or three pairs of shoes throughout the day, especially if you have new shoes.

Things do get inside shoes—pebbles, pennies, buttons, pins, and sharp objects that have been stepped on and have pierced through the sole. So before putting your shoes on, give them a shake and take a quick look inside each shoe.

The most important point about shoes is to wear them! *Never* go barefoot if your feet have lost feeling. Avoid walking barefoot on a lawn or beach or even in your own house—these are all areas where objects on the ground can cause a break in your skin if you step on them. It's not worth the risk. Wear shoes, or at least slippers.

Foot Hygiene

Daily bathing of your feet is an important measure in reducing the risk of infection. Wash them as thoroughly as you wash your hands. Dry carefully between your toes. Bacteria and fungi like moisture. Don't make it easy for them.

Trim your toenails by filing them even with the top of the toes. Round the edges slightly so the nails don't dig into the next toe. The best time is after bathing, when your nails are soft and clean. Using scissors or clippers is not recommended, as any slip could cause a break in the skin and create a point of entry for bacteria.

Some people think of themselves as bathroom surgeons. They'll get out razor blades or knives and try to whittle away at a callus or cut out an ingrown nail. Avoid doing so. It may not cause pain, especially if your foot is numb, but cuts in the foot can lead to serious infections.

It also is not advisable to use chemical agents that promise to make a corn or callus disappear, since they can injure your healthy skin too. If you need care beyond trimming your toenails, see a foot specialist: a podiatrist, a specially trained nurse, or an orthopedist. A corn or callus is an indication of a high-pressure area that should be treated.

Sometimes dry skin is a problem. It can crack, creating an entry for bacteria. You can moisturize dry skin by applying a thin layer of lotion, petroleum jelly, or lanolin after bathing to seal in the moisture. Don't put it between your toes, as this can cause the skin to break down. Soaking your feet is not recommended either. Ironically, soaking the feet actually causes the skin to become *more* dry because it removes the natural protective oils from the skin. If you have sweaty feet, your feet may do better if you use a small amount of foot powder or antiperspirant.

Make sure your socks do not become a source of injury. Socks that are too loose and create wrinkles and socks with holes or seams can all cause sores. Socks should be clean, smooth, without holes, and appropriate for the shoes being worn.

Inspect Your Feet

Daily foot inspection is very important. If you have neuropathy, you can't rely on your feet to tell you that something is wrong. You have to use your eyes (or somebody else's) and hands to check for problems.

Go over your feet systematically: top, bottom, and between your toes. Check for areas of redness, openings, warm or hot spots, overgrown calluses, ingrown toenails, or discoloration. If you can't maneuver to see the bottom of your feet, use a mirror. This only takes a few seconds. Report any worrisome changes to your physician or podiatrist. It's better to treat small problems quickly so they don't turn into big problems. At office visits, take off your shoes and socks as a reminder to your health care professional to inspect your feet; if you need to, *ask* him or her to do so. It's important.

Be aware of what comes in contact with your feet. Test your bath water with a sensitive area on your hands or with a thermometer before stepping into it. Hot water can scald the feet, and very cold water can cause blood vessel constriction. If you have cold feet, wear socks. Heating pads and hot water bottles can cause burns.

Improving Circulation

Narrowing of the arteries is to some extent reversible. The quickest and probably most effective thing you can do is stop smoking. The next most effective thing is exercise, which causes new blood vessels to grow, creating bypass routes around small blockages in the arteries. This is called *collateral circulation*, a remarkable nonsurgical bypass phenomenon.

While massage feels good and may help you relax, it doesn't do anything to promote circulation. Neither does elevating your legs (although putting your feet up can reduce swelling). To encourage new blood vessel growth, you have to create a demand for more oxygen in the muscles by exercising vigorously. That means walking or cycling for a sustained period, stopping if you experience more than mild muscle soreness. Some people whose circulation is seriously reduced won't be able to exercise vigorously because of muscle pain caused by inadequate oxygen delivery. With the development of collateral circulation, the pain of claudication may decrease or go away.

Finally, avoid doing things that squeeze off blood flow. Tight bands at the top of socks or stockings will cause a mechanical constriction of the blood vessels. Crossing your legs or sitting on your leg can temporarily reduce circulation. The tingling sensation you get from a leg "falling asleep" is actually due to compression of a *nerve*, not an artery.

Treatments for Foot Trouble

What do you do if you find a problem when you inspect your feet? It depends on the nature of the problem, its seriousness, and how fast-changing it is. Most people aren't in a very good position to tell how serious a problem is, so our recommendation is *when you see a change that worries you, get professional help quickly*. Specifically, when you first see a foot ulcer, redness suggesting an infection, new loss of color, a significant break in skin, or any other sign of new change, see your health care professional. Treatment will vary depending on what is wrong and how serious it is, but the following are the most commonly prescribed treatments.

Antibiotics

Antibiotics are used for the treatment of infection or inflammation (*cellulitis*) that has resulted from bacteria entering the skin. For preventive care, topical antibiotic creams should be applied to areas of recently injured skin to help stop an infection from developing, until the skin has healed. Antibiotics are most effective if used at the earliest sign of infection (redness, warmth, swelling, tenderness, or fever), by mouth if the infection is not severe or intravenously in the hospital if it is a serious infection. Don't stop the prescribed course of antibiotics too soon, just because things look better. Discontinuing treatment too early can result in an immediate relapse.

Bed Rest and Elevation

This can be the most frustrating recommendation both for you, because of the limitations it places on your usual daytime activities, and for the doctor, because patients don't take it seriously. But when trying to get an infection or ulcer to heal, staying off your feet may be the most important thing you can do. Without question, staying off the affected foot helps it heal.

Debridement

Debridement is the removal of dead (*necrotic*) tissue from around the edge of an infected or ulcerated area. It eliminates a breeding ground for bacteria. For superficial infections, this can be accomplished quite easily. For deep infections, debridement may require anesthesia in an operating room. The procedure cleans up a wound, allowing healing to occur, and may have to be done several times.

Casting

Most of us think of casts only for broken bones. But they are also used very successfully in the treatment of foot ulcers. The rationale is to protect the area from external stress. The cast spreads the pressure and stress around. And because there's no mechanical jarring when moving the foot, the ulcerate area has a chance to grow new tissue and skin. Casts are put on in various ways. Usually they are walking casts, and sometimes they are bivalved (meaning they are in two pieces that are held together and are taken off at night). Be sure you are dealing with someone experienced in treating foot ulcers with casting: a poorly applied cast can do more harm than good.

Special Shoes

Your doctor may suggest special shoes, called *orthotics*, usually with extra depth. The extra room in the shoe is to accommodate an interior that can be molded to the exact shape of your foot. When the shoe makes full contact with the sole of your foot, your weight is more evenly distributed, decreasing the risk of pressure areas and skin breakdown. Sometimes, a shoe with a "rocker bottom" is prescribed, which will take some of the stress off the forefoot that results from normal walking movement. Orthotic shoes are expensive. A prescription from your doctor will let your insurance provider know that the shoes are medically necessary.

Vascular Surgery

In cases where the circulation is severely limited and the foot is not getting enough oxygen and nutrients, vascular surgery may be needed to prevent tissue destruction. An angiogram is the first step and is used to determine which blood vessel is involved, whether the blockage can be corrected, and whether the other vessels seem to be reasonably open. Often, in people with long-term diabetes, many arteries are affected rather than just one. This limits the surgeon's ability to correct the problem. As with so many of these treatment options, finding an experienced surgeon is essential to successful treatment.

Orthopedic Surgery

If you have a bone irregularity that is causing a projection vulnerable to skin breakdown, your doctor may suggest orthopedic surgery. The goal is to make the foot as even as possible so that body weight is more evenly distributed. The surgery may involve removal of bony projections or correction of deformities.

Hyperbaric Oxygen

Some medical centers use a procedure called *hyperbaric oxygen* to treat various nonhealing wounds, particularly of the feet, in people with diabetes. The treatment amounts to being enclosed in a chamber that has a high oxygen concentration at a high pressure. Each treatment takes 90 minutes, and often 20–30 treatment sessions are used. There are certain unusual conditions in which hyperbaric oxygen is a proven therapy, but its use in treating difficult wounds in diabetes is controversial.

Amputation

This chapter has emphasized preventive approaches that will greatly reduce your chance of ever needing an amputation. But amputations still are sometimes necessary, especially for older people with long-term diabetes that hasn't been well taken care of over the years. If doctors have talked to you about the possible need for an amputation, it is important for you to have some background and understanding of what it all means and what the options are. An understanding of the facts should make this less scary for you than worrying about the unknown.

Types of Amputation

There are many kinds of amputations and many surgical approaches. Some are minor, some major. They are always done while you're under either general or local anesthesia, so the procedure itself doesn't hurt. Depending on how large a portion of the foot is involved, the amputations may involve only one toe or just part of one toe, the full toe and its connecting bone in the foot, half the foot (*transmetatarsal amputation*), the whole foot and part of the lower leg (*below the knee amputation*), or the foot and lower leg (*above the knee amputation*).

The amount of disability that follows is related to what is removed. This is important to understand, because the very word *amputation* may be so frightening that its actual significance is blown out of proportion. The amputation of a toe, for example, rarely leaves any disability at all. It's far better to lose a toe than to have the significant risk of a toe infection spreading to your entire foot.

When Is an Amputation Considered?

An amputation may be recommended in two general situations: when an infection is out of control or has no likelihood of healing and when gangrene has set in. Sometimes infections can be aggressive, showing signs of spreading despite repeated debridement and intravenous antibiotics. Sometimes the infection is not so aggressive but still is not curable; in this case, there is more time to consider the options, but one option may be to remove the bone, as mentioned above.

Gangrene occurs when tissues die. The area becomes black, lacks feeling, and cannot "come to life again." Gangrene can also be a breeding ground for infection. Sometimes, a gangrenous toe can just be left to *autoamputate*, just as a deadened fingernail will eventually drop off. More often, surgeons need to amputate a gangrenous toe or even the foot. They may want to wait until it *demarcates*, meaning that a clear border is established between dead and live tissue.

Will One Amputation Lead to Another?

This is a real concern, for the patient and doctor alike. Depending on the seriousness of the underlying problem, there is always the chance that after an operation, the wound will not heal and further amputation will be needed later. The importance of having an experienced surgeon cannot be overemphasized. The object is to remove *all* the diseased tissue to the point where healthy tissue remains that can heal over the wound.

There is really no way for us to generalize about the chances that one amputation will be followed by another—it depends so much on the specific situation. You should talk to your surgeon, get his or her opinion, and remember that no one can be absolutely sure.

Rehabilitation and Life after an Amputation

Without being overly optimistic, we do want to emphasize that life will go on and that life can be very good indeed despite an amputation. After a small amputation—for example, a toe—the scars are psychological more than physical. Normal activities probably won't be affected at all. With more extensive amputations, the opportunities for rehabilitation today—with an artificial limb, for example—are truly extraordinary. People may learn to walk virtually normally, so that those around them may be completely unaware that they have an artificial limb. Some individuals suffer from *phantom limb pain*, in which the nerves continue to give signals that make the brain think there's still a limb there, even though it has actually been removed. This is relatively unusual and generally decreases or goes away over time.

So, amputations are definitely not the end of the line. If this is something you are thinking about, consider the facts of the situation very carefully and talk about it thoroughly with your family members and physician. The right answer will usually become clear. If, for example, it becomes evident that your toe or your foot is just not going to get better and is never going to cause anything but pain and more risk, then there's not much sense in delaying the inevitable. Better to move on to rehabilitation and the rest of your life.

• • •

Diabetes increases the risk of foot problems, but with good self-care, amputations are certainly not inevitable. The underlying problem is that neuropathy can make the foot numb, increasing the chance of undetected trauma, and decreased circulation can slow healing and promote infection. If you have neuropathy and poor circulation, attentive foot care is essential for prevention. You may be used to thinking *on* your feet, but we recommend that you get into the habit of thinking *for* your feet.

The objective is to prevent any breakdown of the skin that could initiate a nonhealing wound. Early detection of problems is critically important so that aggressive treatment measures can be taken to prevent progression. Remember, numb feet won't give you the early warning that a foot problem is starting. You have to be vigilant. When you see a problem, get it taken care of quickly—by your health care professional or even at an emergency room. Prevention and early treatment are the keys to staying on your feet!

Take Home Messages

- Foot problems are among the most common reasons that people who have diabetes are hospitalized.
- Foot problems are more common in people with diabetes for two reasons: nerve damage (peripheral neuropathy) and poor circulation.
- Nerve damage ranges from mild tingling to complete loss of feeling. Loss of feeling makes walking more difficult and foot injuries more likely.
- Poor circulation increases the risk that small infections will not heal well.
- Not smoking, exercising regularly, and controlling cholesterol and blood pressure levels lower your risk for circulatory problems.
- Always wearing well-fitted shoes and washing, carefully drying, and inspecting your feet daily lower your risk for serious foot problems.

27

Diabetes and the Skin

with Laila Tabatabai, M.D.

- "What are those bumps where I take my insulin?"
- "Now that my blood sugars are down, my skin feels better—less itchy and less of those awful fungal infections."
- "My skin gives me fits. Are all my problems due to diabetes?"

People with diabetes often have skin problems, including itching, dryness, and infections. If your skin looks just the way you want it to and doesn't hurt or itch, you probably don't think about it very much. For most people, however, their skin doesn't look or feel just right. And for people who have diabetes, it's often difficult to know which skin problems are due to diabetes and which are due to unrelated conditions. In this chapter we take a closer look at the skin—our most vulnerable as well as our most visible organ. If you have a skin problem that's not mentioned here, see your primary care physician or a dermatologist.

Skin Changes Due to Insulin Injections

Christine has noticed a few things about her skin. At age 55, after 22 years of multiple daily insulin injections, she occasionally gets a bruise where she injects, but that doesn't bother her. She has also noticed, though, that she has a fairly distinct band of fat just below her navel, extending about 10 inches across her abdomen. As much out of curiosity as vanity, Christine wonders why she has gained fat in just this one spot. She also wonders why the skin at the top of her arm, where she used to take her insulin every day, is so tough and has areas of depression.

Christine is noticing some of the most common skin consequences of taking insulin by injection. These include occasional bruising, lipohypertrophy, and lipoatrophy.

Bruising

Insulin injections sometimes cause a small bruise at the site of injection. This is due to a tiny blood vessel being nicked by the needle. It doesn't cause a significant problem unless some of the injected insulin enters right into the bloodstream through the nicked vein, in which case it will have a quicker-than-usual effect on blood glucose. The bruise will heal before long. This problem is avoidable, though. Look to see if a drop of blood appears at the site of injection. If so, apply some pressure right over the site to keep the blood from spreading in the skin, causing the bruise. Taking a blood thinner such as warfarin (Coumadin) or even daily aspirin may increase your tendency to bruise. Bruising is usually not a major problem.

Lipohypertrophy

Lipohypertrophy is the accumulation of fatty tissue where insulin is injected. The cause is thought to be the normal activity of insulin in stimulating the growth of fatty tissue. It may be a fairly large area and is soft and painless. Lipohypertrophy may not be present at all, may be barely noticeable, or may become very obvious if you look at your skin closely. Usually, lipohypertrophy can be avoided simply by changing the sites of injection.

Lipoatrophy

Lipoatrophy is the opposite of lipohypertrophy: it is the loss of the normal fat under the skin due to insulin injections. It appears as a slightly depressed area of skin, with a firm or fibrous feel to it. There is strong evidence that lipoatrophy may be an immunological response to the insulin. It is also partially due to repeated trauma to the skin by injecting insulin in one spot. Lipoatrophy has become uncommon with the use of purified, human insulins. Note that insulin injected directly into an atrophic area is erratically absorbed, so other injection sites should be used.

There is a very unusual form of diabetes called *lipoatrophic diabetes* in which the whole body is lacking in fat tissue. People with this form of diabetes look very muscular, but this is just because they have no fat smoothing out the muscle. They may require very high doses of insulin.

Skin Reactions to Oral Diabetes Medications

Reactions to oral diabetes medication are extremely rare. Metformin has been reported to cause erythema multiforme, an allergic reaction that can cause fever, itching, and many areas of skin that look like hives, bull's-eye sores, or blisters. Metformin can also (rarely) cause a drug rash that resembles psoriasis, causing red plaques with silvery white scales. Sulfonylureas such as glimepiride and glipizide can cause photosensitivity (sensitivity to the sun); the skin becomes more susceptible to sunburn. Sulfonylureas can also cause a lichenoid drug eruption, a rash that resembles shiny, purple papules that can have a network of white lines over them. If any kind of skin rash occurs shortly after you start taking a pill for diabetes, immediately contact the health care provider who prescribed it. Most skin reactions to medications are reversible and will disappear when the pill is stopped.

Dry Skin (Xerosis) and Itching (Pruritus)

More than 25% of people with diabetes have dry skin and itching. High blood glucose levels cause dehydration, which worsens dry skin (xerosis). Dryness can also be caused by decreased sweat gland activity due to autonomic nerve damage. The autonomic nerves are involved in the body's sweating and temperature regulation systems; these nerves are damaged by longstanding high blood glucose. Diabetic neuropathy can also damage nerve fibers, which leads to itching (pruritus).

Whatever the cause, dry and itchy skin can be dangerous because it is susceptible to cracking or breaking, which increases the risk of infection. People with neuropathy or poor circulation in their hands and feet should take special care of their skin, inspecting their feet daily for any cuts, scrapes, or ulcers (see Chapter 26). We recommend the use of mild, moisturizing soaps. Regular moisturizing can also help reduce itching, dryness, and cracks in the skin.

Fungal Infections

Dewayne called us, worried about athlete's foot. He is a 17-year-old high school student and was concerned because of what he's heard about foot infections and diabetes. He takes good care of his blood glucose levels. He is reassured by the information that athlete's foot is responsive to over-the-counter medica-

tions; that since his control has been good, the infection may not be due to his diabetes; and that with proper care, it does not pose a threat to his feet.

A fungal infection of the skin can appear as a red, itchy rash. Fungal infections often develop under the nails or between the toes. These infections are more frequent in people who have diabetes simply because a fungus needs sugar to grow and multiply; the skin's epidermal layer is high in sugar in people with uncontrolled diabetes. Fungi also multiply more in areas high in moisture and for that reason are more typically found in skin folds, such as under the breasts, in the armpits, in the genital and groin area, and between the toes. Candida (also called monilia) is a common yeast that causes skin infections. *Intertrigo* is the name given to a rash due to candida that develops between two skin surfaces in contact with each other.

The best way to prevent and treat fungal infections is by controlling your blood glucose levels and carefully washing and drying your skin. Wearing cotton underwear may help reduce skin irritation, since cotton "breathes" and allows air to circulate better. Vaginal yeast infections are more common in women with diabetes. You should avoid using vaginal douches or feminine hygiene sprays, unless specifically prescribed, because they can alter the pH balance of the vagina and set the stage for increased fungal growth.

As noted in Dewayne's story, superficial fungal infections such as athlete's foot respond very well to over-the-counter medications. If left untreated, however, they can become chronic and more difficult to eradicate. Sometimes fungal infections cause small, invisible fissures to develop in the skin, especially on the feet, which serve as an entrance port for bacteria. This can cause bacterial skin infections (cellulitis) or even infections of bone. If you have any doubts about skin infections, talk with your primary care physician or dermatologist.

Vitiligo

Vitiligo is a patchy depigmentation of the skin. Areas with vitiligo look completely white and do not become tanned when exposed to sun. Vitiligo is an immune problem of the skin, just as Type 1 diabetes is an immune process involving the pancreas. Vitiligo is more common in people with Type 1 diabetes than in those without it. There is presently nothing that can be done to alter its course, though staying out of the sun (so the unaffected skin doesn't get even darker in contrast) will make it less noticeable. It is especially important to have a physician make this diagnosis because vitiligo can be confused with fungal infections.

If you have vitiligo, be sure to cover the depigmented area carefully with a sun block. Skin lacking normal pigmentation is extremely sensitive to sunlight.

Necrobiosis Lipoidica Diabeticorum (NLD)

Necrobiosis lipoidica diabeticorum is a skin condition that is characteristic of diabetes, usually Type 1. NLD has a distinctive appearance: it is usually located on the shins or ankles and appears as a patch, ranging from ½ inch to 3–4 inches in diameter, of brownish-purple to violet skin with clearly demarcated edges. It comes on gradually over weeks, often in people who have had Type 1 diabetes for a short period.

NLD is usually not itchy or painful. Occasionally the skin may become so thin that an ulcer forms. NLD can be treated with steroid creams or injections, phototherapy, or immunosuppressive medications, drugs that block the immune system's action on the skin. It is very important to have NLD examined by a dermatologist periodically because, in some cases, it can undergo changes leading to squamous cell skin cancer.

Shin Spots (Diabetic Dermopathy)

Up to 10% of people with diabetes have *diabetic dermopathy*, the development of pigmented spots, about ½ inch or less in diameter, on the shins. These spots aren't as big as those in NLD and do not go through a phase of being purple. Diabetic dermopathy should raise concern because its presence increases the likelihood that the person also has diabetic complications in the eyes, kidneys, nerves, and blood vessels.

Xanthelasma and Eruptive Xanthomas

Xanthelasma is the name for the small yellow bumps that some people develop on the eyelids or at the inner corner of the eyes, by the nose. This condition can run in families. Xanthelasma may indicate high blood cholesterol, so people who have these spots should have their cholesterol level checked.

Eruptive xanthomas are yellow to red bumps on reddish skin, usually on the buttocks, arms, or legs. These occur when blood lipid levels, specifically triglycerides, are high. Treatment includes eating a healthier diet, exercising more regularly, and taking medications to control high blood glucose and triglyceride levels. Laser therapy can be used to remove xanthomas that remain after these other treatments.

Loss of Hair on the Head (Alopecia)

The condition doctors call *alopecia* is what most people know simply as hair loss, occurring abnormally and often in clumps. It is different from normal male balding. It is seen occasionally in people with Type 1 diabetes, in uncontrolled diabetes of any type, or as a result of other significant stresses. The cause of alopecia is not well understood. Alopecia associated with diabetes is usually mild and tends not to worsen with time.

Skin Tags (Acrochordons)

Skin tags (acrochordons) are soft, skin-colored, benign tumors (growths) of the skin commonly found on the neck, in the armpits, in the groin area, and on the eyelids. High blood glucose levels can lead to increased multiplication of skin cells. In fact, there is a direct correlation between fasting blood glucose level and the number of skin tags: higher blood glucose causes more skin tags to develop. These are completely harmless and can be removed by cryosurgery (freezing) for cosmetic reasons.

Finger Pebbles

Some people with diabetes have thickened skin on their fingers, which can lead to small papules or "pebbles" on the fingers and knuckles. These papules can develop because of higher levels of insulin, which cause the formation of increased amounts of collagen (a protein that makes up the skin). High blood glucose can also bind to collagen, which can lead to skin thickening. When this condition occurs on the neck, upper back, and shoulders, the skin becomes thickened and raised, and the condition is called scleredema diabeticorum. These skin changes are most commonly found in obese men with Type 2 diabetes and can be treated with low-dose steroids or UV light therapy.

Lichen Planus

There is a strong association between diabetes and *lichen planus*, collections of shiny, purple papules (bumps) that may have a network of white lines overlying them. The papules appear on the wrists and ankles. Oral lichen planus affects the mouth and causes whitish plaques to form. Oral lichen planus should be evaluated by a dermatologist because it can (rarely) undergo a malignant change to oral cancer. Lichen planus can be treated with steroids and phototherapy.

Acanthosis Nigricans

Acanthosis nigricans is a skin condition that occurs in people with obesity and Type 2 diabetes. It is a velvety-feeling increase in pigmentation (a darkening of the skin), most often located around the back of the neck and in the armpits; it is more common among African Americans. Acanthosis nigricans can indicate a high level of insulin resistance, a key component of Type 2 diabetes. This benign condition does not require any specific treatment. Prescription creams are used for cosmetic reasons only.

Take Home Messages

- The skin is our most vulnerable as well as our most visible organ. It can be damaged by almost anything, from sunlight to trauma.
- For people who have diabetes, most skin conditions occur infrequently and are not often seriously affected by the diabetes. However, it is important to pay attention to all skin changes because they can indicate poor blood glucose control or the presence of other diabetes complications (such as neuropathy, retinopathy, or nephropathy).
- Some skin conditions, including NLD and oral lichen planus, can lead to skin or oral cancer over time. A dermatologist should examine them. Other skin conditions can be evaluated and treated by a primary care physician or dermatologist.
- Almost all diabetes-related skin conditions improve when blood glucose control is improved through diet, lifestyle changes including exercise, and medications.

PART V

Sexuality, Pregnancy, and Genetics

At one of our first self-management programs at the Johns Hopkins Diabetes Center in 1986, a newly diagnosed, newly married 22-year-old man was sitting next to a 55-year-old man who'd had diabetes for 35 years. The 22-year-old was feeling panicked. He had heard on the street that people with diabetes couldn't have children. Luckily, the man he sat next to had eight children and six, going on seven, grandchildren. So much for rumors about diabetes and fertility!

There is so much emotion, as well as good and bad information, swirling around reproduction and heredity that we decided this topic deserved a section of its own in this book. People beyond their childbearing years won't be so interested in the fine points of managing diabetes during pregnancy, but older people are at least as concerned about the genetics of diabetes: what are the chances that my children and my children's children will get it.

Part V, then, deals with many aspects of sexuality, pregnancy, and genetics. We try to distinguish fact from rumor, we are realistic, and we are optimistic.

28

Diabetes and Sexuality

- "Sex is just not what it used to be. I hardly ever get excited any more, and even when I do, I almost never have an orgasm. I'm disappointed, and my husband is too."
- "When I became impotent it really shook me up. I feel I lost my manhood."
- "I haven't had an erection in four years, but my wife and I have learned there's more to sex than intercourse."

Diabetes can affect a person's libido, or interest in sex, as well as his or her physical ability to engage in sexual activity. What makes sex good or bad is complicated even if you don't have diabetes. When you do have diabetes, it is even more complicated. Some factors that make sexual problems more likely can affect anyone, whether they have diabetes or not—like depression, high blood pressure, being overweight, smoking, being physically inactive, hormonal changes associated with aging or menopause, taking certain medications, and alcohol consumption. All of these factors and others can contribute to sexual problems when you have diabetes, and some of them (depression, being overweight, being physically inactive) are somewhat more common in people with diabetes.

Some physical factors that are much more common in people who have diabetes increase the likelihood of sexual problems. These include high blood glucose levels and damage to nerves and small blood vessels. High blood glucose levels lead to feelings of fatigue and lack of energy. These don't do much for a person's interest in sex—or in most other activities, for that matter. Damage to autonomic nerves, those that signal the body to increase blood flow to the genitals, can hinder normal sexual function (erections in men, vaginal lubrication and sexual response in women). Reduced blood flow resulting from damage to small blood vessels can also contribute to these problems.

So, sexual problems are more common in people who have diabetes. We are not saying that everyone with diabetes has sexual problems, just that these problems are more common in people with diabetes. There are people with diabetes who have no sexual problems at all, and there are people without diabetes who have plenty of sexual problems.

The psychological aspect of sexuality is very important. We mentioned that depression can affect sexual interest and sexual performance. You won't be surprised to hear that sexual problems can affect your psychological well-being. Fortunately, there are things you can do to improve your sexual experiences by paying attention to both the psychological and the physical aspects.

Most people think about their sex life a lot but talk about it rarely, even with their partner. Some people find it hard even to bring up the subject with a health care professional. Sexual experiences are very important but very personal. We hope this chapter faces the issues squarely and helps you understand how diabetes might be affecting your sexual experience and puts you in a position to pursue available remedies.

Physical Consequences of Poorly Controlled Diabetes

As we've seen throughout this book, for people who have diabetes there are direct, immediate effects of high blood glucose. When it comes to sexual functioning, many of these symptoms can get in the way. The immediate effects of high blood glucose usually play out, for women as well as for men, as generalized fatigue, lack of energy, and feelings of whole-body exhaustion. And it doesn't help the mood when a person has to urinate every few minutes and is constantly thirsty. Low blood glucose levels can also lead to a decrease in sexual interest and, for men, difficulty with attaining or maintaining erections.

About Women

Latesha reluctantly mentioned to her doctor that her sex life was not good at all. She wanted to make her husband happy, but she had almost no desire, and when they did try intercourse, it really hurt and she got almost no pleasure. Latesha was not depressed and she did not have neuropathy, but her glucose control was not good, so the doctor told her that improved glucose control could help with her sexual problems. He also suggested she use a vaginal lubricant. By Latesha's next visit her glucose control was much improved and so was her sex life.

There are other problems for women with diabetes. For one thing, dryness in the mouth is often matched by vaginal dryness. In addition, when diabetes is out of control, a woman is very likely to develop vaginal infections (specifically, infections by the yeast candida or monilia—candidiasis or moniliasis). The itching and discomfort caused by these infections naturally make sex less appealing. But all these symptoms will improve when the blood glucose control improves.

High blood glucose levels maintained over months or years may also lower a woman's estrogen levels, which will cause inadequate vaginal lubrication. Diabetes isn't the only thing that can do this. All women have low estrogen levels following menopause or surgical removal of their ovaries (unless they receive hormone replacement therapy), and these women also suffer from reduced vaginal lubrication. You can use topical ointments to improve lubrication or estrogen replacement in the form of pills, patches, or vaginal creams. Internal lubricants, such as Replens, may help maintain a favorable pH balance in the vagina, but they are expensive. An alternative is to use a water-based gel on the outside or, for severe dryness, a vaginal suppository that you can insert before you have intercourse.

Poor glucose control can also cause menstrual irregularity or even absence of menstrual periods. Improving glucose control is the best way to remedy this, although your health care provider may prescribe artificial cycling with birth control pills.

Usually, the physical problems that lessen sexual enjoyment in diabetes are due to the acute, immediate effects of high blood glucose and will resolve when the diabetes is under better control. This is just another reason to get in control of your diabetes. For women, the only long-term complication of diabetes that can occasionally affect sexual function is neuropathy, which can affect the genital region. This condition may prevent adequate lubrication and orgasm.

Psychological factors also play a role. To enjoy sex, it's important to feel sexually attractive. For many women who have diabetes, being overweight can be a barrier to sexual enjoyment, even when it's more of a self-image problem than a lack of desirability in their partner's eyes.

We've mentioned depression and its potentially devastating effect on your sex life. Don't ignore the signs. Even mild depression may be playing a role.

What You Can Do

If you are not satisfied with any aspect of your sexual experience, the first thing to do is recognize that your sexual problems may be related to your diabetes. Knowing this can provide some relief right away. If the problem is high blood glucose, chances are you'll see a substantial improvement with better control—one more major incentive to engage in the work it takes to achieve that goal. If the problem is something else, like hormone issues, some of the suggestions we just offered could help. If neuropathy is contributing to your sexual problems, be sure to ask your physician for advice. If you are depressed, counseling, possibly combined with antidepressant medication, may help.

Whatever factors are contributing to your sexual problems, the key to resolving these problems is to talk about them. If you are in a relationship, talk to your partner. Talk with your health care provider. You'll probably have to bring up the topic yourself, especially if your physician is a man. A survey of physicians (both male and female) showed that 85% of them regularly asked their male patients about sex, but only 33% regularly asked their female patients the same question.

Finally, if you, your partner, and your diabetes health care provider have addressed the emotional and physical components of sex and things still aren't going well, we advise you to seek help from a mental health professional who is specially trained in dealing with sexual problems. It's always important to get a referral from your doctor or from the local teaching or community hospital and to find out about the counselor's background and experience. Many counselors will send you detailed printed information about these matters if you request it, so you can be an informed consumer before you make an appointment.

About Men

At the age of 62, after 20 years of life with diabetes, Joseph began to have a problem getting an erection. The problem was taking a toll on his self-esteem, so he finally brought it up with his doctor. The doctor told him that most men his age who had diabetes shared his problem, and she offered him some treatment options, including pills—Viagra (sildenafil), Levitra (vardenafil), or Cialis (tadalafil)—or a medication taken by injection, or devices that help make and maintain an erection.

Some of the emotional and physical problems caused by diabetes can decrease libido in men, just as they can in women. But for men, sexual problems are often more obvious because of the ability or inability to have an erection. Some men link having an erection to their image of what it means to be "a real man." Others take it much more in their stride, as just another part of the functioning of their anatomy. But there's no getting around it: a common long-term complication of poorly controlled diabetes is deterioration of potency—the inability to have or keep an erection, often referred to as erectile dysfunction.

Erection problems (being unable to achieve an erection or have an erection firm enough for sexual intercourse) are two to three times more common in men who have diabetes than in men who don't have diabetes. Half of all men with diabetes over the age of 50 have erection problems. Men who have diabetes are likely to develop the condition 10–15 years earlier than men who don't have diabetes.

We know the odds of experiencing erection problems increase with the duration of diabetes, high glucose levels, and the presence of autonomic neuropathy. Let's consider some facts.

Having and maintaining an erection is a complex process, involving psychological, hormonal, vascular, and nervous systems. To have an erection, *all* systems must be functioning well. Like most diabetes-related problems, interest in sex is affected by recent blood glucose control. Good control is generally associated with higher levels of libido and well-being, sexual and otherwise.

Erection problems can be permanent or temporary. Temporary problems can be caused by exhaustion, overconsumption of alcohol, ingestion of some prescription drugs, and worry, especially the worry that you might have problems getting or sustaining an erection.

If you have erection problems, you have to determine whether the cause is physical or psychological, or both. Don't shy away from the possibility that it is at least partly "in your head." The strongest, toughest men get just as stressed, depressed, and anxious as anyone else. You can start to find the answer by asking yourself these questions:

—Did the erection problem begin suddenly?

—Is the problem occurring on and off—sometimes or in some situations a complete problem, and in other situations no problem at all?

—Do you get an erection when you masturbate?

—Do you have erections during the night, when you wake up, or when you are especially sleepy or bored?

If your answer to any of these questions is yes, psychological factors are almost certainly at least a part of your problem. This is good to know because counseling and recognition of the psychological roots may lead to their correction. If you essentially never have erections (at night, when bored or sleepy, when fantasizing or masturbating), there is a physical problem. Tests can confirm whether erectile dysfunction is primarily psychological or physical. One test to determine whether you do have erections is relatively simple. You place a device called a snap gauge around your penis before you go to sleep at night. With each erection, the gauge will snap. Normally, a man has an average of four erections a night, each lasting 15–45 minutes. If you want to try the test yourself without buying a snap gauge, you can substitute a strip of postage stamps. Wrap the strip of stamps around your penis and seal it. If the stamps break apart at night, you've had an erection. Try this for several nights to be sure.

If diagnostic tests find a physical cause for your erectile dysfunction, your physician may arrange for other tests to determine whether hormone, blood vessel, or nerve problems are involved. Low blood testosterone (the primary male hormone) is usually not the cause, but if the doctor picks up signs or symptoms that are suggestive, a testosterone level can be measured.

How Diabetes Contributes to Erection Problems

Most men who experience erection problems want to know why. "It's the diabetes" or "It's psychological" usually aren't good enough answers. So let's look more specifically at how diabetes contributes to these problems.

As we noted above, emotional distress can play a role. We suspect that every man, and we do mean every man, has at one time or another questioned his ability to achieve or maintain an erection. Men with diabetes may have more than their share of questions about their ability, and they may find it particularly difficult to let themselves go sexually instead of constantly monitoring the state of their penis. This "performance anxiety" can, and often does, contribute to difficulty getting and sustaining an erection.

More general psychological factors such as anxiety or depression may also play a part. For men with diabetes, estimates of how often erectile dysfunction is caused by psychological factors vary widely. We see figures ranging from 10% to 67%. One reason is that psychological factors can *contribute* to erection problems even when they are not the sole cause.

Neuropathy is the most common *physical* cause of erection problems. The autonomic neuropathy that we discussed in Chapter 25 is usually associated with peripheral neuropathy and is a long-term complication of high blood glucose. Erection problems are partial at first, causing difficulty in maintaining an erection. The problem may fluctuate to some degree but is not particularly related to the situation: you may be very interested and aroused, but "the flesh just isn't willing." Over the years it can progress to complete inability to achieve an erection.

Vascular problems that interrupt blood flow to the penis also play a part. They are more common in older men with diabetes, especially those with heart disease or evidence of poor circulation to their feet. Hardening of the arteries (arteriosclerosis) blocks blood flow to the penis and prevents it from becoming erect and firm. Smoking is a major contributor to this problem.

You should also be aware that many prescription medications can contribute to erection problems, including blood pressure drugs such as beta-blockers and diuretics, some antidepressants, ulcer medications, and drugs to prevent vomiting. Be sure to talk with your physician about the possibility that these medications (or others) might be contributing to your erection problems.

A decrease in the male hormone testosterone may also cause erectile dysfunction, though this is a less common cause. Most men don't have a problem with their hormones, but this is something your doctor can easily check with a blood test.

What You Can Do

Remember that smoking may be the most important contributor to erection problems caused by blood vessel damage. So if you smoke, please stop. While sexual health is only one of many good reasons to quit smoking, maybe it's the one that will finally inspire you. Also be aware that even though alcohol and illicit drugs sometimes increase desire, they almost always decrease sexual performance.

There are several successful approaches to treating erectile dysfunction. Some primary care physicians can explain the options and make recommendations, or you may want to consult a urologist. To some extent the treatment can be based on understanding the specific cause; in other cases, though, it may be worth just trying a given therapy to see if it works.

Men with diabetes who are having erection problems can take oral medications like Viagra, Cialis, or Levitra. But, if you are taking heart medication, especially nitrates or nitroglycerin, using these drugs could be dangerous. Be sure to talk with your doctor before taking any of them.

Another successful approach is treatment with alprostadil, a medicine that causes blood vessels to expand. By increasing blood flow to the penis, this drug helps facilitate an erection. You can take alprostadil either by injection (Caverject, Edex, and Prostin VR), inserting the needle directly into the base of the penis, or as a suppository (MUSE), placing it into the opening at the tip of the penis.

Alprostadil delivered by injection results in an erection firm enough for sexual intercourse in more than 80% of men with erection problems, regardless of their age or the cause of the problem. When the drug is delivered as a suppository, it is about half as effective, with 30%–40% of men benefiting. Given by injection, the drug works within 5–20 minutes, producing an erection that lasts about an hour. The erection may persist after ejaculation. You should not use the drug more than two or three times a week, with at least 24 hours between each use. Side effects can include bruising and priapism (erections that take a long time to go away). You should get the medication through a prescription from your doctor, and you should receive careful instruction on its use.

There are vacuum constriction devices you can use to produce and maintain an erection. These devices look like a large, solid condom. The penis is inserted, and the device generates a vacuum to draw blood into the penis, with a band to prevent the blood from flowing out again until the band is removed. You can have intercourse with the band in place to help maintain the erection. Studies show that about 50%–80% of men are satisfied with the results of using these devices. There are two possible side effects. First, the band can leave a small area of bruising on the penis, though this is usually painless. Second, the band may decrease the force of your ejaculation, though this generally does not interfere with the pleasure of orgasm. If you buy a device without a prescription, make sure it has a "quick release" feature for the band.

Sex therapy may be helpful if you are able to have a normal erection during sleep, are in generally good health, and have a partner who is willing to be part of treatment. In such situations, where erection problems are likely to be caused at least in part by stress, sex therapy may be the best treatment option. In these cases, sex therapy resolves the problem 50%–70% of the time. Sex therapy is usually short-term, 5–20 sessions. During the session the counselor encourages you and your partner to practice better sexual communication skills and suggests exercises to do at home between sessions. When a man goes through counseling alone, the results are usually not as positive as when the therapy includes his partner. Some insurance companies cover sex therapy.

. . .

Feeling good about yourself is important, whether or not you have diabetes. And feeling happy and confident sexually may be an important part of feeling good about yourself. As we've noted here, there are many causes of erection problems in men and of an unsatisfactory sex life for women with diabetes. It is just as true that people's response to less sexual activity varies enormously. So, in your own thinking, be honest with yourself and know the facts. Your sex life does not define you as a person. It does not make you one bit more or less of a man or a woman. If it's important to you to have an active sex life, think of the things we have discussed in this chapter, talk over the issue with the appropriate person, and take action.

Take Home Messages

- Sexual problems are more common in people who have diabetes.
- Diabetes can affect a person's interest in sex and his or her physical ability to engage in sexual activity or enjoy this activity.
- Higher rates of depression, higher blood glucose levels, and higher rates of blood vessel damage and nerve damage contribute to higher rates of sexual problems in people with diabetes.
- Common sexual problems in women who have diabetes include discomfort during intercourse and reduced sexual desire and sexual pleasure.
- The most common sexual issue for men with diabetes is erection problems.
- There are effective treatments for the sexual problems experienced by people who have diabetes.

29

Diabetes and Pregnancy

with Reshmi Srinath, M.D.

- "I never even thought of diabetes until now. But here I am, 32 years old, 8 months pregnant, and now I have diabetes too."
- "Some people say you shouldn't get pregnant if you have diabetes, others say it's no big deal. I just want to know if the baby will be okay."
- "Will having a baby make my complications worse?"
- "I'll tell you what pregnancy with diabetes is like—it's as if the doctors want me to have a nine-month insulin reaction."
- "I think the 3 a.m. blood sugar check they make you do is just to get you ready for middle-of-the-night feedings."

For any woman, the very idea of pregnancy is both exhilarating and frightening. There is greater worry, though, if that pregnancy is complicated by diabetes. In this chapter we want to help you understand what is involved. We give you and your mate the right information so you can make informed decisions and take action to improve your odds. We'll say it again: every pregnancy is both beautiful and scary. We wouldn't dream of taking the wonder out of pregnancy, even if we could.

We also recognize that the pregnant woman isn't the only person who is anxious in a pregnancy: the expectant father is too (not to mention the grandparents-to-be). This chapter focuses on the *mother*, however. Although a father with diabetes may affect, to some degree, the chance of the child eventually developing diabetes (see Chapter 30), the father's diabetes has no effect on the pregnancy itself.

We start with a general description of how diabetes and pregnancy interact, summarizing the reasons for treating diabetes in pregnancy intensively. Then we discuss more specifically what you can expect, what goals to set, and how to take care of yourself. Our overriding message is this: *during pregnancy, you control your diabetes well and see your doctors regularly for two good reasons: your developing baby and yourself.*

First, some definitions are in order. *Gestational diabetes mellitus* (GDM) is diabetes first diagnosed during pregnancy. It is usually a signal that Type 2 diabetes may develop later in the woman's life. *Pregestational diabetes mellitus* refers to diabetes that exists before pregnancy—in other words, when a woman with known Type 1 or Type 2 diabetes becomes pregnant. Now let's take a closer look at these different kinds of diabetes in pregnancy.

Gestational Diabetes Mellitus

Gestational diabetes mellitus usually comes on in the last half of pregnancy, when the fetus is growing larger. Testing for GDM has become routine in the health professional's office, not only by looking for glucose in the urine with a urinalysis but also by doing a screening test with an oral glucose challenge, usually in weeks 24–28 of pregnancy. Urine glucose is a very poor test for diabetes in pregnancy because many women without diabetes show some glucose in their urine when pregnant. Glucose in the urine may serve as a reminder, though, that all women should have the glucose challenge test as a screen during pregnancy. The challenge test uses a smaller amount of glucose (50 grams) than a full oral glucose tolerance test (OGTT), and only a single blood glucose is drawn 1 hour later. The test does not have to be done while fasting; it can be done at any time during the day. If the blood glucose is 140 mg/dl or more an hour after this challenge, a full 3-hour, 100-gram glucose OGTT is recommended.

Gestational diabetes mellitus is by far the most common form of diabetes in pregnancy: between 2% and 5% of all pregnant women in the United States develop it. GDM is usually a shock to the woman who gets it: it comes "out of the blue," in the middle of pregnancy.

Why Is GDM So Common?

In this book, when we talk about Type 2 diabetes we stress that resistance to the actions of insulin is the crux of the problem: the body responds poorly to normal amounts of insulin in the bloodstream. Obesity is perhaps the most common cause of insulin resistance, but pregnancy is another. In the case of pregnancy, the hormones made by the placenta counteract insulin, causing the resistance.

The same sequence that can lead to diabetes with obesity can cause it during pregnancy. If your pancreas is strong enough to increase its insulin output during pregnancy, it overcomes the resistance and you do not develop diabetes. But if the reserve of your pancreas is limited, if it is unable to increase its insulin production in response to the hormones produced during pregnancy, you may develop gestational diabetes.

The good news about developing diabetes during pregnancy is that the cause of the insulin resistance, the pregnancy, ultimately goes away (with delivery). In three out of four cases of GDM, the diabetes disappears at the end of pregnancy. So GDM is one of the few kinds of diabetes that is often temporary. The not-so-good news is that the reason GDM develops in the first place is that the pancreas has a reduced capacity to produce insulin. This is a signal that you are at high risk for developing diabetes later in life. This information should provide a special incentive for you to try to maintain normal body weight so that the insulin resistance caused by obesity does not tip over into diabetes. It also, of course, means that there is a high risk of developing diabetes with subsequent pregnancies. More than a third of women with GDM during one pregnancy will develop it again during their next pregnancy.

How GDM Affects Pregnancy

Gestational diabetes mellitus increases the risks of miscarriage and neonatal complications for the baby (this is discussed in more detail below). It should be taken seriously and should be treated quickly and effectively. The usual medications for Type 2 diabetes (oral antihyperglycemic agents) are not used to treat diabetes in pregnancy, for fear of damaging the fetus. So you will have to check your glucose often to see whether diet and exercise are working. If not, you will have to start injecting insulin.

Pregestational Diabetes Mellitus

Not all women with Type 1 diabetes enter into pregnancy on an equal footing. If you have diabetes and are thinking about becoming pregnant, there are some important questions you should ask yourself. You'll want to consider these questions with your loved one and with your doctor:

—How long have I had diabetes?
—What is my complication status?

—Am I prepared for the hard work involved in being pregnant with diabetes?

Dr. Priscilla White, one of the first practitioners to specialize in the field of diabetic pregnancy, developed a classification of complications and noted that, in general, the more long-term complications of diabetes a woman has at the start of pregnancy, the lower the chance of a successful outcome. Her finding makes sense. If your kidneys are significantly affected by diabetes (nephropathy) at the start of pregnancy, there is an increased chance of hypertension and toxemia (a serious progression of high blood pressure, with protein in the urine; also called preeclampsia). If you have severe retinopathy, vitreous hemorrhages may occur during pregnancy at an increased rate. If you have heart disease, it may become overburdened by pregnancy. Established long-term diabetes complications sometimes worsen during pregnancy. The evidence indicates, however, that the downturn, if any, reverses after the pregnancy is completed, so pregnancy does *not* actually cause a *permanent worsening* of long-term complications. Similarly, pregnancy does not cause new long-term complications where none existed. But if you already have significant or severe long-term complications, even the transient damage done during pregnancy (such as a major retinal bleed or serious toxemia of pregnancy) could affect your long-term health. If you have retinopathy before pregnancy, you'll want an ophthalmologist to examine your eyes before you become pregnant and regularly during your pregnancy.

Our advice generally is that if you have late stage diabetes complications, you need to consider carefully whether starting a pregnancy is really a risk you want to take. We know women who have successfully completed pregnancies despite serious long-term complications of diabetes, but it can be dangerous for the mother. If you are generally healthy and have diabetes, pregnancy is a perfectly viable option.

Healthy Baby, Healthy Mother

There's not much question about what you want out of pregnancy is there? A happy, healthy baby. It's also important for *you* to stay healthy so that you can raise your child and enjoy your grandchildren. These are not trivial matters.

As we mentioned above, every woman is somewhat anxious about pregnancy. Will I carry the pregnancy to term, or will I miscarry? Will the delivery be normal? And, most important of all, will the baby be normal? No person, and certainly no health care professional, can guarantee a normal pregnancy. But we can talk about your chances. To a considerable extent, you and your health care team can work together to improve the odds. Good health care, after all, is about improving your chances and your baby's chances.

No one can ever know the exact odds of having a healthy baby, since so many factors contribute. Some people don't want to know much at all; they accept the mystery of pregnancy and are happy to take the chance, whatever it is. Others want to know all the facts. Our approach to healthy living with diabetes is that the more you know, the better off you'll be. Here, then, are some guidelines.

Spontaneous Miscarriage

About 16% of apparently normal pregnancies (without diabetes) are lost through spontaneous miscarriages. Many miscarriages occur early in pregnancy, often before the woman knows she is pregnant, and in most cases the fetus had a lethal abnormality, meaning that the abnormality was not compatible with life. It's encouraging to know that for women with well-controlled pregestational diabetes, the spontaneous miscarriage rate does not seem to be any higher than for women without diabetes. (GDM doesn't occur until the middle of pregnancy, when the risk of miscarriage is lower.) The chances of losing a pregnancy are much greater if you don't control the diabetes very closely throughout the pregnancy and if you don't get good, regular prenatal care. As we discuss below, the chance of carrying a pregnancy successfully with diabetes increases directly with good blood glucose control.

Congenital Malformations

The other serious issue is whether the child will be born with any malformations, called *congenital anomalies*. These are divided into minor and major anomalies. In the minor category are small skin discolorations or a webbed toe that can easily be corrected. Minor congenital malformations do not require major surgery and have no long-term impact on the child. Major congenital anomalies include such important medical problems as heart or intestinal abnormalities, spina bifida and other vertebral bone abnormalities, or severe cleft lip and cleft palate.

The chance of major congenital abnormalities is in the range of 2%–3% without diabetes but increases to as much as 5%–13% with poorly cared-for pregestational diabetes. Most studies show that good diabetes care before conception reduces the chance of major congenital malformations to a range of 1%–5%. We want to emphasize that such estimates of odds are very inexact and may not apply to a particular individual.

Macrosomia

Macrosomia is the technical term for an abnormally large, fat baby. What does abnormally large mean? To some extent it depends on the size of the parents: big parents normally have big babies. It also depends on whether the delivery is premature. But generally speaking, a baby who weighs more than 10 pounds at birth is considered large. For generations, macrosomia has been known to be a complication of diabetic pregnancy. Now we know not only that it happens and what complications it can cause but also *why* it happens.

When a woman's blood glucose is high during pregnancy, that glucose passes through the placenta to the developing fetus. Because the fetus is constantly bathed in high-glucose blood, its own developing pancreas is constantly stimulated to produce more and more insulin (which stays on the fetal side of the placenta, not passing through to the mother). The high levels of glucose and insulin in the fetal blood cause more fat to develop. The baby is born large and will often have larger shoulders. More specifically, the baby is born *fat*; other than the fat tissue, the baby's organs are not overly large, and in fact may be underdeveloped due to the effects of high glucose levels during pregnancy. However, if the woman's diabetes is well controlled, this cycle never occurs, and the baby is often born with a normal body weight.

Complications during Delivery and in the Neonatal Period

The complication rate is increased in deliveries of a large baby, especially to a small mother. Sometimes the labor is more difficult. Sometimes it takes longer for the actual birthing. And sometimes the baby is just too large to be delivered vaginally, requiring a cesarean section.

There are also more complications than normal in the first few days and weeks of life. These fall into two categories: neonatal hypoglycemia and complications of prematurity. The hypoglycemia results from the activity of the baby's pancreas, which has been producing large amounts of insulin to try to correct the high blood glucose environment experienced throughout gestation. Outside the womb, this pumped-up pancreas can well cause hypoglycemia before it readjusts to the baby's own normal blood glucose levels. This is especially likely if the mother's blood glucose is high at the time of delivery. Hypoglycemia shouldn't be a problem if the mother's diabetes was well controlled during the pregnancy, and even if neonatal hypoglycemia does occur, it can be managed in a modern newborn nursery.

It's often surprising when complications of prematurity develop in the baby of a mother with poorly controlled diabetes, since the baby appears to be large, healthy, and anything but premature. As mentioned above, though, this is not necessarily a mature baby, it is a fat baby. The internal organs may be underdeveloped and underfunctioning at birth; this can include underdeveloped lungs and respiratory distress syndrome.

The Mother's Blood Glucose Control throughout Pregnancy

Very early in the pregnancy (in the first 4–8 weeks), as the fetus's vital organs are developing, high blood glucose levels increase the chance of these organs developing abnormally. There is a relationship between a woman's distinctly poor blood glucose control during early pregnancy and congenital malformations. It is therefore worthwhile to strive for the best blood glucose control possible as the fetal organs are developing and to start this effort even before conception: fetal organs develop very early, often before you know you are pregnant. The recommendation, then, is to *establish excellent blood glucose control before attempting pregnancy*.

In middle and late pregnancy (3–9 months), the mother's blood glucose control has a direct effect on the *size* of the developing fetus. Obstetricians therefore work closely with pregnant women to ensure that their diabetes is well controlled during this period to prevent large-baby complications at delivery. Good control is also good for the mother.

The Healthy Mother

We have described the "odds" of having a successful pregnancy in diabetes. But for any individual woman, the only statistic that matters is her specific pregnancy. There is no doubt that pregnancy can be successful despite diabetes; the odds, overall, are about 95% in your favor. For some couples, especially if the woman has severe long-term complications of diabetes or if other options, such as adoption, are attractive, trying for a pregnancy may seem ill advised. For many others, if the woman does not have established, long-term complications and if she is willing to work hard on her blood glucose control, pregnancy is not only possible but likely to work out well.

Care before conception, or *preconception care*, is important for all women—but for women with diabetes, it is crucial. Plan a pregnancy, establish good blood glucose control *before* pregnancy, and recognize the pregnancy as soon as possible. Then, once you've conceived, prenatal care—caring for you and the fetus during pregnancy—begins.

We know it's a tough road, demanding even more attention to diabetes than you ever thought possible. But the successful pregnancy with the birth of a healthy child is about as great a reward as we can think of. So we'll discuss what to expect, what goals to set, and how to achieve them.

What to Expect in a Pregnancy with Diabetes

Nine months can seem like an eternity when you are going through it: just imagine 2,160 blood glucose tests, 840 snacks, 25 doctor's visits, sonograms, cravings, fatigue, and nausea. But when you stop to consider what happens during that time, it's amazing that it doesn't take longer. In only nine months, a baby develops in your uterus—from two little cells that came together at conception to a baby boy or girl.

There will be profound physical changes in your body to support it all. Obviously, your pregnancy will be apparent in your waistline, your breasts, and your enlarged uterus. There will be an increase in your blood volume and heart rate (this can sometimes stress your heart if it isn't fully well to begin with). And there will be an increase in your body's fat stores, which is nature's adaptation to protect the fetus if a period of starvation should occur during pregnancy.

Huge hormonal changes also take place in pregnancy, regulating the growth of the new body inside your womb and keeping a supply of glucose available for you and your baby. A direct effect of these hormones of pregnancy, however, is the predictable increase in your insulin requirement (if you take insulin) late in pregnancy. We discuss this in more detail later.

Finally, pregnancy puts a stress on your body as a whole. It can change your diabetes complications status: retinopathy may worsen (usually temporarily), and hypertension or toxemia can develop, especially if you had protein in your urine before pregnancy.

Blood Glucose Goals in Pregnancy

All the usual prenatal care guidelines apply to pregnant women with diabetes: regular visits to your health professionals, a healthful diet, vitamins, and so on. But with diabetes you have another area of concern: controlling your blood glucose as tightly as possible. Having very specific control goals can help in this effort.

The ultimate blood glucose goal, of course, amounts to nothing short of perfection: the same glucose levels found in a pregnant woman who doesn't have diabetes (these levels are lower than normal blood glucose levels in the nonpregnant state). Here are the targets:

—Before breakfast: less than 95 mg/dl
—Before lunch, supper, and bedtime snack: 60–100 mg/dl
—One hour after meals: less than 140 mg/dl
—Two hours after meals: less than 120 mg/dl
—2 a.m. to 6 a.m.: 60–100 mg/dl

If you have gestational diabetes, you may be able to achieve these targets fairly regularly. This is because GDM, like Type 2 diabetes, is intrinsically easier to manage, since the pancreas can still make insulin and blood glucose levels are relatively stable. But if you have pregestational diabetes—in other words, if you had Type 1 or Type 2 diabetes before the pregnancy—you may be thinking that these targets are impossible. Our answer is that these are *targets*, not levels required for every successful pregnancy. In fact, brief elevations of blood glucose are unlikely to cause you to lose a pregnancy. Also, tolerance to insulin reactions (low glucose levels) is better during the second and third trimesters, so tight blood glucose control can be achieved more safely. As with all parts of diabetes self-care, we suggest that you do the very best you can.

Avoiding high ketones is also important during pregnancy. Recall that ketones are a by-product of fat breakdown. They increase in the blood and spill into the urine in two situations: when you are not eating enough calories and when you have a seriously inadequate amount of insulin in your body. Pregnancy has been described as a condition of "accelerated starvation" because the developing baby is siphoning off calories from the mother all day. Not eating enough (fasting) causes ketones to show up in the urine more quickly in pregnancy. There is a debate about whether these "ketones of fasting" pose a danger in pregnancies complicated by diabetes; the answer is probably not. However, spilling ketones into the urine because of inadequate insulin treatment—in other words, as a result of poor diabetes control (high blood glucose)—is a serious risk. Ketoacidosis (see Chapter 21) during pregnancy, when ketones not only increase but accumulate in the blood to the point of acid buildup, is associated with a high rate of loss of the pregnancy.

So keep an eye on your ketones by checking your urine daily. If it tests positive, figure out why. If you are not eating enough calories (and you have good blood glucose control), increase your dietary intake. If your blood glucose control is poor, improve it quickly and contact your doctor for guidance.

Prenatal Care with Diabetes

The largest and best-conducted study of blood glucose control in pregnancy made a surprising discovery: early in pregnancy, the mother's blood glucose levels did not have as important an effect as just *getting good medical supervision*. This does not mean that blood glucose doesn't matter; it just means that the whole package of good prenatal care is most important. Good prenatal care improves the chance of a successful pregnancy.

Having a good health care team is always the best way to ensure good diabetes care. During pregnancy the team is even more important. There is no way you can handle diabetes and pregnancy by yourself. You will need professional help—to understand diabetes care if you just developed GDM and to fine-tune your regimen if you have preexisting Type 1 or Type 2 diabetes.

You need to be sure that someone is "quarterbacking" the health care process for you, checking to be sure that you have the appropriate eye exams, urine tests for protein, and so on. Your blood glucose management can be handled by your obstetrician or by your primary care doctor, endocrinologist, or nurse educator team in conjunction with your obstetrician.

Let's consider the role of the new member on the health care team for a woman who has diabetes: the obstetrician. Although many women are well served during pregnancy and delivery by midwives and other health care professionals who are not physicians, for a woman who has diabetes complicating her pregnancy, close involvement of an obstetrician is essential. The medical issues are more complex, unpredictable, and dangerous than in a pregnancy not involving diabetes. A primary role of the obstetrician is to monitor your baby's progress during the pregnancy: most likely, at regular intervals, measuring the size of your abdomen, listening to the heartbeat, and recommending such tests as sonograms, alpha-fetoprotein, amniocentesis, and the contraction stress test. Let's consider each of these commonly done tests.

The sonogram. This is a harmless and painless ultrasound procedure. It amounts to sending sound waves through your skin and picking up their echo—much like a depth finder used in boats—to produce a picture of the fetus (it generally doesn't look much like the full-term infant you have in mind). Sonograms are used to estimate fetal size in comparison to fetal age and to inspect for malformations. Your doctor may also order a special sonogram called an *echocardiogram* to inspect the baby's heart more closely for defects. Like all tests, the sonogram is helpful but not perfect; some abnormalities cannot be picked up by a sonogram or any other test.

The alpha-fetoprotein test. This test is done at 16 weeks' gestation, with a simple blood sample drawn from your arm. The idea of the alpha-fetoprotein test may be scary and emotionally upsetting because its aim is to screen for defects in the baby's spinal column. In some cases the result is positive even in the absence of any defect. If it is positive, an amniocentesis is recommended to confirm or refute the presence of an abnormality in the developing fetus.

Amniocentesis. This procedure involves sampling the fluid surrounding the developing fetus (the *amniotic fluid*) along with cells from the fetus that float around in this fluid. It is done with a needle that looks formidably long, but the procedure is usually not particularly uncomfortable. By examining the fluid and the cells, doctors can determine several things: whether there is evidence of Down syndrome or other chromosomal abnormalities, whether the baby is a boy or a girl, and, near the end of pregnancy, whether the baby's lungs are ready for delivery. You may want to ask your obstetrician whether an amniocentesis would be a good idea; if the obstetrician suggests this test, of course, you'll want to know why. In any case, you choose which of the available results you want to know, including knowing the sex of the baby before birth.

The contraction stress test and nonstress test. These tests are done to assess whether the baby is developing normally and will respond normally to labor. The contraction stress test measures changes in the fetal heart rate during spontaneous or induced mild contractions of the uterus. It is a painless procedure done by attaching an electronic fetal monitor to your abdomen with a belt. The nonstress test is similar, except that the fetal heart rate is measured in response to the fetus's own movements rather than to contractions of the uterus. Other tests are also available to help the obstetrician decide whether the fetus is ready for delivery.

Timing of Delivery

The timing of delivery is the obstetrician's call. Many factors go into the decision, but the general preference is to let a pregnancy continue to term or near term. For a woman with diabetes, the old practice was to deliver the baby early to avoid a late-in-pregnancy death of the fetus. In recent years, however, it has become clear that this practice was misguided—that more problems arose from delivering too early than from letting the pregnancy progress.

Tests of fetal maturity are now quite sophisticated, and obstetricians can determine pretty well when a fetus is ready to be born. Unless an emergency develops, it would be unusual for a baby to be prematurely delivered just because the mother has diabetes; if an elective delivery (either by inducing labor or by cesarean section) is recommended, tests are usually done to be sure the baby is ready. (The ratio of cesarean section to vaginal delivery for women with diabetes is three to five times greater than for women without diabetes.) Again, the decision on the timing of delivery is best left to the obstetrician.

Common Problems in the Management of Diabetes in Pregnancy

Morning sickness, the "will I make it to the bathroom before I throw up?" feeling that is common in early pregnancy, can present a challenge if you have Type 1 diabetes and are trying to maintain your meal plan and control your blood glucose. (Recall that gestational diabetes usually doesn't show up until later in pregnancy.) The nausea may be worsened by high or low blood glucose levels or may *cause* a low blood glucose. Eating crackers or dry toast seems to help. Avoiding spicy and greasy food and eating smaller, more frequent meals may also be helpful.

Constipation plagues many women during pregnancy, whether or not they have diabetes. Your intestinal muscles are more relaxed, and your baby will press on your intestines with increasing intensity as the pregnancy progresses. Increasing your fiber intake along with your fluid intake often takes care of the problem. Gentle, regular exercise helps too.

In later pregnancy, the baby takes up so much room in your abdomen that it will compress the volume of your stomach, forcing some of the acids into your esophagus. The result is a burning sensation in the stomach or throat (heartburn). Again, eating smaller, more frequent meals helps, along with avoiding high-fat foods.

Achieving Tight Blood Glucose Control in Pregnancy

Any attempt at tight blood glucose control is hopeless without close self-monitoring of blood glucose, and this is especially true during pregnancy. For starters, you never really know where your blood glucose is if you don't test. Also, you need to know at what times during the day your glucose is too close to low so you can adjust your regimen to avoid hypoglycemia. Most health care professionals suggest that women test their blood glucose much more often during pregnancy. If you take insulin, it's recommended that you test glucose levels before and after meals, at bedtime, and at 3 a.m. We even advise a test before driving as well, because walking the line of tight control increases the risk of a serious low blood glucose at any time.

There are other ways than self-monitoring to test for average blood glucose control: hemoglobin A1c (glycated or glycosylated hemoglobin) and fructosamine assays (see Chapter 4). Recall that the hemoglobin A1c test assesses blood glucose control for a period of 8–12 weeks, which in pregnancy is too long to make the rapid corrections in treatment. The A1c value is also affected by changes in blood volume and age of the red blood cells during pregnancy. The fructosamine assay may be used to get a better indication of what has happened over the previous 2 weeks or so. In the end, though, self-monitoring of blood glucose is the way to find out about your up-to-the-minute control, day in and day out.

If you find your glucose levels increasing in a certain pattern—for instance, always high before breakfast—call your health care professional and adjust your regimen. If the levels are very high (and by this we mean, in pregnancy, over about 180–200 mg/dl), take corrective action right away. You don't want to go too long with inadequate diabetic control, and you certainly don't want to slip into ketoacidosis. Ketoacidosis can occur during pregnancy with blood glucose levels not much over 200 mg/dl.

Diet

A healthful diet in pregnancy is one that meets your nutritional needs, helps keep your blood glucoses stable, *and* provides for the growth of your baby. Your total weight gain and pattern of weight gain are important measures of the adequacy of your diet, but they are not the only measures.

Calories and weight gain. You will need sufficient calories to support the growth of the baby and maintain nutrient stores in your own body. This means weight gain—about 30 pounds, more or less. Specific weight goals are individualized, depending on whether you are underweight, at ideal weight, or overweight before pregnancy. Set a target with your obstetrician.

Weight gain is usually minimal at first, peaks in mid-pregnancy at about a pound a week, and is a little slower thereafter. Generally, underweight women should gain the most, as they will need to add nutrient stores in the form of fat; overweight women do not need to gain as much because they probably have sufficient fat stores before pregnancy.

In deciding how to control your weight gain, consider that your caloric requirements increase by an average of about 300 calories per day. However, needed intake will vary considerably depending on your physical activity, resting metabolic rate, and pre-pregnancy weight. Your doctor and dietitian will help you estimate caloric requirements for your pregnancy, given your usual intake and activity.

Bear in mind that pregnancy is not the time to lose weight. Some people, especially when confronted with the need to keep their diabetes under especially good control, mistakenly restrict their calorie intake too much, endangering the pregnancy. Although weight loss may be a goal in the treatment of obesity, it is never a goal during pregnancy. Calories must be sufficient to meet the glucose demands of the growing baby. Measuring your urinary ketones in the morning is a good way to determine whether your calorie intake is sufficient to prevent the breakdown of fat. Your urine should be free of ketones.

Changing nutrient requirements during pregnancy. Protein and micronutrient needs increase during pregnancy. You should increase the protein in your diet to include an extra 10 grams per day. This amounts to just an extra ounce and a half of meat (cooked) per day.

Pregnancy significantly increases your requirements for the micronutrients iron, folic acid, and calcium. Iron is needed for the increase in blood production during pregnancy and for production of the baby's blood. It is difficult to meet this need from food alone, so most doctors prescribe an iron supplement.

Folic acid is needed for rapid cell division during pregnancy. It prevents some birth defects. Dark-green leafy vegetables (like kale), dried beans, and whole wheat products are good sources. You will need extra calcium for bone development as well. A daily intake of at least 1,200 mg is recommended. That's equal to a quart of milk or the equivalent in other milk products. You'll also need vitamin D to promote calcium absorption. Milk is usually fortified with vitamin D, or you can get enough through exposure of your skin to sunlight. To be sure you get sufficient amounts of the proper nutrients, your doctor may prescribe a vitamin and mineral supplement. Please don't self-prescribe megadoses of vitamins and minerals, though. They could be harmful to you and your developing baby.

Timing of meals. Your baby will be drawing glucose from you at the same time that your hormones are working to make sure glucose is available. In the end, it will be a balancing act to take in carbohydrate to keep your blood glucose up, but not so much at any one time that your blood glucose goes too high. Eating small, frequent meals often makes this easier to accomplish, especially since large meals may be unappetizing when you are feeling nauseous in early pregnancy and distended in late pregnancy.

You should be especially alert to the composition of breakfast. For many women, glucose is hardest to control just after breakfast, especially if you have not given the mealtime insulin time to be absorbed and start acting. So breakfast is usually not a good time to load up with carbohydrates. Instead, spreading the carbohydrates out with a smaller breakfast meal and a mid-morning snack will often keep your blood glucose from spiking up.

A bedtime snack should be part of your meal plan. Because the fetus will continue to take glucose from you through the night, you're at risk for low blood glucose and ketones if you do not have a snack. Your dietitian will probably recommend that you take some protein along with the carbohydrate to provide slower release of glucose through the night. Cornstarch is sometimes used for this purpose. Some women may need to have a snack in the middle of the night as well.

Exercise

Activity during pregnancy has real benefits: relaxation, improved fitness, good overall body image, a sense of well-being, and relief of constipation.

But stabilizing blood glucose may be the most significant feature of exercise in pregnancies complicated by diabetes.

We have heard it all: some women have run marathons during pregnancy (though not at our suggestion!); others have taken up residence in an easy chair for the duration, despite normal health (the nineteenth-century model). What's best? Ideally, you should engage in safe exercise in moderation. As usual, individualization is the key. Some conditions, such as premature labor or mid-pregnancy spotting, specifically rule out any exercise whatsoever, and some women have a level of fitness perfectly compatible with heavy exercise remarkably far into pregnancy.

In general, safe exercise is any type of activity that gets you moving but prevents injury to your baby and your changing body structure. Injury can come in the form of direct trauma (from falling down) or straining ligaments and joints. Whatever your self-image, pregnancy does change your center of gravity and may make you more likely to tumble. It may be best to avoid water skiing or snow skiing, for example, since a fall at high speed could be harmful to you and your baby. Activities that involve twists and turns, such as racquetball, volleyball, and basketball, can also damage ligaments and joints that are loosened up in preparation for childbirth. Jogging up to a certain point in your pregnancy may be okay if you're already used to it before pregnancy. Swimming and water aerobics are, on the whole, safe activities during pregnancy, as the buoyancy eases the strain on joints. Walking should be safe as well.

Again, moderation is recommended. If you were not used to exercising beforehand, pregnancy is not the time to start a strenuous activity regimen. If you were a regular exerciser before, you may be able to continue.

There are further precautions for pregnant women with diabetes. First, as with activity at any time, hypoglycemia is a danger. Test your blood glucose before you exercise. Prepare for exercise by eating an appropriate snack, and carry a source of quick-acting carbohydrate. Skip the exercise altogether if your glucose is very high—over 200 mg/dl, for example—since exercise at this time can raise the blood glucose higher, rather than lower it, if not enough insulin is circulating. Treat high blood glucose right away, preferably with insulin rather than by not eating or by exercising, as you might do if you weren't pregnant.

We are often asked whether repeated insulin reactions (hypoglycemia) can harm the developing fetus—a natural question, given that the very tight control we are talking about in pregnancy often causes more hypoglycemic reactions. The fetus can grow normally in a relatively low-glucose environment, and there is evidence that the placenta maintains a certain glucose level even when the mother's blood glucose is very low. So the answer is no; no studies have shown that hypoglycemia damages the fetus. But that does not minimize the effect on you, the carrier of the baby. It does not help the pregnancy if you have repeated dangerous insulin reactions.

A final concern with exercise during pregnancy has to do with complications. Some types of exercise can exacerbate unstable retinopathy—for example, weight training. Don't get us wrong: we're all for exercise. But when you're pregnant you have to be a little more careful. Seek the guidance of your health care team.

Insulin and Oral Antihyperglycemic Agents

Let's start with oral antihyperglycemic agents. Their potential for doing damage is not well established, but neither is their safety. Some data suggest that continuing metformin may be okay in the first trimester for women with pregestational diabetes that was well controlled with metformin previously, but studies are limited. The pills glyburide, metformin, and acarbose have all been studied in women with GDM. When compared with insulin, glyburide and metformin have shown similar degrees of good diabetes control during pregnancy. None of these three medications have been shown to increase adverse outcomes in either mothers or babies. However, none of these drugs are approved for use during pregnancy by the Food and Drug Administration, and no major medical society has advocated for the use of any of these agents over insulin. For now, as with so many other drugs during pregnancy, we recommend you avoid starting oral antihyperglycemic agents when you are pregnant.

There are limited other options for treating diabetes in pregnancy: diet, exercise, and insulin. Given that the blood glucose has a strong tendency to rise as pregnancy progresses, many women with diabetes in pregnancy are well advised to use insulin shots, so don't be upset if this is the recommendation. Keep telling yourself that using insulin is for the good of your baby. Remind yourself that if you didn't need insulin before pregnancy, the chances are good that you won't need it afterward.

Insulin treatment during pregnancy usually means an intensive regimen, generally three or four shots a day, although two doses may be adequate if you have GDM. First, you want to have adequate insulin circulating throughout the 24-hour day to avoid uncovered gaps of insulin in your blood. Second, you want to cover the carbohydrates you ingest and to provide for rapid correction of high blood glucose levels. (Refer to Chapters 11 and 12 if you are unclear about specific insulins, their duration of action, and so on.) Your physician may prescribe one or two of several available insulins. Intermediate-acting NPH and short-acting Regular insulins have been prescribed the longest in pregnancy and have the best safety record. Thus far, studies using the rapid-acting insulins aspart and lispro show they are safe and effective and do not have any harmful effects on the baby. Because these two insulins act more rapidly than Regular insulin, they control after-meal glucose levels better. And since aspart and lispro also have a shorter duration of action, they lead to less hypoglycemia many hours after injection when compared with Regular insulin.

Twice-a-day regimens. In a basic twice-a-day regimen of mixed NPH and Regular insulin, the Regular covers the meal that's eaten right after the injection, and the morning NPH dose covers lunch. The evening NPH helps keep blood glucose levels down overnight. For some women, however, the NPH can wear off before the next injection, resulting in high blood glucose levels before dinner, overnight, or in the morning. And for some women, increasing the amount of NPH may lead to *hypoglycemia* as the NPH peaks to get the glucose into a good range later on. In other words, an insulin reaction may happen in the afternoon or in the middle of the night in order to get blood glucose levels down at suppertime or before breakfast. If this occurs, the twice-a-day schedule won't work for you, and you'd better move to at least three insulin doses a day.

Three- or four-dose regimens. The object of these intensified insulin regimens is to mimic the normal pancreas's output of a little insulin all through the day and night (basal insulin) and to provide a brisk increase in insulin level (bolus) at mealtime. This involves multiple insulin injections and close blood glucose monitoring. Of the longer-acting insulins we prefer to prescribe NPH in two doses to cover insulin needs over the course of the day. The basal insulin glargine is usually discontinued at the start of pregnancy due to its unclear safety for the fetus, but new data indicate that it may be safe to start or continue once- or twice-daily basal insulin detemir in pregnancy. The rapid-acting insulins lispro or aspart can be used before meals to match carbohydrate intake and to help lower high pre-meal blood glucose levels when they occur.

Insulin pumps. Our practice is to discuss the use of external insulin pumps with anyone who requires three or four shots of insulin a day, since on the whole we find pumps to be a more stable, more effective, and much more convenient approach to intensive insulin delivery (see Chapter 13). They are especially useful in pregnancy, when intensive regimens are more common and blood glucose goals are tighter. One cautionary note is the danger of ketoacidosis if there's an interruption in the flow of insulin from the pump, since only short-acting insulin is used in the pumps. We tend to recommend continuing the use of an insulin pump during pregnancy if the woman has used it effectively before the pregnancy. Your health care team may recommend starting an insulin pump for diabetes control during pregnancy; we prefer our patients to start the therapy before pregnancy so that they can become experienced in problem solving and can effectively prevent ketones from appearing in the blood or urine.

Matching your insulin to your intake. This is especially important in pregnancy because your intake may vary, as you may not feel like eating if you are experiencing nausea. The thing to remember is that you need insulin to cover the carbohydrate ingested. Adjusting the insulin not only to blood glucose but also to actual grams of carbohydrate eaten is the most precise way to accomplish this match. Remember that the carbohydrate will raise your blood glucose faster than the insulin can work to lower it, so you'll need to inject the insulin a good 15–20 minutes before eating. Your physician and nurse educator team will assist you in insulin dosing.

Correcting the highs. The final element of the day-to-day insulin regimen is the relatively quick correction of highs and lows. Your team should advise you on what adjustments of your insulin doses are reasonable for a given elevated blood glucose. For example, you may learn to inject 1 unit of insulin for every 40 mg/dl above 100 mg/dl pre-meal and 1 unit for every 80 mg/dl above 100 mg/dl after meals.

The pattern of blood glucose and insulin. There is a predictable pattern of blood glucose during pregnancy. In early pregnancy, around 8–12 weeks after conception, there's a tendency to have more hypoglycemic reactions and to require *less* insulin. This may be because nausea can reduce your appetite so that you eat less or because you and your health care professionals are working so hard to obtain tight control. But there is also evidence that hormonal changes are involved. For whatever reason, if you had pregestational diabetes, you are well advised to be alert to a possible decrease in insulin requirement during this phase of pregnancy.

From about week 12 to week 35, near the end of pregnancy, the insulin requirement marches steadily upward. By the last weeks of pregnancy, the insulin requirements, on average, double for women with Type 1 diabetes and may even triple for those with pregestational Type 2 diabetes. To maintain good control, you can count on needing more insulin.

One warning: this very much increased insulin requirement by the end of pregnancy will drop right back to the pre-pregnancy level as soon as the baby is delivered. The increased insulin requirement is purely a function of the pregnancy. Consider, for example, the case of Lauren.

Lauren is a 32-year-old woman who has had diabetes since the age of 14. She's always done pretty well caring for her diabetes and has very few long-term complications: the ophthalmologist mentioned just a few spots on the retina but was very pleased with how minor the retinopathy is. Lauren and her husband decide to have a child. She is referred to an obstetrician experienced in managing high-risk pregnancies and is told to establish very tight control of her blood glucose even before discontinuing contraceptive methods. This is difficult, but Lauren is reasonably successful, and she becomes pregnant. Her usual insulin requirement is 42 units per day, which is split into three doses of NPH and aspart insulin after she becomes pregnant. Unfortunately, she has serious problems with nausea and vomiting in the first trimester, leading to difficulty in keeping her food down. She learns to compensate with her insulin dose, which falls to 28 units per day total. At week 15, Lauren feels like a new person. Her amniocentesis and blood tests are all fine, her nausea is subdued, and her abdomen is starting to bulge. To keep her blood glucose in range, though, she requires more and more insulin. By the last month of pregnancy, she is astounded by the fact that she takes 80 units of insulin a day, 24 units of it in the morning—much more than she's ever taken in her life. Lauren's delivery is vaginal, with labor induced after her obstetrician determines that the baby is ready. After delivering a healthy baby girl on a Friday, she's told she will be sent home on Saturday morning. Her doctor is away for the weekend, and the covering doctor hasn't made rounds yet. Lauren, not thinking much about it, takes 24 units of insulin that morning. All afternoon, as the family gathers to see the new arrival, Lauren is fighting serious low blood glucose reactions.

The bottom line. Excellent blood glucose control is the day-to-day goal in pregnancy. If you can demonstrate, first to yourself, then to your health care provider, that your glucose levels are really in the range you want on a simple regimen, more power to you. Remember, though: if you aren't checking often, you don't know how high or low your glucose levels are running. Usually it is hard to maintain tight control during pregnancy without a more intensive insulin regimen, especially if you have preexisting Type 1 diabetes.

Delivery and Postpartum

When the time comes, you'll deliver your baby in one of three ways: *spontaneous vaginal* (through the vagina after labor has started spontaneously), *induced vaginal* (through the vagina after labor is started by taking a medication), and planned or emergency *cesarean section*. As we said, your doctor will keep you updated on your and your baby's progress during pregnancy and will make a decision that's safest for both of you. Factors to consider will be the baby's health (is the baby still surviving well in your uterus?) and your health (are your blood glucose and blood pressure well controlled, and are there any changes in complications status?).

Your blood glucose control during labor and delivery, regardless of the method chosen, is important in controlling the baby's blood glucose as well. If your blood glucose goes too high, your baby will overproduce insulin and have a low blood glucose immediately after delivery. If your glucose goes too low or if you don't get enough glucose, your body could start to produce ketones. So the balance is delicate. Although practice trends vary, a method commonly used is an intravenous infusion of insulin and glucose along with frequent blood glucose monitoring during delivery. The intravenous route has the advantage of acting immediately. But be sure to alert your doctor if you took long-acting insulin earlier on the day of delivery.

During labor, your insulin needs may dramatically *decrease*, presumably due, at least in part, to the extreme exertion of labor. Upon delivery, as mentioned, you will have an almost immediate return to your pre-pregnancy insulin requirements. After loss of the hormones made by the placenta that raised glucose during the pregnancy, the body becomes much more sensitive to insulin. Some women won't require any insulin for several hours after delivery. Most women with GDM see the diabetes disappear altogether, at least for the time being. Failing to reduce your insulin dose even the day after delivery can cause serious hypoglycemia, as we saw in Lauren's case.

Breastfeeding is good for your baby, and women with diabetes are encouraged to breastfeed if possible. Breast milk has all the nutrients that your baby needs, is pre-packaged at just the right temperature, and has antibodies that fight certain infections. Best of all is the closeness you'll feel with your infant. Your own and your baby's nutrient needs for breastfeeding can usually be met by your pre-pregnancy diet, provided it is adequate in calcium, fluids, and protein. If you have Type 1 diabetes, however, you may need to rearrange your calories and insulin regimen to compensate for the lowering of blood glucose that can occur as the baby takes glucose from you. Middle-of-the-night feedings may require an extra snack at that time or before retiring.

In the immediate postpartum period, you're likely to be exhausted. Seek out and accept help from those who can be genuinely supportive of your and your baby's needs. Preparing a meal, changing a diaper, helping you give your baby a bath: this kind of assistance can give you the support you need to recuperate.

It is well recognized that some women have bouts of depression after childbirth. With diabetes in the picture, you may feel especially down. Do not feel you are alone, do not feel ashamed. Be candid with your doctor about any blue feeling that persists day after day, any difficulties with sleep (besides disturbances for feeding the baby), or any feeling of bringing harm to yourself. If it becomes a significant problem, seek professional help. Sometimes a change in thyroid function can be involved.

From the instant your baby is born, you and your partner become parents and have the responsibility and joy of meeting your child's every need. In some ways, having diabetes or developing GDM in the pregnancy, you are better prepared than most parents. The discipline and perseverance required to get through a pregnancy with diabetes will serve you well in dealing with middle-of-the-night feedings and figuring out a crying baby's needs, not to mention dealing with all the joys—and, yes, traumas—of parenthood to come.

. . .

Becoming pregnant when you have pregestational diabetes or developing GDM when you are pregnant is traumatic. You will be pushed by your health care provider and by your own conscience to test your blood glucose levels frequently and to keep them as close to normal as possible. All this is an effort to improve the chances you'll have a normal pregnancy and a healthy child.

If you have diabetes, think carefully about whether you want to become pregnant. If you do, get your diabetes under control, preferably before conception. Enter into good prenatal care immediately, and stay in close touch with your health care team throughout the pregnancy. You will probably have to use insulin, and if you've already been using it, you'll probably have to intensify your regimen. And your insulin requirements will increase late in pregnancy. But you can do it, as have many before you.

One final point. For nine months you've focused on taking good care of your health. Maybe you were able to sustain the motivation because of the baby. Don't let it stop. Continue it for your own good, and remember that your baby is still dependent on your health. If you are sick a lot or develop complications of diabetes, it will be difficult for you to care for your child.

As you take good care of yourself, give yourself a big round of applause. You have set a wonderful example for your child to see.

Take Home Messages

- Good blood glucose control during pregnancy is good for your developing baby and good for you.
- Some women develop gestational diabetes mellitus (GDM) during pregnancy. This is a sign that Type 2 diabetes may develop later in your life. GDM increases the risk of problems for the developing baby, so it should be treated with diet and exercise to control blood glucose levels, and with insulin if necessary.
- If you already have diabetes, it is important to plan your pregnancy. Establishing close to normal blood glucose levels in the months before you become pregnant and throughout your pregnancy dramatically increase the likelihood you will deliver a healthy baby.
- Frequent blood glucose monitoring, a healthful diet (including additional protein and micronutrients), and exercise that gets you moving without risking harm to yourself or your developing baby are the keys to keeping your blood glucose levels as close to normal as possible.
- Your health care providers will help you establish the best diabetes medication regimen for your pregnancy.

30

The Genetics of Diabetes

- "There's lots of diabetes in my family. What are my chances?"
- "I couldn't believe that my child would get diabetes. They say it's genetic, but there is absolutely no history of diabetes on either side of our family. I just don't understand it."
- "Naturally, my first thought when I learned that one of my children had diabetes was, Will his brothers get it too?"
- "I love my boyfriend, John, and I have no problem whatever with his diabetes. But frankly, I'm worried about whether any children we might have would get diabetes. Should I be worried about that?"

We live in the midst of a revolution in human genetics. Genes are the basic pieces of DNA that determine all of a person's genetic characteristics, and every day, new genes are being identified, analyzed, and even *sequenced* (a process that defines their exact structure). But in terms of practical knowledge, we are really just at the beginning. If you think of the effort to understand all the human genes as being like mapmaking, then genetic research is about at the stage of seventeenth-century explorers groping their way down the coast of Maine in the fog. We have a long way to go. We have a lot to discover. And genetics will be profoundly important in understanding and ultimately curing diabetes.

What do genes have to do with diabetes? We already know that it is to some extent inherited, but there are still many questions we can't answer. We can talk about the *chances*—that is, the risk or the odds—of getting diabetes, but we can't tell you whether you or your child *will* get diabetes, and we can't tell you precisely why one person gets it while another does not. When all the genes that cause diabetes are discovered (and there will probably be many of them), scientists not only will be able to predict diabetes but will also be in a position to discover how to modify or correct the gene

431

abnormality responsible for diabetes. This might prevent diabetes altogether. Knowing the genetic causes for someone's diabetes should also allow physicians to better select the treatments to which a person is most likely to respond.

At the moment, we still have only the most general notions about the genetics of diabetes. One of these observations is that Type 1 and Type 2 diabetes are two different diseases, not only clinically (as discussed in Chapter 2) but also genetically. It is clear that these two major kinds of diabetes run through families independently. If the family has a large number of people with Type 2 diabetes, that doesn't increase the chance of family members having Type 1 diabetes, and families with individuals with Type 1 won't necessarily have family members with Type 2. So we'll consider the genetics of Type 1 and Type 2 diabetes separately.

Type 1 Diabetes

Is Type 1 diabetes caused by your genetic makeup or by something in your environment? The answer is both. Some people start off with a genetic predisposition to Type 1 diabetes. If they meet up with the environmental trigger, the causative factor in the environment, they get diabetes; if they don't meet up with the trigger, they never get diabetes.

By analogy, you could think of the tendency to get badly sunburned. If you have dark skin genetically, bad sunburn may never be a problem. But even if you are genetically susceptible to sunburn by having very fair skin, the sunburn will happen only if your skin is exposed to the environmental trigger (the sun). So sunburn is the result of both a genetic predisposition and an environmental exposure.

The trouble is, unlike sunburn (which obviously is more likely in genetically fair-skinned people and is triggered by an overdose of sun), for Type 1 diabetes, little is known about the genetic predisposition and almost nothing is known about the environmental trigger. Certain genetic characteristics, called *haplotypes* or *HLA types*, are known to be associated with a greater or lesser chance of developing Type 1 diabetes, but little else is known about the actual genetic abnormality for Type 1. Likewise, it has long been speculated that the environmental trigger is a virus or early infant exposure to cow's milk, but these ideas remain unproven. Some studies support each of these environmental causes, while others do not. We do know that an illness or stress that occurs shortly before a diagnosis of Type 1 diabetes often brings it out, but these stresses are *not* likely to be the cause; evidence of the autoimmune process can be seen years before the onset of Type 1 diabetes.

As more of the basic genetics is understood, we think it will become possible not only to predict who will get diabetes but also to replace genes or prevent environmental exposures or take other approaches to prevent diabetes from developing. In the meantime, we have to rely on relatively crude information, such as that derived from twin studies.

Twin Studies

Identical twins have exactly the same genes; non-identical (fraternal) twins have just a partial sharing of genes, like brothers or sisters who are not twins. If a characteristic is entirely determined by genetics, both individuals in a pair of identical twins will be identical for that characteristic. Eye color is an example of this: both twins in identical twins always have the same eye color. If something is not genetic, it will not be identical in both twins—for example, identical twins won't both break their arms at the same time (unless they fall out of the same tree at the same time).

When one identical twin has Type 1 diabetes, there is about a 50% chance that the other twin will develop it too, although the onsets may be many years apart. This simple number tells a lot. It shows that there is a strong genetic component to Type 1 diabetes (otherwise the second twin would not have nearly such a high chance of getting diabetes), but it also shows that heredity is not the whole story, since about 50% of identical twins whose twin has Type 1 diabetes never do develop the disease. So there is also a strong nongenetic component, whether viral or something else. If the disease were entirely genetic, like eye color, the second identical twin would always have diabetes if the first one did.

That's why it's said that the cause of Type 1 diabetes is both genetic and environmental. But where does this leave you, personally, in terms of planning for yourself and your family?

What Are the Odds?

As discussed in Chapter 2, there are laboratory tests, including islet cell antibodies or GAD (glutamic acid decarboxylase) antibodies, that can detect—years before any apparent illness—that a person is undergoing immune destruction of the pancreatic beta cells and will probably get clinical Type 1 diabetes. But the test results are not always positive in people who do get Type 1 diabetes (false negatives), and sometimes they are mistaken in predicting who will get it (false positives). Furthermore, the tests don't yield positive results until the diabetic process is already under way, so they cannot be used to predict who will get Type 1 diabetes before any damage is done.

Because we can't predict with certainty who will get diabetes, we can only talk about the odds, or risk. Odds, as any card player will tell you, don't tell you what *is* going to happen, they just tell you what is *more likely or less likely* to happen. And sometimes the odds (or relative risk, as it is called) can be deceiving.

As an example of calculating the odds, consider that if you live on a farm instead of in a city, there may be a much greater *relative risk* of your being hit by a bale of hay falling from a silo. But hay falling from a silo is not very common, so the *actual risk* is still very small. Similarly, the chance of Type 1 diabetes recurring in a family that already has one case is greater than if no one in the family had the disease. But the chance is still small.

If no one in the family has Type 1 diabetes, the chance of a non-Hispanic/Latino white child getting it is about 0.2%, or a 2 in 1,000 chance; the risk is much less for children of other races/ethnicities. So what are the odds of getting diabetes if you do have it in the family? If one parent has Type 1 diabetes, the chance that a given child will get it is about 3%–6% (about 3% if the mother has it and about 6% if the father has it). If one child (but neither parent) has Type 1 diabetes, the chance that a brother or sister will get it is about 5%. These odds hold true over the whole population, but there are certain unusual families that have Type 1 diabetes much more frequently, often associated with other endocrine deficiencies such as thyroid disease or adrenal insufficiency. If you have this sort of family, you probably know it, because there will be a lot of family members with diabetes.

On the whole, these are pretty good odds. They also explain why, in most cases, Type 1 diabetes seems to come out of the blue, with no family history. That does not mean it isn't inherited; it just means that the gene never *showed itself* in living memory (wasn't "expressed," the geneticists would say). Someone in the family probably carried the gene but didn't develop the disease.

What Can I Do to Tip the Odds in My Favor?

Unfortunately, with Type 1 diabetes, there are few things you can do to tip the odds in your favor. Unlike Type 2 diabetes, which is so closely related to body weight, for Type 1 diabetes there's nothing we know about for sure in diet, exercise, or any other activity that changes your chance of getting it. The amount of sugar in a child's diet may cause dental cavities, but it has nothing to do with causing diabetes. As we noted earlier, some researchers have proposed that exposure to cow's milk at a young age (as opposed to breastfeeding) is a major factor in causing Type 1 diabetes, but so far this lacks solid confirmation. Some more recent research studies suggest that vitamin D supplements and diets high in omega-3 fatty acids may be protective against Type 1 diabetes, but there are currently no guidelines for supplementing the diet of children with either of these to prevent the development of diabetes. More studies that look into the benefits of vitamin D and omega-3 fatty acid supplements in higher-risk children are needed to confirm these early findings. We have mentioned the lab tests that can tell when Type 1 diabetes is developing, but unless we can do something to interrupt progression of the disease—and so far we cannot—the information is not of much use. The Diabetes Prevention Trial, Type 1, sponsored by the National Institutes of Health, showed that using low-dose insulin injections or oral insulin did not prevent diabetes from developing in persons at high risk of developing the disease. Drugs that are used to suppress the immune system can slow the loss of insulin-producing beta cells in individuals with new-onset Type 1 diabetes, but the side effects of current drugs are too great to warrant their use in the long term, and short-term use is not effective. However, there is great hope that the mystery of why the immune system attacks its own beta cells can be solved, and this information should lead to treatments that will prevent the attacks from occurring.

Many diabetes centers in the United States and around the world, including ours, are participating in TrialNet, also sponsored by the National Institutes of Health. TrialNet is a multinational network of diabetes centers dedicated to the study, prevention, and early treatment of Type 1 diabetes. One of the studies is screening family members of persons with Type 1 diabetes for antibodies. First-degree relatives (children, siblings, or parents) aged 1–45 years and second-degree relatives (grandchildren, nieces, nephews, aunts, uncles, or cousins) aged 1–20 years are eligible to participate. Persons who test positive for one or more antibodies will be closely followed up, checking for a decline in insulin production or for the development of high glucose levels. Individuals who have multiple positive antibodies and are at highest risk for developing Type 1 diabetes may qualify to participate in studies of oral insulin or new immune-regulating drugs. If you have family members who would like to participate in this study, you can see whether there is a TrialNet study site close to you by going to the website www.diabetestrialnet.org.

Type 2 Diabetes

Type 2 diabetes is much more strongly determined by genetics than is Type 1. The results of identical twin studies strikingly prove this point. If one identical twin has Type 2 diabetes, there is a very high chance, perhaps 90% or more, that the other twin will get it as well.

In studies of the genetics of Type 2 diabetes, the majority of clues have come from certain very high-risk populations. About half of the Pima Indians of Arizona develop diabetes, for instance, and up to 80% of people over age 55 in the Nauruan tribes of the South Pacific have diabetes. Type 2 diabetes is also more common in African Americans and Hispanic/Latino Americans than in Caucasians. By studying individuals and families with these backgrounds, investigators are slowly piecing together "candidate genes" that may explain the inheritance of Type 2 diabetes. All gene abnormalities (variants) identified thus far as contributing to diabetes are involved in beta cell development, beta cell survival, or insulin production.

An interesting line of research has emphasized the role of the environment, particularly the diet, in bringing out Type 2 diabetes in susceptible individuals. Investigators studied groups of people as they moved from one lifestyle to another. Natives of Japan who move to the United States, for example, with all the changes in diet, activity, and stress that such a move demands, are much more likely to develop Type 2 diabetes than are Japanese people who remain in Japan—so there clearly is an environmental effect. Similar studies have been done as other groups of people, whether Native Americans, Pacific islanders, or Arabian peninsula nomads, are introduced to Western civilization.

With less exercise and more high-calorie foods, obesity is more likely to occur. Obesity is the factor most closely related to Type 2 diabetes. Any way you look at it—whether in the whole population of a nation or in a single individual—the more fat you carry, the more likely it is that you'll get Type 2 diabetes.

When we put all these factors together we find that the individual at highest risk of developing Type 2 diabetes is a middle-aged woman of Native American, African American, or Hispanic/Latino descent whose family has many cases of Type 2 diabetes and who is overweight and has a history of diabetes during pregnancy.

What Are the Odds?

The odds of developing Type 2 diabetes are difficult to calculate because they depend so heavily on *how many* of the risk factors you have. But considering family members alone, if one parent has Type 2 diabetes, the chance is about 20% that a child will develop it (usually in adulthood, of course). If both parents have it, the risk doubles.

What Can I Do to Tip the Odds in My Favor?

The most important thing you can do to tip the odds against developing Type 2 diabetes is to *maintain a normal body weight*. There is some evidence that reducing your dietary fat intake will help, even if you don't reduce your body weight. Exercise appears to be another effective preventive approach.

The Diabetes Prevention Program, funded by the National Institutes of Health, investigated whether Type 2 diabetes can be prevented and, if so, how. More than 3,000 obese people at very high risk for Type 2 diabetes were enrolled in the study and assigned randomly to one of several study treatments. After three years of follow-up, researchers found that lifestyle leading to a 7% weight loss (through a low-fat diet and exercise for 150 minutes per week) was more effective at preventing diabetes (58% reduced risk) than taking the diabetes medication metformin (31% reduced risk). Other studies have since shown similar benefits of weight loss and regular exercise in reducing the risk for developing diabetes. In addition to metformin, treatment of people at high risk for diabetes with the medications rosiglitazone, pioglitazone, or acarbose was shown to reduce the rates of diabetes when compared with a placebo (non-drug) pill. However, all individuals treated with these drugs had more frequent side effects.

· · ·

The genetics of diabetes is extraordinarily complex. One of the few certainties is that Type 1 and Type 2 diabetes are inherited independently—having one type in the family doesn't increase the chances of having the other type. In Type 1 diabetes, there is often no family history of diabetes; even in families where one member has it, the chance that another person will develop Type 1 diabetes is about 1 in 25. There is no way to predict accurately who will get Type 1 diabetes unless the immune process that destroys the pancreas is already under way; attempts to prevent Type 1 are an area of active research.

Type 2 diabetes is more strongly influenced by heredity, with family history usually revealing multiple cases. There are clear features that mark someone as being at especially high risk for getting Type 2 diabetes: obesity (especially abdominal), certain minority racial/ethnic heritages, and a history of diabetes during pregnancy. Maintaining normal body weight is the best thing you can do to prevent Type 2 diabetes. In some cases, persons with prediabetes are given metformin to help prevent the progression to diabetes.

Take Home Messages

- We still have only the most general notion of the genetics of diabetes.
- Type 1 diabetes is caused by your genetic makeup triggered by something in your environment, though we don't know what the environmental trigger or triggers might be.
- If a man has Type 1 diabetes, the chance a given child of his will develop it is 6%. If a woman has Type 1 diabetes, the chance a given child of hers will develop it is 3%.
- Type 2 diabetes is much more strongly determined by genetics than is Type 1. If one parent has Type 2 diabetes there is a 20% chance that a child will develop it (usually in adulthood). If both parents have Type 2 diabetes, the risk doubles.
- The most important thing you can do to reduce your risk of developing Type 2 diabetes is to maintain a normal weight.

The Future of Care

Recognizing that no one knows for sure what diabetes care will be like in the future, we do know three things for certain: it will be different, it will be better, and it will depend on research. In Part VI we try to describe what the future of care for people with diabetes may be like. We don't describe diabetes research just to satisfy your curiosity or to solicit your support for a good cause. We write about diabetes research because it is exciting, it is fascinating, and it is ultimately the only way that diabetes and its complications will be stamped out.

Browse through the research topics that we talk about here, and use the resources we mention to stay abreast of new work. There is a strong link between the research being done now and the prognosis for people with diabetes: the more and faster the research, the better the outlook.

31

Diabetes Research

- "I just read in the newspaper that they cured diabetes in mice. Does that mean they can cure it in people too?"
- "Is there a way to monitor glucose that doesn't require a finger stick?"
- "I saw an ad for a diabetes research study at the local hospital. Should I volunteer for it?"
- "Why do some people in research studies have to take a placebo?"
- "I want to contribute money to diabetes research, but I want to get it in the right hands."
- "Who pays for most diabetes research?"

Diabetes research is such an enormous topic that it could easily fill an entire book. But since we have to limit ourselves to a single chapter, we start with a general discussion of the research process and the types of research, make some suggestions about how to read and interpret accounts of research that you may come across, and give specific examples of current diabetes research and how you can get involved.

The Research Process and the Broad Areas of Diabetes Research

First, the researcher asks a question. To get funding for the project, the question has to be a good one—one that's important and one to which the answer isn't already known.

The research question also must be *answerable* within the time frame and the budget of the proposed study. If it would take 1,000 people and a five-year study to answer a particular question, there's no point in starting if you can't afford such a study. Full-time investigators are highly trained and must meet rigorous intellectual and ethical standards. Competition is tough if you want to make a career doing research. It is not a part-time hobby.

Young people go through many years of education and training, with long apprenticeships, to become independent researchers.

Diabetes research can be broadly categorized into three types—basic, applied, and clinical research—all of which are essential to the greater goal of making progress in the treatment and prevention of diabetes.

- "A number of groups, including our own, are now able to make insulin-producing beta cells. We hope to move to human trials in the next few years."—Michael German, M.D., University of California, San Francisco.

Basic Research

Basic research is designed to answer questions about fundamental processes, questions such as "How does the cell respond to insulin?" or "Which genes cause fat cells to multiply?" Basic research is the first step toward developing effective treatments. Often, several basic research questions must be answered in the process of developing a new treatment.

A good example is the discovery of insulin, which we described in Chapter 11. First it was discovered that the pancreas has some sort of antidiabetic factor. Then it was discovered that the factor resides in the islets of Langerhans. Finally, a technique was worked out to extract islets from a pancreas without damaging them. To the public, insulin was "discovered" in this last step, but to those who understood the process, it was the climactic conclusion of a long chain of basic research discoveries.

In the same logical way, the reality of human insulin started with basic research. First, basic scientists found that DNA is the genetic material that regulates all proteins (including insulin) made in a cell. Then methods were developed to cut up DNA into smaller pieces and to splice pieces that are known to cause cells to produce insulin into cells, like bacteria, that don't normally make insulin. With this basic understanding of how insulin is made and the ability to splice insulin-producing DNA into bacteria, pharmaceutical companies could *apply* this basic research to insulin production.

Applied Research

Applied research is the effort to bring together the discoveries of basic science and apply them to a defined need. It is based on and builds on basic research. In the first edition of this book, we illustrated applied research with the story of implanted insulin infusion pumps, developed at the Johns Hopkins University.

This development was made possible by earlier technological break-throughs pioneered by NASA, including the creation of computer micro-chips and a small pump that was developed to deliver tiny pulses of culture medium onto samples from the surface of Mars to see whether anything would grow.

It took a major effort in applied diabetes research, though, to make the system a reality. A sophisticated engineering team was assembled at the Johns Hopkins University Applied Physics Laboratory, involving the collab-oration of mechanical and electrical engineers, software experts, telemetry specialists, insulin chemists, and diabetologists. A prototype device was fabricated, and in 1982 it was ready for four years of testing in dogs with diabetes, before being tested in people. The pump worked in humans.

Now, many years later, the implantable pump is available in France and a few other European countries, but not in the United States. The company that sponsored the research in this country decided not to pursue approval of the device, for a number of reasons—including that the device required meticulous care and refilling in a hospital setting and that the original for-mulation of the concentrated insulin used in the pump was no longer avail-able. The company also decided to invest in other products it was develop-ing. Not every good idea eventually reaches people with diabetes.

The use of animals in medical research. We are well aware that people have very strong opinions about this subject, and they have a perfect right to their opinions. It is a complex subject, ethically and practically. We would say, first, that the ethical use of animals in diabetes research has allowed in-numerable advances in the treatment of humans. The very fact that some-thing in the pancreas (insulin) could prevent diabetes was discovered in dogs. Every treatment advance you can think of required testing in animals before its use in humans. It is impossible to imagine how backward our treatment of diabetes would be today, how many people who are living and well today would be dead or dying, without animal research.

We also want to emphasize that there are now well-established standards and review processes to ensure that animals are ethically cared for in re-search, just as human research subjects are. We support the ethical use of animals in diabetes research. It is absolutely essential.

Clinical Research

Clinical research is research conducted in people. It is designed to test new treatments such as new pills, devices, or procedures (like weight loss surgery).

Clinical research trials are conducted with participants' full knowledge and consent. This research is highly regulated, governed by a carefully developed set of rules and ethical considerations. If a scientist wants to do a research project involving people, the proposal is subjected to a detailed scientific and ethical review to be sure that it is sound and that it is in the proposed research subjects' best interests to take part.

The institutional review board (IRB) of the institution where the research is planned conducts this review process. Made up of independent scientists, ethicists, lawyers, and community members, the IRB is designed to look out for the rights and safety of the research subjects, making sure the project is as safe as possible, with a reasonable *risk-benefit ratio*. A minimal-risk project, such as one that involves just drawing a tube of blood, does not have to give much benefit, but research that involves any real risk has to have substantial potential benefit to be approved. Issues of compensation are considered carefully. People may be offered monetary or other compensation (such as free medical evaluations). But compensation can't be so high that participants might be induced to join a study that would otherwise not be in their interest.

Most of all, the IRB makes sure that a potential research subject knows what he or she is getting into. Potential study participants are asked beforehand if they are interested in taking part; all aspects of the study are explained in understandable language; participants have a chance to ask questions before or during their participation; they have the right to withdraw from the study at any time; and they sign a consent form This series of safeguards ensures that participants' rights are protected.

We discuss the benefits of taking part in research studies later in the chapter.

Understanding Diabetes Research from the Outside

Whether they take part in clinical research or not, people are often confused and even misled by reports they read in the newspaper or see on television or the Internet. If you are not trained in diabetes research but are eager to follow what's happening, it can be a problem. There is no easy answer to how to keep up with diabetes research, but our responses to some frequently asked questions may help.

Where do I go for information? There are several reliable sources of information designed specifically to describe diabetes research to the public. The American Diabetes Association's *Diabetes Forecast*, the Juvenile Diabetes Research Foundation's *Research Report*, and publications from the National Institutes of Health's National Institute of Diabetes and Digestive and Kidney Diseases (NIDDK) come to mind. Each of these organizations has a website where you can find additional, up-to-date information.

If you belong to a club, fraternal organization, or religious group, ask diabetes researchers from a local academic institution to speak at one of your meetings. Researchers are more and more eager to take part in these outreach programs, recognizing that public support is fostered by public understanding of research. So ask a researcher to talk about current research with your group, and get it straight from the horse's mouth.

What sources of information are less reliable? You will probably first hear about most new diabetes research on the television or the Internet or in a newspaper or magazine. Some of this information may be reliable, especially if it refers to a study in a reputable scientific journal and you can find it discussed in one of the sources we mentioned above. Other information may be less reliable, especially if it's in the form of a paid advertisement, a company press release, or another source that could be biased.

What will this new finding mean to my diabetes? First, find out whether the study was done in animals or in humans. Animal research is very important, but as one of our colleagues said, "Diabetes has been cured hundreds of times in mice, but not yet once in humans." Animals and people are not identical. Then try to figure out what stage the research is at. Is it just an idea that may or may not turn out to be practical? Is it a basic research finding that may translate into a therapy years down the road? Finally, if it was a human study, was it done in a large enough group of people for the results to be truly meaningful?

Your health care professional may be able to help you understand the relevance of a particular research study, but some words of caution here. First, the press usually gets a look at journals before practitioners do, so there could be a time gap before your health care professional sees an article. Second, no professional can read or understand all the articles that are published, and it is unrealistic to expect him or her to have an expert opinion on every research finding reported in the press.

The bottom line. Valid research is necessary to test whether any given treatment works. We run into claims about all sorts of treatment, from seaweed to herbal teas, that will cure (or reverse) diabetes. Many claims are simply untrue, based on testimonials and backed by no real evidence. So get your information from well-established sources, figure out where each research advance fits into the larger picture of diabetes, and take advantage of the long-range improvements in care options.

Active Diabetes Research

You may be wondering what areas are "hot" in diabetes research. Ask any researcher, and you'll hear about his or her own work, of course. Indeed, if we all knew and agreed on exactly what research would prove most fruitful in the long run, that would be the only research done. But we can only make educated guesses. Here are our thoughts on some areas of diabetes research that are especially active and could be especially important. It is by no means a complete list and is intended only to give an idea of how broad the field of diabetes research really is.

Basic Research

Insulin action. There is still much mystery surrounding how insulin acts on the cell, allowing glucose in and affecting so many of the cell's crucial actions. If the process always worked perfectly, maybe it would be less important to understand it in detail. But as you know from reading about Type 2 diabetes, insulin resistance—when cells are unable to respond normally to insulin—is a fundamental part of that very common and very serious kind of diabetes.

We know that insulin resistance is closely linked to obesity, but we don't know why. We know that insulin receptors on the cell surface seem to be present in adequate numbers and that once they do their job, the biochemical pathways inside the cell don't respond normally. If we fully understood insulin action and insulin resistance, treatments could probably be developed to reverse that resistance. The benefits of being able to control Type 2 diabetes would be enormous. Basic research into insulin action is extremely active and important.

The genetics of diabetes. Studying the genetics of diabetes goes way beyond drawing family trees. Since the 1950s, genes have been recognized as the central determinant of how an organism develops; in humans, genes determine height, hair and eye color, and many of the diseases to which a person is susceptible. In Chapter 30 we described a "genetics revolution," and it's true that scientists' understanding of genetics is progressing very quickly. In the research laboratory, this means identifying and examining genes that make people susceptible to diabetes, either Type 1 or Type 2. It means looking at how these genes are "expressed"—that is, how they function.

The research problem is made far more difficult by the certainty that there's no *single* gene responsible for causing either Type 1 or Type 2 diabetes. Both kinds of diabetes undoubtedly involve multiple genes as well as important nongenetic factors, such as the amount of food a person eats or his or her exposure to particular viruses. Still, there are specific genetic factors with very practical implications. A new field of basic research has been studying obesity genes.

There is a kind of mouse, called the ObOb mouse, that gets enormously fat and develops a disease very much like Type 2 diabetes. Obesity in these mice is an entirely inherited trait. In 1994–95, some investigators found the gene that goes awry in these mice and described the problem this gene has in making its protein, called *leptin*. Furthermore, the same gene and the same protein, leptin, are present in humans. Before anyone concludes that the "obesity gene" solves all human weight problems, we must point out that most of the genes in a mouse are also found in humans, and they may or may not play important roles in human disease. While the ObOb mouse's problem is entirely genetic and is inherited in a straightforward way, human obesity is anything but straightforward. And human Type 2 diabetes involves factors other than obesity.

But this discovery of an obesity gene in the mid-1990s illustrates the power of medical genetics. Over the coming years, at the pace genetic research is moving, it is likely that new insights into diabetes-related genes will be in store.

The dream is that researchers will be able to identify a major gene defect that is modifiable or correctable. Gene therapy has already had some success for certain unusual diseases caused by relatively simple, single-gene defects. It will be much harder to apply gene therapy to a disease like diabetes. But genetic research may ultimately find the cure.

The immunology of Type 1 diabetes. In describing the causes of Type 1 diabetes earlier in the book, we described how the insulin-producing pancreatic islet cells are destroyed by an immune process in which the body's defense mechanisms turn against its own beta cells. Immunology as a science has progressed rapidly in recent years, but it is fair to say that the immune process that attacks the pancreas in Type 1 diabetes remains poorly understood.

If the cause of the immune attack on the beta cells were known, it would be possible to try to block that response. For example, if scientists could identify an antibody that is causing the damage, they could work on a "blocking antibody" to neutralize the offender. Our basic understanding of how this immune process works is still inadequate, and jumping to clinical trials before building the basic knowledge base is rarely productive.

Basic research into the immune processes causing Type 1 diabetes is an important area of basic research today, one that could lead to the prevention or cure of Type 1 diabetes.

Behavioral and Psychosocial Research

- "We helped people integrate diabetes care into everything else that was going on in their lives. We helped them understand that diabetes care can be a priority, and that problem solving lets us meet them where they are."—Felicia Hill-Briggs, Ph.D., Johns Hopkins University, on her research to help low-income patients with diabetes take better care of their health.

Behavioral and psychosocial research in diabetes focuses on understanding what influences people's behavior, especially their diabetes self-care behavior, and how to facilitate diabetes self-care. This research also tries to understand the emotional side of diabetes and how to improve the coping skills of people living with diabetes.

Your behavior is the key to your health and well-being. Your chances of living a longer, healthier life go way up when you stick to your diabetes management plan—take your medication as prescribed, monitor your blood glucose regularly, eat a healthy diet, and exercise regularly. Behavioral and psychosocial researchers are trying to understand what helps people "do the right thing" when it comes to diabetes management and how to help more people do the right thing more often.

As we mentioned in Chapter 14, emotional well-being can play a role because diabetes distress and depression can make it harder for people to do the things they want to do and need to do, including taking the best possible care of their diabetes. As a consequence, people with diabetes who suffer from diabetes distress or depression tend to have higher blood glucose levels, more diabetes complications, and higher mortality rates. The treatments we discussed in Chapters 14 and 16 can help improve emotional well-being and create a positive spiral of more active self-care, lower blood glucose levels, fewer complications, and lower mortality rates. Researchers are constantly searching for new medications and counseling techniques to relieve symptoms of distress and depression in people who have diabetes.

In the past decade other researchers have found that depression can increase a person's risk for developing Type 2 diabetes in the first place. This could be the result of behaviors associated with depression (such as unhealthy eating and a sedentary lifestyle) that increase a person's risk for developing Type 2 diabetes, or it could be the result of hormonal changes associated with depression that also increase blood glucose levels. In addition, in the past few years we have seen research showing that taking antidepressant medication may also increase a person's risk of developing Type 2 diabetes. We don't know why, and more research must be done to be confident this association is valid. We certainly don't suggest that people stop taking antidepressant medication, but if they don't have diagnosed diabetes, they might want to ask their doctor to check their blood glucose levels.

Several large, long-term, NIH-funded studies are looking at the effect of lifestyle changes designed to help people lose weight. The Diabetes Prevention Program (DPP) study, which we mentioned in Chapter 30, found that people with "prediabetes" who were part of a lifestyle intervention designed to help them lose weight—by cutting calories and increasing physical activity—lost an average of 14 pounds and cut their risk of developing Type 2 diabetes during the study by 58% compared with study participants in the placebo group. Pretty amazing results!

In another study, the Look AHEAD trial, which we've talked about throughout the book, participants with Type 2 diabetes in the lifestyle intervention group, who were encouraged to make lifestyle changes similar to those in the DPP, lost an average of 20 pounds in the first year of the study and enjoyed dramatic improvements in blood glucose, blood pressure, cholesterol control, and fitness, as well as a decrease in the use of medications. Both the DPP study and the Look AHEAD trial are being conducted at Hopkins.

New treatments for diabetes—medications, devices, and procedures—are being studied and introduced every year. All research on potential new treatments looks at the safety and benefits of these treatments. Now more and more studies are also considering behavioral and psychosocial issues, including the effects of new treatments on patients' quality of life, treatment satisfaction, and treatment preferences. This makes sense; new treatments will be widely used only if they have no substantial adverse effects (and have, it's to be hoped, positive effects) on quality of life and if they improve treatment satisfaction and are preferred to existing treatments. The FDA is interested in hearing about these effects when companies apply for approval of new treatments.

Research to Improve Blood Glucose Control

- "I've had diabetes long enough to remember the days when glucose monitoring meant testing urine. The blood glucose strips (Chemstrips) were introduced, with glucose monitors just a few years later. Now I use a CGM. It's amazing how much technology—and my glucose control— has improved over the past 30 years. I can hardly wait for what comes next."

A huge amount of research is directed toward investigating various ways to improve blood glucose control. We describe some of these efforts here.

New oral antihyperglycemic agents. As described in Chapter 10, the mid-1990s were landmark years in the availability of oral antihyperglycemic agents. Two new types of antidiabetes pills became available in the United States: metformin and acarbose. Since then, many more drug classes have become available that are helpful in controlling diabetes. These include the thiazolidinediones, DPP-4 inhibitors, GLP-1 agonists, amylin analogs, and SGLT2 inhibitors. Research studies were performed on all these drugs, and they were approved by the FDA only after study results showed them to be effective and safe to use. Many studies done after these drugs were approved have confirmed that since the drug classes work differently, they have additive effects to lower blood glucose levels when used together.

New insulins. Building on the advances in basic science, it has become possible to make new kinds of insulin. If bacteria can be "programmed" to make insulin that is exactly like human insulin, they can also be programmed to make insulin that is slightly different and has slightly different absorption characteristics. New insulins are in development that will be absorbed through the skin even more quickly, so they can be taken right before meals and still control after-meal glucose levels well. Other modifications of insulin are being developed that will allow it to be absorbed more slowly and more consistently, to lower the risk of hypoglycemia even more.

The artificial pancreas. In January 2012, a teenager with Type 1 diabetes walked into a hospital in Boston to begin her participation in a clinical trial. Doctors fitted her with an "artificial pancreas" hooked up to a laptop. For three days, while she was observed at the hospital, the device kept her blood glucose levels close to normal. In the future, the artificial pancreas could be the size of a cellphone, and this teenager and millions of other people with diabetes will use it all the time.

An artificial pancreas is the "holy grail" of diabetes care—a device that adjusts insulin (and glucagon) levels continuously to keep blood glucose levels in the normal range all the time, just as a normally functioning pancreas does. Scientists have taken some steps toward this goal, and more progress is likely to follow in the next few years.

An artificial pancreas consists of three elements: an insulin pump, a glucose sensor, and a computer, as shown in Figure 35. Many people already use insulin pumps and continuous glucose monitors (CGMs). The algorithms that drive the computer's commands to the pump are the most challenging and least well-developed part of a potential artificial pancreas. As you can imagine, creating algorithms that safely and effectively account for all the factors that affect blood glucose control is a mighty task.

The FDA has established guidelines for scientists working toward creation of an artificial pancreas to be sure these devices are safe. The first-generation device will be only partially automated. If blood glucose levels are headed too high or too low, the system will respond by increasing insulin flow or cutting it off temporarily. The user will still have to calculate boluses and deliver these manually.

Glucose sensing. Continuous glucose monitoring is here. Stand-alone CGMs and those integrated with insulin pumps are currently available, but these systems don't completely free people from the need to monitor blood glucose levels the old-fashioned way—by sticking their fingers. When it's time to insert a new sensor (every three to seven days, depending on the device), a finger-stick check is required for calibrating it. And all CGM manufacturers recommend a verification finger-stick check whenever the CGM shows the blood glucose level is high or low.

The next few years should bring advances in CGMs, including approv-

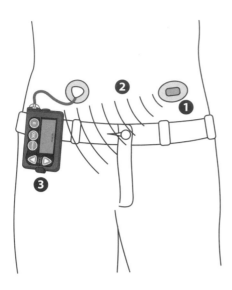

Figure 35. An artificial pancreas consists of three elements: (1) a continuous glucose monitor (CGM)—a hand-held blood glucose device (BGD) may be necessary to calibrate the CGM; (2) continuous glucose signal transmission; and (3) an insulin pump with internalized algorithm to deliver insulin based on glucose level and rate of change of glucose.

al of devices that are reliable enough to use without backup finger-stick monitoring and devices that are smaller, easier to wear, and more accurate. Farther down the road we could see implantable glucose sensors that could work for up to a year without replacement. One device currently in development uses a sensor only about three-quarters of an inch long that is inserted under the skin in a short outpatient procedure. The sensor communicates wirelessly with a monitor that looks like a watch and can be worn on the user's wrist. The monitor can be programmed to sound an alarm when glucose levels are headed toward hypoglycemic or hyperglycemic levels. Initial trials of this system have shown that it provides fairly accurate data. Subsequent trials could lead to FDA approval of this device or similar devices under development.

Islet cell transplantation. The notion of pancreas transplantation is hardly new. Frederick Banting, the discoverer of insulin, wanted to try it within two weeks of demonstrating that his extract of dog pancreas lowered blood glucose. Transplantation of a whole pancreas is now a generally available procedure for people who need a transplanted kidney (see Chapter 24). But much less extensive surgery would be required if the specific insulin-producing cells, the beta cells of the islets of Langerhans, could be separated and transplanted without the rest of the pancreas. Islet cell transplantation has been the subject of extensive research over the past 20 years or so and has been successfully accomplished for several years. The transplant recipients need to take immunosuppressive medications to prevent the islets from being rejected, but the transplanted islet cells still fail in large numbers after one or more years, requiring individuals to start taking insulin again. Researchers are working on ways to make the transplanted islet cells last longer, including better and safer drugs to prevent rejection.

The barriers to islet cell transplantation are formidable. To begin with, a great many islets must be gathered without damaging their viability or their sterility. This generally involves nonhuman sources. When the islets are implanted, they must survive in sufficient quantity to secrete enough insulin. The cross-species origin of the islets poses a particularly difficult rejection problem. Nevertheless, techniques have been developed to harvest large numbers of islets from pig (and other animal) pancreases, and by using modern immunosuppressive medications to prevent rejection, as we noted above, some successful islet cell transplantations have been carried out. The work has led to another research approach, called the biohybrid artificial pancreas.

The biohybrid artificial pancreas. Since a major problem in transplanting pancreatic islets is that they are so vulnerable to immune rejection, some investigators have come up with the interesting idea of putting live islets into a device that gives them exposure to the blood glucose and allows them to secrete insulin into the bloodstream, but does not allow the immune response that would destroy the islets. The islets are put inside a tube or bag made of a highly selective membrane: one that has pores that are the right size to keep the islet cells inside, allow the blood glucose to equilibrate across the membrane, and allow the insulin to flow out, *but* to keep out the cells and antibodies that make up the body's immune response to foreign tissue. Several designs have been developed to insert the tubing, with the contained islets, inside the body and position it into a blood vessel. Hybrid artificial pancreases are essentially a protected islet cell transplant.

Like other approaches to establishing better, simpler insulin delivery, hybrid artificial pancreases have potential advantages as well as problems. Their biggest plus is that they would function in a "closed loop" fashion, with insulin delivery turning on in response to increasing blood glucose and turning off when the glucose gets low. But the technical problems are significant too. Most important, the device requires a large number of islets to remain alive and well for quite awhile (although it might be possible to replace the islets occasionally).

Hybrid artificial pancreases have been used successfully in dog experiments, and reports suggest they will soon be tried experimentally in humans.

Approaches to the Prevention of Diabetes

- "Almost everyone in my family eventually develops Type 2 diabetes. When my doctor told me I had 'prediabetes' I figured my time had just about come. Then I read about a study that showed people with prediabetes could delay or even prevent diabetes by losing weight. I decided to give it a try. I lost 15 pounds, and now, five years later, I still don't have diabetes. It takes quite a bit of work to keep the weight off, but it's worth it. Every day I delay getting diabetes is a good day."

The best approach to diabetes is to prevent it. Once we understood the basic causes of both Type 1 and Type 2 diabetes, it was time to try to prevent it. Two large, government-sponsored trials are under way, one trying to prevent Type 1 diabetes and the other working on prevention of Type 2 diabetes.

Prevention of Type 1 diabetes. Given that Type 1 diabetes is caused by the body's immune destruction of its own pancreatic beta cells, the first step would be to prevent this immune response. To do that we would have to know when and in whom the beta cell destruction is happening. If a single virus or a single toxin were found to be the cause of Type 1 diabetes, it might be possible to develop a vaccine for that virus or a way to avoid that toxin. But there is little evidence at this point that such a single cause is likely.

In the 1980s, a series of studies were done using the immunosuppressive drug cyclosporine to knock down a person's immune response as soon as he or she showed signs of Type 1 diabetes—within weeks of the initial diagnosis, during the "honeymoon period." But these studies had limited success, both because the drug has serious side effects and because the disease had probably already damaged the islet cells irreparably by the time the diabetes was apparent.

Tests for circulating antibodies against the pancreas have allowed this research to enter a new phase. The antibodies are rare in the population as a whole but common in people who will soon get Type 1 diabetes. This opens the window of opportunity for prevention before diabetes actually develops. TrialNet, which we mentioned in Chapter 30, has a large clinical trial now in progress that is screening large numbers of high-risk people (mainly first-degree and young second-degree relatives of people with Type 1 diabetes) to find those who are positive for the antibodies and likely to develop Type 1 diabetes.

Once an individual is identified as likely to get Type 1 diabetes in the near future, several prevention approaches are being tested. One is to use oral insulin (insulin pills), which in the Diabetes Prevention Trial, Type 1, appeared to show prevention or delay in onset of Type 1 diabetes in participants who had higher levels of antibodies. It's believed that oral insulin "seen" by the immune system in the intestine may lead to the immune system becoming more "tolerant" to insulin and making fewer antibodies against islet cells. Oral insulin was not effective for participants with low levels of antibodies. Individuals found to have positive antibodies in Trial-Net may also qualify to be in studies of other investigational drugs that target the immune system, drugs now being studied or new ones that become available in the future.

Prevention of Type 2 diabetes. As we mentioned earlier, the Diabetes Prevention Program showed that an intensive lifestyle intervention that produced an average 14-pound weight loss cut the risk of developing Type 2 diabetes during the DPP study by 58%. Participants in the same study who took the diabetes drug metformin cut their risk by 31%. Most DPP participants are continuing to take part in a study called DPP-OS (DPP Outcomes Study), which is looking at how the original interventions affect the ongoing risk of developing diabetes in participants who did not develop diabetes during the DPP. The DPP-OS will also assess the effects of the original interventions on participants' risk of developing diabetes complications. Ten years after the beginning of the original DPP, fewer people in the lifestyle and metformin groups than in the placebo group had developed diabetes. In a few years we'll know the results for diabetes complications.

Treatment of Complications

So many advances are occurring in the treatment of diabetes complications that describing this field of clinical research would take far more than a few paragraphs, so a couple of examples will have to suffice.

Following up on a previous study showing that laser therapy is highly effective in slowing the progression of severe retinopathy, a large ophthalmology trial called the Early Treatment of Diabetic Retinopathy Study asked whether treatment at earlier stages would be even more beneficial. In the course of this more recent trial, researchers found that a condition called macular edema should be treated early but that, otherwise, laser therapy at early stages of retinopathy gave no additional benefit.

Another study compared coronary bypass surgery with angioplasty in treating coronary heart disease. The study found that the bypass surgery gave a better long-term result in treating certain stages of the disease.

How You Can Help

- "I signed up for the Look AHEAD trial, a study designed to see if losing weight reduced the risk of heart attack and stroke in people with Type 2 diabetes. I knew this would be a big commitment because the study lasts 12 years. I was hoping to get into the weight loss group, but I didn't; I was randomized to the group that got only support and education classes four times a year. I was pretty disappointed at first, but the meetings are interesting and I learn a lot from them. Plus the checkups every six months are good, and the staff is very friendly. Put it all together and what I get from the study is well worth my time. I am more aware of my diabetes and what I can do to stay healthy."

Most people understand that diabetes research is the key to progress in treating and ultimately preventing or curing diabetes. But to many people it seems like another world, one that's technical, remote, and inaccessible. Researchers sometimes don't do a good job of bridging this gap by explaining in plain language what they're up to and helping people take part. We want to show you how to get involved, how to do whatever you can to advance diabetes research. There are three broad areas that need your help: personal participation in research trials, financial support, and advocacy. Each takes some explaining.

Participating in Research Trials

Clinical research requires research subjects, or participants, people who volunteer to take part. We think of the people enrolling in our research as partners, as well as heroes, in the advancement of medicine. They may benefit personally by getting a new treatment before anyone else, or they may benefit just from the knowledge that they are helping others. Their participation may be quite simple (one of us was a research subject, taking a pill every morning for 12 years) or may be very demanding, requiring multiple visits or rigorous training. Being a research participant, of course, is not for everyone, but many people find it a thoroughly rewarding experience.

When we talk to people about taking part in clinical research, several questions often come up, which we'll try to address here.

What does it mean to say that I will be "randomized" to one treatment or another? The term *randomization* refers to the assignment of research participants, as if by the flip of a coin, to one of the treatments being tested. Randomization may be crucial in a study, because if you are consciously assigned to one group or the other, bias may creep in. For example, if the investigator really wants experimental pill A to work better than pill B, he or she could consciously or unconsciously see to it that the least sick people are assigned to pill A.

What does it mean to use placebos? A placebo is an inactive treatment; if it's a pill, it is made to look exactly like the active pill but doesn't have the active ingredient. Placebos are used in order to have a comparison group. If pill A is active and pill B is a placebo, the study compares pill A with pill B. If pill A, being active, were already known to be safe and effective, the research trial would not be worth doing. It is very possible that pill A won't work or will have some side effects that are worse than any benefit, so it has to be compared against the inactive pill. You may ask, why not just compare taking pill A to taking nothing? The answer is that pill A may *seem* to work but actually provide only a "placebo effect." Most people feel better if they are taking a pill, any pill, even a placebo. The point of a trial that uses a placebo comparison is to see whether the active drug is really effective, not just having a placebo effect.

What does "double-blind" mean, and why is it part of a study? The term *double-blind*, or *double-masked*, means that neither you nor the researcher knows what pill you are taking. Sound strange? Of course, there *are* people who know which pill it is, and in an emergency it's always possible to find out. But double blinding is another important part of answering a research question fairly. If the doctor or nurse who sees you is unmasked—knows that you are taking, let's say, pill A, the active pill—and is really hopeful about pill A, bias can creep in. The health professional may consciously or unconsciously let you know that he or she expects you to be feeling better taking pill A—or, if you're in the pill B (placebo) group, expects that you aren't feeling better. Body language, winks of the eye, even the phrasing of questions can make all the difference: "You're feeling better today on those pills, aren't you, Mrs. Jones?" "Not noticing much difference on those pills today, Mrs. Jones?" Double masking keeps the investigator from influencing the results unfairly.

How can I be sure I am getting the treatment that works? The answer is, in short, you can't. A principle of clinical investigation is that *no one* knows if the treatment works. If the answer were known, it would be unethical to do the study. Sometimes, in fact, a research study should *not* be done. For example, when the new insulin extracts were first shown to save children dying of diabetes in Toronto in 1922, no one then and no one now would suggest there should have been a large clinical study giving insulin to only half the dying children on that ward. The answer was obvious—the material worked—and the question immediately turned to how more insulin could be produced. But results are seldom that spectacular. If a study is being done, it is because the answer to the question is simply not known.

Looking at all drug trials, we see that the majority of experimental drugs are never proven safe and effective; either they don't work or they have side effects that are worse than the benefits. So whichever pill you take, A or B, active or placebo, you're doing good for people with diabetes by helping find out what works and what doesn't.

How long will the study go on, and when will I know the results? In principle, the study goes on until an answer is found or until it is clear that an answer won't ever be found by this study. For instance, if it turns out that pill or treatment A is dramatically better than pill or treatment B, as soon as this becomes clear, the study will be stopped. This happened in the DPP study. The study was designed to last four years, but before the time was up, it was clear that people in the lifestyle group and the metformin group were developing diabetes at a significantly lower rate than people in the placebo group. The study question was answered, so the study was stopped. Most often, studies are planned for a specified period of time—six months, two years, or whatever—so that any difference should be found within that time. Usually, the results of the study are not revealed to the investigators or the research participants until the study is over and the results completely analyzed. This is often a frustration for everyone involved, since they naturally want to know as soon as possible how the study turned out.

How to Become Involved as a Research Participant

Becoming a participant in a research study may not be as easy as you'd expect. There are several barriers to getting involved. First of all, studies take place in a limited number of settings—often at universities or in specialists' offices. Second, to have a relatively comparable group of people in the study, investigators have to set up a very specific set of *inclusion* and *exclusion criteria*. For example, there may be an age range (such as 20–60 years old); a certain kind of diabetes (for example, Type 2 diabetes) may be required; or maybe anyone taking insulin is excluded. The sad part to investigators and potential participants alike is that many people have to be excluded who would be terrific participants in all respects and are eager to take part. All we can say is keep up the interest. Don't feel rejected or sad. Keep in touch. Maybe you'll be right for the next study. (As an aside here, "Leaving my body to research" usually refers to the use of cadavers for the training of medical students and is very different from signing an organ donor card. The widespread use of organ donation cards is absolutely essential to organ availability for transplantation and is recommended for everyone.)

How do you find out what studies are available in your area? You may want to ask the American Diabetes Association or call your local medical center. Read the papers and look for advertisements. The website ClinicalTrials .gov provides information about current research studies.

In summary, it can be rewarding and satisfying to take part in diabetes research. It can keep you in touch with the latest advances, provide some good contacts for you, and even offer personal benefit from trying a new approach to diabetes care. It can also be rewarding to support research financially.

Supporting Diabetes Research Financially

- "We're not going to be allowed a U-Haul behind the hearse when our time comes. We want to be sure we leave a legacy that reaches beyond. Planned giving makes that possible."—American Diabetes Association planned-giving donor.

In our opinion, there is no more noble, effective, or satisfying place to put your charitable donations than into diabetes research and education. If you are fortunate enough to have substantial assets, you will find associations and university groups especially eager to demonstrate the need. But small donations, annual giving, planned giving (leaving something in your will), and even in-kind support such as helping organize fundraisers all make important contributions.

You may want to give but feel unsure how and to whom you should give. It is reasonable to ask questions, to want assurance that your money goes exactly where you want it to go. Here are some guidelines:

—The two large, national, volunteer-driven diabetes organizations, the *American Diabetes Association* (ADA) and the *Juvenile Diabetes Research Foundation, International* (JDRF), are rock solid. Organizations such as the *Lions Club International* and the *Shriners* also donate generously to diabetes research. Each group has its own distinct characteristics and priorities, as well as its own fundraising campaigns. But you can be sure that contributions to the ADA, the JDRF, the Lions Club, or the Shriners, earmarked for research, will be used to extremely good purpose.

—*Established universities and nonprofit medical centers* usually have diabetes research projects that represent excellent opportunities if you are eager to contribute to a local activity. Call the development office or the people involved in diabetes research.

—*Various private foundations* and even medical practices accept donations for diabetes research. These may be perfectly good choices, but you would be wise to check into them carefully.

Planned giving (your written decision to donate some portion of your assets to diabetes research upon your death) is a popular approach these days. Experts from the larger organizations and universities can explain all varieties of tax-saving mechanisms. This is strongly recommended.

In sum, diabetes research needs individual charitable giving, and many families with diabetes in their midst, or even people who just understand the need, are willing and eager to give. The established nonprofit organizations, such as the ADA, the JDRF, or universities, are ready and eager to receive donations and manage them responsibly. They have the experience and mechanisms to see that the money is well spent. There really is no reason to go outside these established routes when you consider charitable giving.

Being an Advocate for Diabetes Research

- "Every year our whole family takes a vacation to Washington, DC. We drive and stay in an inexpensive hotel to save money. We visit the monuments and the museums. And we always go to Capitol Hill to tell our Congress members how important it is for them to support funding for diabetes research and education. Our 6-year-old, who has had diabetes for four years, is a veteran, and she is really good at making our case."

Most funding for diabetes research comes from the federal National Institutes of Health, particularly through the NIDDK. Hundreds of millions of dollars are devoted to diabetes research each year, but this is not enough. Fewer than one in four approved grant applications from qualified investigators receive funding. The competition for NIH grants is fierce.

One way to increase diabetes research is to keep up the pressure for funding at the federal level. This is what we call advocacy, and it works. The Diabetes Research and Training Centers around the country and the NIDDK were founded, and the Diabetes Control and Complications Trial and many other important studies were funded, as a result of effective advocacy.

Both the ADA and the JDRF organize specific, targeted public campaigns to advocate for diabetes research. Through them, you can target your letters or your visits to the right people at just the right time. But it is up to you. We do live in a democracy, and both federal and state governments respond to pressure. Rest assured that if you don't put on the heat for biomedical research, whatever funding is available will go to other types of projects

The world of diabetes research is vast and exciting. It stretches all the way from laboratory attempts to understand the most fundamental questions about insulin action to psychosocial research on how to get whole populations to lead a healthier life. There's no way to tell for sure which research approaches—for instance, islet cell transplantation, mechanical insulin delivery systems, or prevention trials—are the best way to go. A broad-based, well-balanced, and well-funded research effort is necessary to optimize our chances for improving the lives of people with diabetes today and, ultimately, for curing the disease.

You can make a difference. It is enormously important to the effort as a whole for you to understand the process and support it. You may be able to promote diabetes research through a letter to the editor of a newspaper or to a member of Congress. You may meet someone tomorrow who can give substantially. You may get more involved yourself. We believe that an educated, supportive population is the key to a healthy, strong diabetes research effort. And only through such a research effort will the future of diabetes be as bright as we think it can be.

Take Home Messages

- Research is the key to continuing advances in diabetes care.
- Reliable sources for information on diabetes include the American Diabetes Association, the Juvenile Diabetes Research Foundation, and the National Institutes of Health's National Institute of Diabetes and Digestive and Kidney Diseases.
- Important areas of basic diabetes research include studies of insulin action, diabetes genetics, and the immunology of Type 1 diabetes.
- Important areas of behavioral and psychosocial research include studies of ways to facilitate diabetes self-care, the effects of weight loss on the risk of developing Type 2 diabetes or diabetes complications, and the effects of new treatments on quality of life and treatment satisfaction.
- Important areas to improve blood glucose control include studies of new diabetes drugs, the artificial pancreas, and new glucose-sensing technology.
- Studies are under way to test approaches to preventing Type 1 and Type 2 diabetes.
- You can help advance diabetes research by participating in research studies, giving money for research, and advocating for increased diabetes research funding.

32

The Prognosis

- "I'm really hopeful about my future. I hear about all these advances in diabetes, and I realize I won't have the same problems as my mother did."
- "I often let things slide when it comes to managing my diabetes. Then I pull myself together and get with the program again."
- "Every day, I go on the Internet looking for a breakthrough in diabetes. When something hits the news, though, I try to figure out what it means for me."

This book is full of explanations, suggestions, and factual information about how to live life to the fullest with diabetes. We didn't write it for someone who manages diabetes perfectly. We wrote this book for everyone living with diabetes day to day. We wrote this book for you. You will take from it what you need, use what you can, and leave aside what does not apply to you now.

The prognosis, or outlook, for people who have diabetes is excellent. That is not just wishful thinking—it's a scientific fact. Using what is available today, using your best understanding of diabetes and controlling it to the best of your ability, there is every reason to think that you can avoid long-term complications and lead a long and healthy life.

"How good do I have to be?" you're probably asking. We don't know the answer, but we do know that good blood glucose control is achievable. Since we wrote the first edition of this book more than 15 years ago, the average hemoglobin A1c level of people with diabetes in the United States has steadily improved; now almost half of U.S. adults with diabetes have reached the American Diabetes Association's goal of an A1c level below 7.0%. This achievement is a testament to better diabetes treatments, better education, and the hard work of people who have diabetes. Whatever your

463

A1c level, keep in mind that every improvement in your A1c (down to levels even lower than the ADA goal) cuts your risk of diabetes-related eye, nerve, and kidney disease. Lowering your A1c level by 0.5% cuts that risk by 20%, and lowering your A1c by 1.0% doubles that benefit.

Several themes recur throughout this book, reflecting our own beliefs and our thoughts about how to help you improve your own prognosis. First, we strongly believe in people's *ability to get back on track*, and this is one of the most important skills you will learn. Everyone, and we do mean *everyone*, slips from time to time. What matters is how quickly you get back on track. Whether it is watching your diet, exercising, visiting your health care professionals, or even taking your medication, think hard about how to get yourself back on track if you have strayed. It will help your prognosis immensely. We hope some of the suggestions we offered in this book will help you stay on track more of the time.

We believe in *knowledge*. We believe that it's vitally important for you to understand *your* diabetes and what works for *you* in managing it effectively. Pay attention to what affects your blood glucose control and what affects your motivation for self-care. Experiment to find what works best for you. Search for new ideas in the reliable sources we mentioned in this book. Talk with your health care providers and with other people who have diabetes.

You need to be able to *separate the more important things from the less important*. Let's say that in thinking about how to improve the circulation to your feet, you read that you should try to walk upstairs at work to improve your activity, quit smoking, and try not to cross your legs when you sit. Which of these is most important? We'll give you a hint—it's not uncrossing your legs. Or let's say you live alone and are getting hypoglycemic reactions. It's most important to make note of the timing. Feeling a little low before lunch, a time of day when you can readily take a snack if the meal is delayed, pales in comparison with the seriousness of having significant hypoglycemia in the middle of the night and waking up confused. Understanding your diabetes will help you in more ways than you can imagine.

We believe in *communication*. Your health care visits can be more productive if you communicate well. So can your interactions with friends and family. Your diabetes affects everyone who cares about you, and how they relate to your diabetes affects how well you manage it. Finding the balance that works best for you between keeping your diabetes completely to yourself and letting it get in the way of your relationships is so important.

We also believe in the *gradual* cure of diabetes. Does this sound odd? Do you like to think that a day will dawn when diabetes is just—poof!—gone? We'd all like to think that, but it may not happen quite that way. Therapies are constantly being developed that make the disease more and more "forgettable," requiring less and less of your own input to achieve good control. In the future, various approaches to the different kinds of diabetes will move at varying rates.

We have emphasized that the real challenge is not so much to eliminate diabetes as to eliminate the personal burden it places on people and, of course, to eliminate the complications. If you could have just one procedure, whether it's a gene transfer or a transplant or a pump, and never again have to think about diabetes, that would be tantamount to a cure. But it may come gradually, not as a single flash of glory.

Finally, we believe in *taking advantage of what is available to you*. This book describes many ways to help control your diabetes today. Many of these options were not available when we wrote the first edition of this book. And new treatments will continue to emerge. So it is up to you to stay on top of things, to follow the advances, not just in research or theory but in practical, available tools that can help you manage your own diabetes.

Diabetes care is not a fixed, static set of rules but a wave that moves steadily forward. Care has advanced, is advancing, and will advance. If you ride the wave, taking advantage of what is available as you go along, you put yourself in the best possible position to be strong and healthy when diabetes is ultimately cured. That is the promise of having diabetes today. That is what makes the prognosis excellent.

Index

A1c. *See* hemoglobin A1c

acanthosis nigricans, 396

acarbose, 81, 166–68, 172, 175, 177, 424, 450

acesulfame K, 101, 102

acrochordons, 395

acromegaly, 34

Actos. *See* pioglitazone

actuary, 301

adrenaline, 47, 72, 75, 83, 310, 360

adult onset diabetes, 26, 32. *See also* Type 2 diabetes

adverse selection, 301

advocacy, 309, 313, 456, 461, 462

Affordable Care Act, 288, 300, 303, 307

African Americans: acanthosis nigricans in, 396; diet of, 139; hypertension in, 140; maturity onset diabetes of the young in, 32; Type 1 diabetes in, 21, 24; Type 2 diabetes in, 26, 27, 30, 35, 436

age/aging, 32; arteriosclerosis and, 340; exercise and, 157, 162–63; latent autoimmune diabetes in adults and, 32; Type 1 diabetes and, 20, 21, 35; Type 2 diabetes and, 26–28, 29, 35. *See also* older adults

air hunger, 328

alcohol use, 104–5, 121; hypoglycemia and, 80–81, 104; in pregnancy, 105

allergies: to foods, 146–47; to hyperglycemic agents, 169–70, 177, 392; to insulin, 193, 195; to sulfa drugs, 165, 170, 177

alopecia, 395

alpha-fetoprotein test, 418

alpha-glucosidase inhibitors, 81, 166–68, 172, 177

alpha lipoic acid, 370

alprostadil, 406

Amaryl. *See* glimepiride

American Association of Diabetes Educators, 101

American College of Sports Medicine, 150

American Diabetes Association (ADA), 5, 42, 51, 64, 255, 286, 289, 462; cholesterol recommendations, 144; Diabetes Forecast, 286, 445; diet recommendations, 91, 94, 101, 117; employment advocacy by, 309, 313; exercise recommendations, 150, 154, 155, 164; goal for hemoglobin A1c, 65, 66, 463–64; research funding by, 459, 461; weight loss surgery recommendations, 137

American Dietetic Association, 101

Americans with Disabilities Act, 306–7, 312, 314

amino acids, 98, 183

amitriptyline, 370

amniocentesis, 410

amputation, 371, 376, 380, 386–88

amylin analogs, 169, 173, 179, 450

anaphylactic reaction, 146

anemia, 99, 362; sulfonylurea-induced, 176–77

anger, 243–44, 245, 253; at diagnosis, 8, 16; due to too little insulin, 327; family and, 46, 256; of health care professional, 282; hypoglycemia and, 74; related to blood glucose levels, 55

angina, 163, 334, 336, 338, 341

angioedema, 359